FLIP
the
SWITCH

FLIP
the
SWITCH

Proven Strategies to
**Fuel Your Metabolism and
Burn Fat 24 Hours a Day**

Robert K. Cooper, PhD
Recipes by Leslie L. Cooper

RODALE

© 2005 by Advanced Excellence Systems LLC

Printed in the United States of America
Rodale Inc. makes every effort to use acid-free ∞, recycled paper ♻.

Book design by Drew Frantzen
Illustrations by Karen Kuchar

Library of Congress Cataloging-in-Publication Data

Cooper, Robert K.
    Flip the switch : proven strategies to fuel your metabolism and burn fat 24 hours a day / Robert K. Cooper, recipes by Leslie L. Cooper.
        p.   cm.
    Includes bibliographical references and index.
    ISBN-13 978–1–57954–979–4 hardcover
    ISBN-10 1–57954–979–9 hardcover
    1. Weight loss.   2. Weight loss—Psychological aspects.   3. Reducing diets.
    4. Reducing exercises.   I. Cooper, Leslie L.   II. Title.
    RM222.2.C6169   2005
    613.2'5—dc22
                                             2005019325

Distributed to the book trade by Holtzbrinck Publishers

    4 6 8 10 9 7 5 3   hardcover

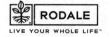

RODALE
LIVE YOUR WHOLE LIFE™

We inspire and enable people to improve their lives and the world around them
For more of our products visit **rodalestore.com** or call 800-848-4735

To all who realize that
the next frontier is not only in front of us,
it is also inside of us.

"It is useless to close the gates against new ideas;
they overleap them."
—*Prince Clemens Wenzel Nepomuk Lothar Metternich,*
Austrian diplomat (1773–1839)

CONTENTS

Acknowledgments ix
Introduction: Maximize Fat Loss and Energy Automatically xi

PART ONE. THE META-STAT SOLUTION

Chapter 1. The New Science of Fat Loss 3
Chapter 2. Hormones: Your Meta-Stat's Master Regulators 19
Chapter 3. Turn On Your Meta-Stat,
              Turn Off Fat Gain and Fatigue. 31

PART TWO. THE MSON SWITCHES

Chapter 4. MSON Switch #1: Wake Up on the Right Side
                          of the Bed 41
Chapter 5. MSON Switch #2: Create Activity Momentum 55
Chapter 6. MSON Switch #3: Catch Light to Boost Energy 67
Chapter 7. MSON Switch #4: Take In More Oxygen 71
Chapter 8. MSON Switch #5: Seek Ideal Fluid Intake. 75
Chapter 9. MSON Switch #6: Rise Up and Stand Tall 85
Chapter 10. MSON Switch #7: Turn Down the Heat,
                          Turn Up Your Energy 94
Chapter 11. MSON Switch #8: Improve Hormone Balance,
                          Hour after Hour 97
Chapter 12. MSON Switch #9: Stay Calm in an Uptight World . 106
Chapter 13. MSON Switch #10: Stop the Stress Response 122
Chapter 14. MSON Switch #11: Ramp Up Your Evening
                          Meta-Stat Setting 136
Chapter 15. MSON Switch #12: Get Plenty of Good-Quality Rest . 151

PART THREE. THE MSON WORKOUT

Chapter 16. A Cardio Kick for Your Meta-Stat 161
Chapter 17. Anytime Muscle Tone-Ups 164
Chapter 18. Lower-Body Strength: Abs and Legs 177
Chapter 19. Upper-Body Strength: Chest,
                          Back, Shoulders, and Arms 188
Chapter 20. Balance and Flexibility. 194

PART FOUR. THE MSOn EATING PLAN

Chapter 21. Rethinking Mealtimes 201
Chapter 22. Protein Principles. 211
Chapter 23. Right Carbs, Right Times. 219
Chapter 24. Good Fats Aren't Fattening 232
Chapter 25. Calories Still Count 240

PART FIVE. SET YOUR COURSE FOR SUCCESS

Chapter 26. The Meta-Stat Success Map 245
Chapter 27. Choosing the Right Goals for You 254
Chapter 28. Guide Your Success Instincts 262

PART SIX. META-STAT RECIPES

Starters and Snacks. 269
Bakery-Fresh Breads and More 279
Sumptuous Salads. 287
Soups by the Spoonful 304
Poultry Entrées. 325
Seafood Favorites 337
On the Side 353
Sweet Endings 361

Notes. 379
Index 411

ACKNOWLEDGMENTS

With enduring gratitude to:

- Our children, Chris, Chelsea, and Shanna

- Our editor, Susan Berg, and the leadership team at Rodale Books

- Our independent editor, Ed Claflin

- Our many friends who served as recipe testers and early reviewers for *Flip the Switch*

INTRODUCTION

MAXIMIZE FAT LOSS AND ENERGY
AUTOMATICALLY

hat if I said I have a system that will steadily awaken your natural, hidden powers to slim down and tone up, 24 hours a day? A system that becomes automatic, so you can't fail? A system that sets you up for success from day one?

You just might say that it sounds too good to be true. And I wouldn't blame you. After all, literally hundreds of books offer weight-loss programs of one sort or another. You probably have read some of them. And more than likely, they probably didn't produce the results you expected.

How many people do you know who have gone on a diet and lost some weight, only to regain what they lost—and possibly a few extra pounds for good measure? They fret over every last calorie or every last minute of exercise, only to end up heavier than when they started! The problem, in my opinion, is that far too many of these weight-loss programs rob people of their sense of control. Put them in control, and they'll succeed.

That is what this book is all about. It's a revolutionary, one-of-a-kind approach to turning up your body's metabolic thermostat, or Meta-Stat. I'm convinced that the Meta-Stat is the most overlooked yet most powerful secret to lifelong fat loss and energy.

IT'S EASIER THAN YOU THINK

The Meta-Stat approach is a breakthrough that draws on the very latest scientific research. You can apply its principles right away, anywhere, anytime—even in the midst of your hectic life. You'll be amazed at how the results grow and last. By the time you finish this book, you'll be able to:

- Easily activate your MSOn Switches so that they're second nature

- Forget about dieting

- Forget about willpower, guilt, and frustration

- Determine your goals and chart your own course for success

There are many reasons that the Meta-Stat approach works so well. To get a sense of how you might benefit from it, think for a moment of a perfect day. You wake up feeling refreshed and ready to go. Your mind is sharp. Your energy is high. You're focused yet calm, at ease yet confident. You feel ready for anything that might happen. Laughter comes easily. You're connected with the people and the world around you.

On a day like this, you probably sail through stressful situations more easily. You look forward to exercise rather than dreading it. Come day's end, you're ready to wind down and recharge. You sleep deeply and well. A great day ends with a great night.

Guess what? This kind of day doesn't happen by chance! Rather, it's the result of a series of simple, specific actions that we engage in, perhaps without even realizing it. This is the foundation of the Meta-Stat approach.

IT'S AS SIMPLE AS TURNING ON A LIGHT

The Meta-Stat approach is so simple that once you start practicing it, it will become second nature. Your body's own signals will guide you, hour by hour and day by day. You activate your Meta-Stat with science-based skills so easy and straightforward that I call them switches—like light switches. Each time you turn on one of these switches, you'll more easily turn on the next one, and the next . . . increasing fat-burning and energy-producing power every step of the way.

While the Meta-Stat approach is simple, it's based on a wide range of research not just in nutrition and exercise science but also in physiology, psychology, chronobiology (the study of daily biological rhythms in the body and brain), neuroscience, stress dynamics, and much more. Throughout this book, I'll share scientific insights from a host of specialists—as well as hundreds of scientific and medical studies—that support each specific switch as a means of burning off excess body fat and generating energy.

In recent years, scientists have done so much groundbreaking work to understand the biochemical intricacies of the human body that we have an unprecedented wealth of information about what causes fat gain and fatigue and how to reverse them. For instance, we now understand:

- How a few easy moves can jump-start metabolism and build muscle

- Why momentary pauses ramp up energy levels

- How sipping ice water can elevate metabolism by 30 percent for 1½ hours

- How deep breathing can short-circuit stress

- How light instantly revs up fat-burning power

The Meta-Stat approach is the first to formulate all of this cutting-edge information into a comprehensive, integrated program that fits your lifestyle.

IT WORKED FOR ME—AND IT CAN WORK FOR YOU!

On a personal note, the Meta-Stat approach is the same one that my family and I have followed for more than a decade. It transformed our weight-control efforts so that rather than struggling to make healthy choices, we followed through on them without a second thought. They became almost automatic.

My wife, Leslie, has experienced a number of lasting benefits. Between 1984 and 1986, her dress size dropped from a 12 to a 5. Even after a traumatic miscarriage and two successful pregnancies, she has maintained her natural weight and figure—and, more important, her energy level and stamina.

Leslie created every one of the Meta-Stat recipes right here in our kitchen. Every one is rich in protein, modest in carbs and good fats, low in bad fats, and high in fiber and nutrients. Most require only a minimum amount of prep time. And they're delicious, as our kids—ages 24, 13, and 10—will attest.

TAKE ACTION NOW!

This book is written to be highly interactive. You can't learn the Meta-Stat approach just by reading. You need to take action and then make observations about your preferences and outcomes. That's how the Meta-Stat approach becomes automatic, prompted by your own instincts and awareness of what enhances your fat-burning and energy-producing power and what doesn't. If you're wondering whether something will work for you, the only way to find out is to try it!

For example, each Meta-Stat switch comes with its own collection of Meta-Stat Starters. They flip the switch to "on" mode, so your body keeps burning fat and generating energy. As you come across these Meta-Stat Starters, feel free to experiment with them. Most take only a few minutes. For switch #5, "Seek Ideal Fluid Intake," I suggest getting a glass of ice water and sipping it while you continue reading. Obviously, this requires very little effort. But I have a compelling reason for recommending it: A new German study has shown that slowly sipping 17 ounces of ice water increases metabolism by 30 percent for 90 straight minutes!

Many of the other Meta-Stat Starters are just as easy. They're perfect for those occasions when you need a quick burst of energy or a steady revving-up of your fat-burning furnace. Others may require more planning and concentration, especially as you start to incorporate the Meta-Stat approach into your lifestyle.

Incidentally, while I hope that you'll try all of the switches, you may decide to use only some of them on a day-to-day basis. That's fine. Your objective is to stimulate your Meta-Stat every 15 to 30 minutes throughout the day. How you choose to do that is entirely up to you.

To help track your efforts and progress, I've provided a Meta-Stat Success Map. It's a modified version of the one that I distribute in my workshops and seminars. With the success map, you can integrate the switches of your choice with the MSOn Workout and the Meta-Stat Eating Plan—the foundation of the Meta-Stat approach—to build your very own version of the program. In no time at all, you'll see how this approach taps into your innate ability to lose fat and replenish energy 24 hours a day, even while you sleep.

SUCCESS IS WITHIN YOUR REACH

The Meta-Stat approach isn't wishful thinking. It works. In the chapters ahead, you'll not only find out how, you'll find out why. You'll develop the skills to raise your body's metabolism, and over time, you'll notice the effects—burning off excess fat, generating energy, and experiencing a vitality you might not have thought possible. Day after day, the momentum builds in exactly the direction you choose.

The Meta-Stat principles are simple and scientific. The Meta-Stat switches awaken natural biochemical processes that produce the results you want. Permanent fat loss and lasting energy can be yours now.

So why wait?

PART

The Meta-Stat Solution

ONE

CHAPTER 1

■ ■ ■

The New Science of Fat Loss

Armed with the latest advancements of the modern world, our society is fighting an all-out war against body fat and fatigue. And we're losing.

Right now, nearly 8 out of 10 Americans are overweight.[1] Millions of good, decent, motivated people are giving all they've got to get in shape and make it last. Huge amounts of time, effort, and hard-earned money are going into this monumental effort. Yet people are falling far short of the results they hope for.[2]

We've never had more diets. Or more technology, pills, fitness clubs, and advice columns. Yet even when weight loss seems to work, looking "thinner" in the mirror is invariably the result of losing pounds of vital fluids and healthy muscle tissue, not excess body fat. Inside, people's health and vitality are going down the drain. With all that dieting and deprivation, those on highly restrictive programs are effectively getting weaker by the day. Sooner or later they sense this, and their frustration grows.

We need to revise, radically and rapidly, our view of fat loss. We need to enlist the very latest insights from neuroscience, evolutionary biology, metabolic research, and a host of other fields. Instead of watching our weight, we need to get really smart about the most effective ways to burn off excess fat automatically and continually by enlisting the natural "engine" of energy production as any ally, not an afterthought.

The focal point of this revolutionary new approach is an integrated group of areas in the brain that I've dubbed the Meta-Stat—"meta" as in *metabolic,* and "stat" as in *thermostat.* The Meta-Stat governs fat burning and energy production. It's the key to fat loss that lasts.

MASTER YOUR META-STAT

Right now, you have between 25 and 30 billion fat cells in your body. Each one of those cells is like a little water balloon waiting to be filled up. Except, as you know, it fills not with water but with fat. In fact, unless you take preventive action, each of these fat cells can easily grow to a thousand times its original volume.

And what happens when those fat cells expand to many times their original size? Well, that's the reason for the weight crisis that we're having today. As the fat cells swell, the entire body gets heavier.

The good news is, just as fat cells swell, they can shrink. In fact, that will start to happen as soon as you begin to understand your natural metabolism and support the genius of that system. Because, as you know, you're a lot more than billions of fat cells. In fact, your body is a complete fat-burning, energy-producing, life-generating power plant.

Let me be clear that not all fat cells are bad. Some are amazingly dynamic and are vital to dispatching dozens of potent chemical signals throughout the body, influencing not only metabolism and muscle strength but also cognition and immune function. As University of Pennsylvania endocrinologist Rexford S. Ahima, MD, PhD, points out, certain body fat cells help "coordinate how much we eat, signaling muscles when they can burn fat, and helping control the flow of energy in and out of cells."[3] So keep in mind that the goal is not getting rid of all fat. It's getting rid of excess fat, both from your body and from your plate. That's where your Meta-Stat comes in.

Twenty-four hours a day, your Meta-Stat is hot-wiring signals to cellular structures known as mitochondria. The root of the word *mitochondria* is "little bean," and that's literally what they look like—tiny, bean-shaped energy factories inside every one of your body's cells. The mitochondria contain enzymes that convert food into energy for health and healing. And since fat is part of the food that they convert, your mitochondria need to be working fast, safely, and efficiently if you're going to burn off excess body fat.

Every one of the mitochondria are listening to, and responding to, metabolic signals that you give them—or, more likely, fail to give them. Not once a week or once a day, but *every 15 to 30 minutes all day long*.

These little cellular furnaces await your signals. Depending on the signal they get, they'll either fire up—which results in growth and renewal—or dampen down. Good things happen when they're fired up. But when they dampen down, or are even extinguished altogether, the cells shift toward fat storage or fatigue. When that happens, they underproduce energy and lapse into disuse.

Researchers at Northwestern University and the Howard Hughes Medical Institute have confirmed that wide-ranging molecular and behavioral changes can occur when people fail to regularly and consistently "spark" their metabolism,[4] which in turn prevents the mitochondria from doing their job. "Timing is critical to keep the metabolic symphony in tune," says study coauthor Joseph Bass, assistant professor of medicine and neurobiology at Northwestern University.

WORKING WITH YOUR BODY, NOT AGAINST IT

So how, exactly, do you keep your mitochondria firing at an optimal level all day long? Why don't you have to strain with heroic intensity to do it? Will your body really cooperate, without telling you to stop, sit down, and take a rest? To answer these questions, let's take a moment to discuss two closely related physiological processes that guarantee the success of the Meta-Stat approach by outsmarting your fat cells' natural tendency to weigh you down and wear you out.

Metabolism. Your body's trillions of cells are designed to function as energy factories. They are programmed to undergo continual chemical reactions that produce a power-generating component called adenosine triphosphate, or ATP. You need ATP to make your heart beat. You also need it to breathe, move, see, hear, think, sleep, sense, and respond productively in every aspect of your life.

Cells regularly produce ATP and constantly use it. According to some estimates, in an average energetic day, the human body makes and burns up over 100 pounds of this fuel. If we ever allow ATP production to fall, it will result in lower energy and a fall-off in fat-burning power. Among the key "ingredients" that aid ATP production are oxygen from respiration; water and other fluids; dietary proteins, fats, and carbohydrates; and micronutrients such as vitamins and minerals.

ATP doesn't work alone. Other stimulators of metabolism include muscle activity, exposure to natural light, cool temperatures, controlled reactions to stress, a positive mental outlook, and good-quality sleep. (As you'll see, all of these factors are partially or fully under your control, using the MSOn Switches.) Studies suggest that a consistently elevated metabolic rate can increase daily calorie expenditure by 17 percent, and sometimes more.[5]

To summarize, the following are the most important factors in determining whether your metabolism is high or low.

- The timing and availability of key metabolism-enhancing nutrients such as protein.

- Your muscle tone. Your muscles are the prime site for fat burning and energy production. If you allow them to weaken—with age, inactivity, or disuse—your metabolism declines. You can, and must, turn this around.

- Your muscle activity from hour to hour and day to day, not just once in a while.

- A number of key metabolic stimulants.

Thermogenesis. The term *thermogenesis* refers to the heat-producing effects of metabolism. It is the inner furnace that keeps our core temperature just right 24 hours a day.[6]

To measure the results of thermogenesis, just stick an oral thermometer in your mouth. There it is—constant heat, hovering around 98.6°F, generated by your cellular activity. But producing that heat, as you know, requires a lot of fuel. That's good news when it comes to burning off excess body fat to provide more body heat and natural energy. If you know how to turn on thermogenesis and keep it on—not just once a day but throughout the day and night—you have a big advantage. Fuel burning remains constant rather than sporadic.

All the benefits that come from thermogenesis, including constant fat burning and increased energy, are under your 24-hour management . . . if you know how to turn on and keep on the appropriate Meta-Stat switches. The four most vital are:

- Physical activity that engages your muscles frequently throughout the day

- A sensible diet of small but frequent meals, with a focus on key thermogenesis-generating nutrients such as high-quality protein[7]

- Cool temperatures that stimulate heat production

- Increased exposure to bright light, either from the sun or from indoor lighting

The more fat you have inside your body, the less thermogenesis you create. In part, that's because body fat seals in heat. Think of wearing a full-body warmup suit 24 hours a day! Your body needs to burn less fat to stay warm. The leaner you become, on the other hand, the more heat your body must produce on a continual basis. It does this by burning off calories from food and from stored fat.

YOUR FOREBEARS AND THEIR META-STATS

Over thousands of years of evolution, our ancestors developed a collage of ways to adapt to the world. While one generation was begetting another, they were also developing exquisitely precise routines. Some of those routines involved action and rest. Others had to do with exposure to light.

Those who survived and thrived were the ones who could maintain their energy. And they had the greatest strength, not only for carrying loads and hurling rocks but also for resisting disease, healing wounds, and coming up with creative solutions when they were in a pickle.

According to Emory University researcher S. Boyd Eaton, MD, over 99.9 percent of our genetic makeup was formed prior to the beginning of the agricultural age—which was 500 generations, or 10,000 years, ago.[8] In exact terms, the human genome has changed less than 0.02 percent in the past 40,000 years. Our genes and biochemistry are deeply, even stubbornly, designed to function just as they did long ago, based on ancient cycles of feast and famine, energy and survival.[9]

You and I inherited this master system. As part of our genes, we have a complete blueprint for optimal activity and nutrition to be lean, energetic, and fit. Yet, in a matter of a few recent generations, most of us have all but lost our awareness of it or the ability to use it.

Mind you, we're not to blame for a bit of evolutionary regression. When we can ride in a car or bus, we don't need the energy once required to flee from predators or stay one step ahead of other natural risks. Turning lights on and off at will has made us far less conscious of how our bodies respond to light and darkness and has also disrupted the natural wake-and-sleep patterns (controlled by darkness and daylight) that regulated our energy reserves for so many millennia. Food comes from the grocery shelf or fast-food window, not from hunting and foraging, so the ratio of energy expended to energy consumed is way out of whack. And the advent of powerful medicines has even altered our immune systems—definitely extending our life expectancy but also making us rely more on pills than on body-generated disease fighters.

But despite all these changes in lifestyle, the truth is that your metabolic physiology has been designed to respond with exquisite precision to your signals. Your actions still govern the choices those cellular furnaces make. The ancient metabolic programming is still in place. If you try to ignore that programming, you do so at your own peril.

The fact is, you and I are so highly evolved that our minds and bodies have everything we need to influence and control the Meta-Stat. But to do that, we need to use the skills we've been given (as human beings) rather than the conveniences we've been given (as a prospering society).

Your Meta-Stat has been intricately programmed over endless generations to carefully monitor and respond to whatever signals it receives or fails to receive throughout the day. All you need to do is practice using those signals, and then get in the habit of using them!

CHECK OUT THOSE FAMILY PHOTOS

By now you may be wondering whether I'm throwing away all the evidence that many genetic factors are involved in metabolism and body type. Of course I'm not. We're all different from each other in a variety of ways, and obviously my genetic makeup is different from yours. But that said, I urge you to do a quick family study.

A century ago, a much higher percentage of people—indeed, nearly all people—stayed trim and fit despite having relatively meager diets. Their idea of fast food was an occasional hot sausage at the fairgrounds. Further, they had no modern exercise equipment for strengthening abs or shaping the gluteus maximus.

Now, look back at the pictures of your great-grandparents, uncles, and aunts. Were they overweight? Rarely.

Well, you might argue that they lived at such a pace, with so much deprivation and duress, that they didn't have the luxuries that we now enjoy—laborsaving devices, leisure time, and the chance to relish life's little pleasures. But in your heart of hearts, you know that's not quite right. In fact, I'll bet you're asking yourself right now: What leisure time?

Actually, there's evidence that those folks may have been far less stressed out than we are. And if you get into the old letters, gifts, and mementoes, you may find evidence that they felt, in many ways, more fully alive. They met the pressures and hardships of their daily life in much the same way that we do. But I would suggest—at least from my own reading of their legacy—that many of my ancestors had a greater appreciation for life's simple pleasures and amazing mysteries. Instinctively, they continuously renewed their own vigor. They sensed how much it mattered.

They didn't fume while sitting in traffic or collapse near-comatose for hours in front of a television or computer screen. Actually, they rarely sat for more than 10 or 15 minutes at a time. They climbed stairs, carried wood, took short walks, cleaned the dishes by hand, swept the floors, shook out rugs instead of vacuuming them, made meals without a microwave or takeout, did manual work and active daily chores. Interestingly enough, all these regular activities accumulated into a series of effective, small actions that were accomplished every half hour or so, all day long.

There were other obvious differences, of course, between their lifestyle and ours. They slept deeply in cool bedrooms with the windows open, played physical games instead of computer games, used their inventive minds instead of sitting while a media center beamed passive programming at them. I also suspect, very strongly, that they laughed (far more often than most of us do today) at life's simple wonders and don't-miss-it moments.

If you were to plot out a typical day in your ancestors' lives, it would include very simple and brief muscle-toning, lung-expanding, light-stimulating, alertness-boosting actions every 15 to 30 minutes all day long. Not too intense, either, because they noticed whenever some action blunted their senses or made them tired. Even with streaks of overeating or nonideal diets, they consumed enough nutritious food to keep the Meta-Stat firing, so they stayed trim, active, and amazingly vigorous.

Necessity may have dictated our ancestors' actions, but we can learn volumes from the life patterns that they followed more instinctively. Today's scientists have come to the very interesting conclusion that we need those regular intervals of action as surely as we need to eat, breathe, and sleep. And, with all of their recent research, scientists also know that if we can add high-quality nutrition to this proven pattern of "sparking" metabolism upward, we gain lasting fat loss and energy.

MAKE IT AUTOMATIC: SOME PRACTICE WITH YOUR META-STAT

In the chapters ahead, I'll offer some guidelines for turning on the biochemical "switches" that control your Meta-Stat. I'll also identify the actions and behaviors that drain energy and cause fat gain. For now, I'd like you to get acquainted with your own Meta-Stat by trying the following exercise. It will take just a few minutes; in fact, you can do it right now. The important thing is to give your full attention to the exercise while you're doing it.

Focus for a moment on your posture. Imagine that a magnet is pulling the top of your head, gently lifting your head, neck, and spine, all the way down to your waist. Don't strain. Just let that magnet pull . . . and pull . . . and pull . . . gently lifting the top of your head as high as it will go. After a few moments, you can mentally turn off the magnet. But stay in the natural, upright, aligned position into which it pulled you.

In this position, shift your focus to your breathing. Instead of filling your lungs and raising your shoulders, fill your diaphragm by expanding your belly. To make sure you're doing it right, rest your hand on the soft part of your stomach. As you do, gently expand your diaphragm, pulling air into your lungs. You should feel your hand going out and in with the rhythm of your breath. If you want, close your eyes while you're doing this. Repeat five or six times.

Now stand up, with your feet about shoulder width apart, and place your hands on your hips. Without any effort at all, you should be able to maintain the upright posture that you just practiced. Continue with the "belly breathing," just as you've been doing. When inhaling, slowly rotate your upper torso to the right without moving your feet. Return to the forward position as you exhale. Repeat, turning your upper torso to the left. Repeat a total of three times to each side, maintaining your breathing throughout. Again, you can close your eyes while you do this if you wish.

That's all there is to it!

At this point, I won't go into a lot of detail about the impact of this simple exercise on your nervous, muscular, and cardiovascular systems. Suffice it to say that this simple three-step sequence has turned on numerous switches critical to your Meta-Stat. Note that you didn't need to set aside a block of time, join a health club, or subscribe to a special weight-loss program. All the necessary resources for activating your Meta-Stat are right there in your own body.

While the effects of exercises like this one—which appear throughout the book as Meta-Stat Starters—will vary, you can feel the switches. They do bring about subtle physical and psychological changes. By consciously turning on a switch, you alter the way you relate to your body and the environment. Of course, a change in metabolism is something that you can't feel right away. But you'll become aware of it over time, after repeated and customary use of the switches.

BURNING BRIGHTER

One of the most fascinating, beneficial characteristics of the Meta-Stat switches, or MSOn Switches, is that they have a cumulative effect. If you activate one, you will feel noticeably stronger and sharper. Activate another switch—or even the same one—after 15 to 30 minutes, and the difference will be even more pronounced.

As you get into a pattern of jump-starting your Meta-Stat every 15 to 30 minutes throughout the day, you take your entire physiology to a very high plateau of fat loss and energy maintenance. Yet the effort required to achieve that high level of metabolic function is no more strenuous or stressful than the most normal actions like breathing, stretching, or daydreaming. It is remarkable that such simple actions and behaviors—if they assume a regular pattern—can have such a cumulative power of transformation.

How much benefit do you want from your daily routine of Meta-Stat

Starters? To a large extent, it's up to you. You might think of your Meta-Stat as a biochemical lightbulb that burns off excess fat and generates energy 24 hours a day. Every day, you need to turn it on at regular intervals. Each click of the switch adds a single watt of illumination for fat burning and energy production, so the light—that is, your metabolism—shines brighter and brighter. But you must turn it on for it to work.

META-STAT VERSUS "STATIC":
TIMING IS EVERYTHING

So how does the Meta-Stat approach compare with conventional diet-and-exercise programs? Even the most advanced, "breakthrough" weight-loss programs emphasize tight dietary controls and sometimes intense physical activity. This sort of program may deliver measurable results, at least at first. You actually experience some weight loss. You might even feel better for a while, if the diet is not depriving you of key nutrients and the exercise builds aerobic capacity and strength. Almost inevitably, though, there is a fall-off in results, accompanied by diminished enthusiasm for the program.

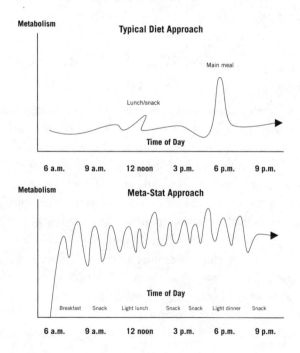

THE META-STAT SOLUTION

Why? If it's a great program, why is sticking with it so difficult? If it shows some immediate results, why do you reach a plateau? If it seems easy at first, why does it require more determination and willpower over time, as days turn into weeks and weeks drag on into months?

As you may already have guessed, it's because these programs do not become automatic, as the Meta-Stat approach does. And they leave out the most crucial factor: timing. They outline what you should eat and how much, they recommend types of exercise and number of repetitions, but they neglect your body's ancient, intricate biological rhythms, and not just the typical sleep-wake cycles. A host of recent research indicates the power and influence of these rhythms, which occur every 60 to 90 minutes during the day.[10]

Let's take a closer look at two key timing factors: nutrition and physical activity. Similar patterns apply to other Meta-Stat switches.

Nutrition and your Meta-Stat. First, if you eat infrequently, as shown in the top diagram on the opposite page, your body slows down fat burning while ramping up fat storage. Similar problems occur when you eat foods that turn off the Meta-Stat. Essentially, your body begins to sense that you are starving (for lack of nutrients in general or lack of the right, energy-producing foods) and "locks" your fat cells so you can put more fat in but you can't get the fat out. On the other hand, when you eat ideal, delicious light meals and snacks at the right times, you dramatically increase your fat burning and energy production all day long, as shown in the bottom diagram.

Physical activity and your Meta-Stat. Similarly, it's simply bad strategy to count on infrequent bouts of (sometimes intense) physical activity. At every gap of more than 15 minutes where there's no "spark" to boost and sustain metabolism, your energy-producing, fat-burning rate plummets. Then it stays at a near-hibernation rate for the day, with only a single upward spike or two. Not nearly enough.

To see the contrast between the Meta-Stat approach and other kinds of weight-loss programs, look at the two diagrams on page 14. In both diagrams, the vertical axis represents metabolism. That's the amount of fuel-burning activity that's going on in your body as you turn food into energy all day long.

In the top diagram, I've charted the metabolism patterns for three

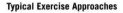

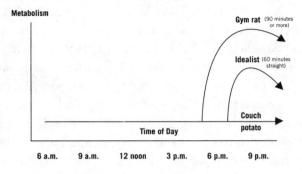

Typical Exercise Approaches

Metabolism

Gym rat (90 minutes or more)

Idealist (60 minutes straight)

Couch potato

Time of Day

6 a.m.   9 a.m.   12 noon   3 p.m.   6 p.m.   9 p.m.

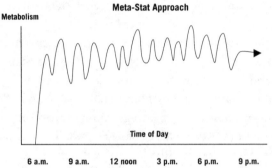

Meta-Stat Approach

Metabolism

Time of Day

6 a.m.   9 a.m.   12 noon   3 p.m.   6 p.m.   9 p.m.

different activity levels. The "couch potato"—well, we're all familiar with that term. That's anyone who spends a lot of time sitting down (in the car, on the couch, in front of the computer screen) and very little time moving around. The couch potato doesn't need much fuel and doesn't burn much, naturally. So metabolism remains on a day-long plateau.

Compare that daily lifestyle with that of the second person on the chart—the "idealist." Most likely, this is someone who's following a traditional weight-loss program. Though daily activities are fairly sedentary—hence, with a low metabolic rate—energy is expended at the end of the day in a burst of conscientious, strenuous activity lasting 30 to 60 minutes.

Also shown in the top chart is the metabolic pattern of the "gym rat"—the person who works out intensively for up to an hour and a half every day. Like the idealist, the gym rat has a concentrated period of strenuous activity, during which a lot of calories are burned. But in many other respects, the balance of the day requires a low level of activity, so metabolism is all but dormant throughout most waking hours.

Skillpower, Not Willpower

Losing fat while maintaining energy could be easier than you think it is. But you will need to make a sequence of specific changes in your daily habits. Many people rely on willpower—doing more of the same, but with greater effort—to make change and stick with it. But willpower works only for a while. The real solution is what I call skillpower.

Simply put, skillpower is the ability to adopt a set of ultrapractical, scientifically sound strategies that are tailored to your own unique needs. These strategies are effective and safe. And they don't require you to list enough New Year's resolutions to rival the length of the US Constitution. When you use skillpower, the results come automatically.

According to more than 50 research studies involving over 30,000 men and women, *effective self-change depends on doing the right things at the right times.*[11] It makes little sense to fight fat by going off on a tangent, as diet-only and exercise-only programs do. According to one study, for example, most people who watch their diets are physically inactive, while many exercisers disregard the need to eat a modest-carb, moderate-fat, higher-protein, higher-fiber diet.[12]

Another review of more than 80 research articles indicates that one of the most important elements in successful self-change is perceived control,[13] a sense that you can take charge of the requisite steps required. According to one leading research team, "People who rely solely upon willpower set themselves up for failure."[14] That's why the Meta-Stat approach adheres to the fundamental principle of "skillpower, not willpower."

Now turn your attention to the bottom chart. This is a graph of day-long metabolism—the key measure of energy—if you take the Meta-Stat approach. Rather than remaining relatively inactive for much of the day, you're constantly jump-starting your metabolism, using the simple, adaptable MSOn Switches. You don't need to plan for—or dread!—that ferociously challenging workout at the end of the day. You don't need to count calories or grams of fat or plan your meals with meticulous care to make sure you adhere to a particular program. When your body is in the rhythm of its most favorable pattern, energy production continues all day long, and your "fueling requirements"—small snacks and modest meals—are satisfying rather than restrictive.

DRIVEN BY REWARDS, NOT GUILT

If you have ever followed a restrictive diet, you know what it means to be on a "guilt-driven program." These programs usually require you to eat certain kinds of foods while severely limiting your intake of others. But what happens if you're on one of these programs and you eat the "wrong" foods? You're likely to feel instant remorse. It's like falling off the wagon. You probably feel as if you're backsliding or (to repeat an oft-quoted phrase) "getting into bad habits" again.

With the Meta-Stat approach, your outlook is quite different. Food is not something that makes you "put on" or helps you "take off" weight. The Meta-Stat approach emphasizes the bigger picture. I ask you to consider all the factors relevant to your eating habits, such as the timing of meals and snacks, the fluids you drink, and how energized, satisfied, or restful you feel. That way, you can discover your personal preferences for certain eating patterns and types of food. With the Meta-Stat approach, you constantly reward yourself in ways that really count—by taking pleasure in what you eat and by timing your meals and snacks for maximum energy, so you end up feeling healthier, more energetic, and more alive.

Or compare the exercise component of the Meta-Stat approach to that of guilt-based programs. In a guilt-based program, you feel remorse if you skip the health club for a few days, cut short your workout time, or do fewer than usual repetitions. These programs rely on firm discipline and self-denial. Some people start to view themselves as complete failures if they backslide in the slightest way.

With the Meta-Stat approach, there are no stringent measurements, no such thing as backsliding. You are not punishing your body into achieving better performance or chastising yourself for missing an appointment at the gym. Instead, you have a constant range of options, some providing immediate rewards, others benefiting your long-term health and sense of well-being. However you use your personal options to integrate the switches into your lifestyle, you'll feel the benefits and reap the rewards.

The Meta-Stat approach is rhythmic, instinctive, and natural. It respects your physical and mental requirements for regular sustenance, periodic relaxation, sensory change, and stress release. Your body and mind can fully accommodate the pressures and constraints of any lifestyle. Once you broaden your range of skills by adopting MSOn Switches and the Meta-Stat Starters, creating cycles of relaxation and tension, you have all the resources you need for energy, strength, and weight loss. Your daily cycles become easy and automatic rather than challenging and guilt-making.

With the Meta-Stat approach, stress is not even a factor. In fact, the focus is on stress *relief,* which is far better for your health and longevity. You simply answer your mental and physical needs in the most natural way possible.

START A POSITIVE CHAIN REACTION

One smart new move—something as simple as an extra few seconds of muscle toning here and there throughout the day, sipping some ice water, or eating a small, higher-protein snack instead of going hours until the next meal—can set off a domino effect that ramps up your fat-burning, energy-boosting power, and does it naturally. With a bit of practice, it becomes automatic. Your body's senses will detect a slight dip in energy and prompt you to raise it. In this way, you unconsciously begin to master keeping your Meta-Stat setting on "high."

And it makes lots of scientific sense. As biologist George Land reminded us, every day of our lives, we are either growing or dying.[15] There is no middle ground. "Life is but a mass of habits—practical, emotional, and intellectual . . . systematically organized for our greatness or grief," concurred psychologist and philosopher William James.[16] Can these habits be changed? he was asked. Yes, he replied, we can change these small habits that press us through each day. And then he added that we must recognize that, whether changed or ignored, "these habits bear us irresistibly toward our destiny."

For years now, many of us have been busy attacking fat with well-intended but ultimately ineffective tactics or in a piecemeal fashion that, biochemically speaking, has doomed us to failure. Despite heroic efforts and all the recent popularity of low-carb and no-carb diets, conventional weight-loss programs can actually increase the body's fat-making and fat-storing activities.

In an editorial that appeared in the *Journal of the American Medical Association,* F. Xavier Pi-Sunyer, MD, director of the Obesity Research Center at St. Luke's–Roosevelt Hospital in New York City, sounded the medical alarm, pointing out that nationwide increases in average adult levels of body fat put millions of Americans at increased risk for heart disease, hypertension, diabetes, stroke, gout, arthritis, and some forms of cancer.[17] In his words, excess body fat is now at "epidemic" levels in the United States—and being overweight may have as much impact on health as smoking.

So what's the best way to begin turning things around? With a single choice you can make right now, wherever you are in your weight-loss efforts: Quit trying harder.

Research shows that doing more of the same, only harder—more exercise, more deprivation, more dieting, more willpower, more guilt—isn't the way to succeed. In fact, it can make the problem even bigger. You become blind to better pathways, and you start accomplishing less and less. Besides, sooner or later, you're going to reach the point where you just can't try any harder—where your physical and mental resources are pushed to the breaking point or your spirit wanes. More effort isn't the answer. It's time to shift gears and break out of old routines.

CHAPTER 2

■   ■   ■

Hormones: Your Meta-Stat's Master Regulators

Asingle moment in time. That's what today's world is from an evolutionary perspective. We humans are genetically designed to function best if we respect the diet, exercise, and stress management principles that evolved a very long time ago.

Remember, the human genome has changed less than 0.02 percent in the past 40,000 years.[1] Our genes and biochemistry are deeply, even stubbornly, designed to function just as they did long ago, based on ancient cycles of feast and famine, energy and survival.

Geneticists estimate that it takes perhaps 200,000 years to significantly shift our genetic makeup as a human race. So the signals that most effectively spark our Meta-Stats are deeply wired into our metabolism today. We ignore them at our own risk.

I've heard some people say, "How can something so old be so important? Weren't our ancestors suffering and barely surviving?" Nothing could be further from the truth. According to virtually all of the in-depth studies, these men and women were free of most diseases, healthy, fit, strong, and filled with vitality.[2] The medical evidence indicates that their body fat levels, strength, aerobic capacity, blood pressure, blood cholesterol, and metabolism were vastly superior to those of the average man or woman today.

Why does it matter so much? Look at our modern society. We're completely out of touch with our genetic needs for specific kinds of nutrition, exercise, light, temperature, and rest.

But fortunately, we now have the scientific knowledge and the research to understand a great deal about how the ancient genetic code works. That also gives us greater power to adapt ourselves, and our daily lives, in such a way that we enjoy the healthiest lifestyle possible. The Meta-Stat approach taps into the body's powerful instinctive wisdom and metabolic mechanisms.[3] It mobilizes your inner power to stop fat gain and fatigue and promote the vigor and strength that millions of people have been desperately seeking but cannot find.

As I've indicated, you can take practical steps to make the most of your genetically inherited power to be vibrant and healthy. All you need to do is activate the MSOn Switches that I'll discuss a bit later in the book. In those chapters, I'll introduce many more techniques that will help control those switches to maximize energy and fat burning.

But right now, you may be wondering about the scientific basis for these guidelines. Just how much do scientists know about what happens inside the body when a particular switch is turned on or off?

While there are—and probably always will be—some gaps in the information, recent discoveries related to the Meta-Stat are as fascinating as any of the newest breakthroughs in science. Much of this research has concentrated on hormones, which appear to influence the Meta-Stat in ways that scientists never imagined.

MEET THE KEY PLAYERS

Hormones are potent chemical messengers generated by the body in response to a wide range of signals. Which hormones you produce, and in what quantities, depends on your eating habits, your activity level, your ability to handle stress, the amount of light to which you're exposed, the temperature of the air and your body, your fluid balance, your sleep pattern, and your capacity for energy renewal.

Hormones relay information about your body and its needs to the brain and to millions of receptor sites around the body. Those sites in turn send out messages that cause your body to either burn or store fat. In other words, hormones have the power to make your body's fat stores available as fuel—or to prevent that from happening, instead stimulating more fat storage. The good news is, you have control over your hormones, perhaps more than you think.

Insulin: The Carb-Control Hormone

One of the most important hormones directly affecting fat burning or fat storage is insulin. It is secreted by your pancreas in response to elevated blood sugar levels, most often after a meal or snack. This hormone deposits blood sugar and proteins into muscle tissues so you can move and function well. Further, insulin helps synthesize proteins inside the body for use in generating other hormones, enzymes, and muscle.

The main challenge posed by insulin is its supersensitivity to carbohydrates. It is especially sensitive to so-called high-glycemic carbs such as refined sugar, fructose syrup, flour, potatoes, and more. These shock your biochemistry into producing lots of insulin. Low-glycemic carbs, on the other hand, have a much gentler effect on blood sugar. They break down much more slowly, over a longer period of time.

Unless you have diabetes—which is an insulin-related health issue—your entire bloodstream requires a whopping total of 1 teaspoon (5 grams) of sugar at any moment. Yet the average American consumes over 20 teaspoons of sugar a day. Our society is filled with carbohydrate addicts who eat more than half of their daily calories as refined or starchy carbs, the high-glycemic foods that shock the system. With this kind of diet, insulin is almost continually produced and dumped into the bloodstream in an attempt to lower, and stabilize, blood sugar levels.

Now, it's true that we need carbohydrates. They are the brain's principal energy source. In fact, of a single teaspoon of blood sugar circulating in your system at any given moment, your brain requires about two-thirds. But the brain and body can use only a very limited amount of carbohydrate. When there are more carbs in the bloodstream than are necessary for fuel, your body tries to store them for future use in the form of a string of glucose molecules called glycogen.

Glycogen is deposited first in the muscles and liver. But there's not very much storage room in those cells, and the carbs that overflow this small storage capacity go immediately into body fat.

By some estimates, the average American consumes 156 pounds of sugar in a year. Now, consider what happens to this overabundance of sugar, plus many hundreds of pounds of other refined or high-glycemic carbohydrates. This quantity so far exceeds the body's requirements that about three-fourths of this carbohydrate goes directly to body fat.

Meanwhile, high insulin levels stimulate the release of the single most powerful fat-storing hormone, lipoprotein lipase (LPL). This is the hormone that sets up your 25 billion fat cells to do two things that, taken to extremes, are detrimental to your health. First, LPL tells those cells to store more fat, starting immediately. Second, it helps protect that fat from being released or burned as fuel in the future.

Most of us have learned that the more fat we eat, the fatter we become. But thanks to the combined effects of insulin and LPL, we also become fatter every time we consume high-glycemic carbohydrates.

The truth is, we vitally need a variety of carbohydrates every day. But we need them in limited quantities—and most people consume way more than they need.

Under optimal conditions, your body was designed to produce about three-fourths of its daily energy primarily by burning stored body fat reserves, not sugar. But when insulin and LPL levels are high, they effectively block your body from using stored fat as the main fuel source.

When you overeat sweet or salty refined carbohydrate foods, lots of insulin gets produced. This causes blood sugar to plummet, which triggers low blood sugar (hypoglycemic) reactions. It also triggers cravings, because the brain wants to make sure there's enough blood sugar for fuel. It's a vicious cycle.

Glucagon: Triggering Fat Release

Glucagon is the hormone that counterbalances insulin. Where insulin production is stimulated by carbohydrates, glucagon production is stimulated by proteins. While insulin works to make sure blood sugar levels don't get too high, glucagon works to make sure they don't fall too low—as happens when you skip meals or snacks altogether in an attempt to reduce calories.

Insulin sets you up for fat gain through its partnership with LPL. Glucagon is dedicated to triggering the release of stored fat from fat cells by producing an enzyme known as hormone-sensitive lipase (HSL).

HSL activity increases after meals or snacks high in lean protein and low-glycemic carbs and moderate to low in healthy fats. Once liberated from the body's fat cells, this free fatty acid can be burned as fuel for energy.

But our bodies have evolved in such a way that whenever glucagon and insulin are present together in the bloodstream in equal amounts, the insulin always wins. By changing the way you eat and implementing the other MSOn Switches, you can turn that tide away from fat storage and toward fat burning.

T3: The Thermostat Setter

Another important factor in Meta-Stat function is your thyroid gland. This gland essentially regulates the Meta-Stat, controlling the rate at which your metabolism hums along and body fat is burned. Triiodothyronine, or T3, is by far the most active of the thyroid hormones.

One of the ways the body synthesizes T3 is from an enzyme called 5-deiodinanse. This process requires the mineral selenium. Many Americans are not getting enough selenium in their diets,[4] which may be hampering their ability to produce the thyroid hormones that help turn up the Meta-Stat and burn off excess fat.

Cortisol and Epinephrine: Partners in Stress

Let's face it: Stress is everywhere. Naturally, your Meta-Stat monitors the hormones that are produced by physical and psychological stress. But the greatest influence on the Meta-Stat is not how much stress you have in your life but how you respond to it.[5] If you handle pressure well, your metabolism can stay high and, with it, your fat-burning power. But if you let stress eat away at you and clutch you like a fog, the Meta-Stat gets turned way down. Chronic anger, frustration, guilt, and worry are all fattening. Here's why.

The body responds to stressful conditions by releasing a cascade of hormones from the adrenal glands. The most powerful of these hormones are epinephrine (which we used to call adrenaline) and cortisol.

Both are designed to give you a quick burst of energy to fight or flee. Epinephrine puts the body's systems on full alert. Cortisol breaks down dietary protein, fats, and carbohydrates into blood sugar for immediate availability to the brain, muscles, and senses.

But here's the sticking point: If you don't have enough readily available protein in the bloodstream from your most recent meal or snack, cortisol extracts it from your healthy muscle tissue. This extraction creates a backward, toxic emergency process known as hepatic gluconeogenesis, which means, literally, "making new glucose in the liver." Each time this happens, the stress reaction robs you of healthy muscle tissue that is supposed to be giving you energy, keeping your Meta-Stat on high, and burning excess body fat. (This is one of the major problems with diets: You gain back weight because you've lost a vital part of your body's fat-burning power.)

There's another reason why you'll gain body fat if you mismanage stress. When you're chronically feeling overstressed or stressed out, your body may stimulate the cortisol to produce even more LPL, the fat-storing enzyme. That in turn ramps up the ability of your 25 to 30 billion fat cells to plump up even more. Some evidence indicates that this stress–fat storage link is even more of a problem in women than in men.

Mismanaged stress also depletes your reserves of a number of key brain chemicals, such as dopamine and serotonin.

Dopamine and Norepinephrine: The Alertness Boosters

In the brain, messages are sent from cell to cell by way of electrical impulses and chemicals called neurotransmitters.[6] A number of the neurotransmitters are manufactured in the brain from components of the foods you eat.

Dopamine and norepinephrine are two of the key alertness neurotransmitters. They immediately increase your level of attentiveness. At the same time, they rev up fat burning and give you a heightened sense of energy and motivation. They help you manage stress and make big problems feel more manageable (as opposed to stress hormones that make little problems feel like mountains).

Certain amino acids—the building blocks of proteins—enable the brain to make these neurotransmitters. The principal ingredient in dopamine and norepinephrine is the amino acid tyrosine. Almost any high-quality food source (not pill source) of protein—my favorites include fish, shellfish, skinless chicken or turkey, low fat dairy products, dried beans, lentils, and soy—makes tyrosine available to your brain. And you reap the benefits.

Serotonin: The Mood Connection

Serotonin is one of the brain's primary mood chemicals. It influences your sleep patterns, hunger, anxiety levels, and temperature regulation. When your brain lacks serotonin, you are likely to become more anxious, and you may be unable to fall into a deep sleep. Also, your appetite soars.

Unfortunately, one of the simplest ways to keep serotonin levels high is to consume high-glycemic carbohydrates, which, as you've learned, are fatiguing and fattening. What's more, after you've eaten high-glycemic carbs, it takes about 20 minutes for the brain to send the satiety signal, "I'm full." So you keep eating those empty-calorie foods that raise insulin levels and create even more cravings for sweet, refined foods.

Luckily, there's a better way to naturally raise serotonin levels. The amino acid tryptophan is essential for the manufacture of serotonin. When you eat enough low-glycemic carbohydrates, a greater supply of tryptophan gets transported to the brain, where it generates serotonin. Foods naturally high in tryptophan can also help. These include low-fat or fat-free milk, turkey or chicken breast, low-fat or fat-free yogurt, soy, whey protein, and even bananas.

Galanin: It's a Downer

In the evenings, it's crucial to avoid high-glycemic, high-fat foods that can cause another brain chemical to wreak havoc. That chemical is the hormone galanin.

The trouble with galanin is that it's an antagonist to serotonin. Similar to the way insulin wins out when competing with glucagon, galanin wins out when competing with serotonin. Galanin creates feelings of fatigue, confusion, and vulnerability, along with cravings for more high-fat, highly sweetened foods.[7] Worse, it not only turns up the taste for fat, it also affects other hormones in such a way as to virtually ensure that any excess dietary fat gets stored as body fat.[8]

Galanin levels crest in the evening, at the very time many of us eat our largest meal of the day. If your evening meals and snacks contain lots of high-glycemic foods with fat—such as chips, high-fat dips, ice cream, doughnuts, cookies, or high-fat crackers—galanin drives this dietary fat directly into your body's fat cells. Some people begin snacking early in the evening, then find they can't stop. The culprit is galanin.

CCK: A Hormone against Hunger

Cholecystokinin, or CCK, is a natural and most powerful anti-hunger hormone. Its environment is the gastrointestinal tract. One of its roles is to trigger the release of a host of enzymes from the pancreas that increase the natural absorption of nutrients from your intestines and the natural movement of waste products through the colon.

But CCK has another job. It signals the brain that you are full. Research indicates that a rise in CCK corresponds with reduced food intake. So when CCK is high, you'll probably eat less at a single sitting.[9]

CCK seems to be strongly stimulated by specialized small protein peptides called glycomacropeptides (GMPs), which also provide antibacterial protection for the body. Small amounts of high-quality protein at meals and snacks, as recommended in the Meta-Stat approach, may support this effect.

Melatonin and Prolactin: The Body Clock Regulators

Good-quality sleep is a major ally in the quest for fat burning and energy building. Getting excellent rest—the kind that builds up your reserves for the next day—requires the right balance of hormones. This comes about naturally (if you let it) when the sun sets. The ancient pre-optic areas of the brain shift your neurochemistry toward sleep by triggering the production and release of the hormone melatonin (which also happens to have a vital antiaging effect on the brain and body).

After a steady stretch of at least 3 hours of melatonin production, another neurochemical, prolactin, joins the mix. It further strengthens the function of your immune system. A few critical sleep factors, including total darkness, are essential if you want to get the most beneficial mix of melatonin and prolactin.

Calcitrol: The Calcium Beacon

In the absence of enough calcium, levels of the hormone calcitrol increase. Among other changes, calcitrol turns off the mechanisms that break down fat and burn it, and it activates the mechanisms that make more body fat.[10]

Leptin, Agouti, and Ghrelin: Antagonists in the Fight for Fat Loss

One of the best ways to resist unhealthy foods and burn more body fat is to enlist the help of leptin. The name comes from the Greek *leptos,* which means "thin." Inside the brain, leptin's job is to regulate the intensity of your appetite and to influence the speed at which your body burns calories.

Leptin is produced in abundance by your natural fat cells whenever your metabolism is naturally high and fat loss is necessary. Leptin levels fall whenever the body thinks you need to conserve existing body fat or make extra fat to survive.[11]

Researchers report that a diet rich in natural plant foods, with healthy amounts of protein and moderate amounts of carbohydrates and good fats—consistent with the Meta-Stat approach—helps keep leptin levels high. Where high-fat foods suppress leptin,[12] low-fat foods not only increase leptin levels but also boost the hormone's effectiveness, helping each molecule of leptin to attach to cells and improve fat burning.[13]

A Harvard study showed that regular exercise can dramatically increase leptin levels.[14] Even 15- to 20-minute cardio workouts or muscle-toning sessions can have a significant effect on the hormone.

Scientists have discovered that leptin acts on certain key brain areas to stimulate the production of antioxidants known as melanocortins. These melanocortins—the same chemicals produced by the skin in response to even brief, safe exposure to sunshine—also suppress the appetite centers in the brain, aiding metabolism and the loss of excess body fat.[15]

Another hormone, agouti, is present in the same parts of the brain as melanocortin and competes with it.[16] Agouti counterbalances melanocortin to keep appetite high when body fat levels drop. With too much agouti and not enough melanocortin, you become hungry and burn less fat. Fat cells have special receptors for agouti and respond to increases in it by creating more fat inside the cell and decreasing fat loss.[17]

Whenever you skip meals or snacks, a hormone called ghrelin is secreted by the stomach and triggers a voracious appetite, so you overeat. At the same time, leptin drops to very low levels, slowing your metabolism so that you convert extra calories to body fat and "lock in" the fat cells you already have. This is an ancient survival instinct. Combined result: The falling levels of leptin stimulate the body to make and store new body fat even when it feels as if you're "starving"; you stop burning off excess body fat because the fat cell "doors" are locked; and you're constantly hungry because there's too much ghrelin. The likely outcome? It's easier than ever to feel overwhelmed with hunger and discouragement.

Adiponectin: Fat-Burning Accelerator

Here's a protein that strongly affects the liver and muscles. According to Harvey Lodish, professor of biology at MIT. "Adiponectin lowers blood sugar by blocking its production in the liver and by increasing the burning by muscles to make energy. It activates part of the same signaling pathway in muscles that is activated by exercise."[18] But adiponectin levels fall as body fat levels rise. The various elements of the Meta-Stat approach work collectively to help keep adiponectin levels higher.

HGH: The Vital Human Growth Hormone

During deep, high-quality sleep, when enough melatonin is being produced, another key hormone is secreted by your pituitary gland. It's human growth hormone, or HGH, which is the body's most powerful natural revitalizer.

One of the most important roles of HGH is to free up stored body fat, so you can burn it to produce energy. It also stimulates an increase in muscle tissue. HGH finds a way to reach all of your body's billions of fat cells. Attaching to specialized receptors on those cells, HGH triggers the signal that will induce the cells to release stored fat. The good news is that you can naturally stimulate the production of HGH at any age. The Meta-Stat approach helps you achieve this optimal activation of HGH in a variety of ways, including:

- Very deep rest during what researchers call the critical healing period between midnight and 3:00 A.M.

- Regular muscle-toning exercise

- A diet that keeps insulin levels in check

The "Sex Hormones": Decoding the Difference

It's a fact that women tend to gain excess body fat faster than men.[19] Not fair, of course, but this is where evolution has led us. The female body was engineered to ensure the optimal birth and well-being of human offspring. This meant women needed more body fat than men. As a result, men and women differ in how they produce energy and burn excess fat—processes driven in part by the so-called sex hormones.

Both the male and female bodies contain the two primary sex hormones, estrogen and testosterone, but in varying percentages. Testosterone is a crucial fat-burning hormone. Human beings can't build any muscle tissue or muscle tone without it.

In contrast, estrogen generally encourages the deposit of extra fat throughout the body. Estrogen-stimulated fat cells tend to more stubbornly hold on to their fat reserves. But there are good estrogens and bad estrogens. The bad estrogens—such as estradiol and 16-hydroxyl estrone—ramp up fat storage. The good estrogens, called 2-hydroxyl estrogens, encourage the release of stored body fat for burning during exercise.

Women tend to lose muscle tone even faster than men as the years go by, apparently due to a biological signal that developed through evolution. This is one reason women need to become very focused on building and sustaining muscle tone, which also helps protect the bones against calcium loss and osteoporosis.

Men are lucky to have extra testosterone, at least for a while. It increases oxygen uptake, which is vital for thermogenesis and fat burning. Testosterone also helps balance blood sugar and keep insulin release in check. That makes it harder to produce and store body fat. But testosterone levels also decline rapidly after age 30. Along with the loss of the hormone comes the loss of vital muscle tissue and an increase in body fat and fatigue.

Mismanaged stress virtually guarantees a loss of testosterone. During a single bout of peak stress, a man's testosterone levels can plunge by 50 percent or more.

For both sexes, metabolism of the sex hormones slowly but steadily changes, starting between ages 25 and 30. But no matter what your age or gender, you can revitalize fat burning and minimize fat storage. Just use the practical methods incorporated in the MSOn Switches. First, try the strength-training exercises, which significantly raise levels of testosterone at every age. Second, get adequate quantities of high-quality protein in your meals and snacks, so you increase fat-burning hormones.[20] Third, stay on top of stress. And fourth, make sure your diet has moderate amounts of soy protein. (Phytoestrogens in soy appear to parallel the natural impact of estrogen, but without the fat-storing side effects.)

There are other strategies that can significantly improve balance among the sex hormones. For one thing, it's important to get enough zinc, a vital ally of testosterone. In addition, make sure you're eating plenty of cruciferous vegetables, a family that includes broccoli, cauliflower, brussels sprouts, kale, rutabaga, and turnips. In women especially, they may tip the balance of estrogens in favor of the good ones—that is, the kind that contribute to fat burning rather than fat storage.

CHAPTER 3

■ ■ ■

Turn On Your Meta-Stat, Turn Off Fat Gain and Fatigue

Now that you have a basic understanding of how and why the Meta-Stat approach works, you're ready to learn how to take control of your Meta-Stat by turning on and off specific switches. Please don't feel that you need to master all of them. The beauty of the Meta-Stat approach is that it's completely flexible, so you can tailor it to your goals, needs, and lifestyle.

My suggestion is to read through the descriptions of the switches in this chapter to get a general idea of how they affect your Meta-Stat. If you see one that piques your interest, you might want to jump ahead to that chapter so you can find out more about it. Maybe you'll give it a test run by trying one or more of the Meta-Stat Starters. But do get acquainted with all of the switches; later on, you'll combine your choice of switches with the MSOn Workout and MSOn Eating Plan to create your very own Meta-Stat program. All the details—including the Meta-Stat Success Map, a handy tool to guide and track your efforts—appear in Part 5.

THE MSOn SWITCHES

The MSOn Switches use simple actions to provide continual boosts to your metabolism and thermogenesis, the key biochemical processes for optimal Meta-Stat function. Individually and collectively, these switches tap into your hidden reserves of fat-burning, energy-boosting power. And their effects last around the clock, even while you sleep.

As you read through the MSOn Switches, please keep in mind that no single switch is a solution in and of itself. Rather, the cumulative effects of the switches make the difference.

1. Wake up on the right side of the bed. What you do first thing in the morning has a tremendous impact on your Meta-Stat the rest of the day. You raise your Meta-Stat setting with the signals you send it. With six simple start-your-day strategies, you convey the message "This is going to be an active, energetic day." (See page 41.)

2. Create activity momentum. With every physical action that makes use of your major muscle groups, your Meta-Stat cranks up a little higher. Just getting up and moving every 30 minutes may not build muscle or aerobic fitness, but it's enough to produce a spike in fat burning and energy. (See page 55.)

3. Catch light to boost energy. More than you might imagine, light is an "on" switch for the brain and senses.[1] It elevates metabolism while providing a burst of energy. With that energy, you're more active and vital. (See page 67.)

4. Take in more oxygen. Oxygen molecules are the primary fuel for adenosine triphosphate, a key energy source in the metabolic process. Fat burning just doesn't happen unless you get enough oxygen.[2] Overcoming the typical shallow-breathing pattern takes practice, but deep, relaxed respiration not only supports fat burning, it helps counteract stress. (See page 71.)

5. Seek ideal fluid intake. There's increasing evidence that fat-loss efforts often fail because of dehydration.[3] Without enough water, your body's fat-burning mechanisms slow down, and appetite increases. Fluids enable your circulatory system to move hormones into exactly the right places for incinerating excess fat. (See page 75.)

6. Rise up and stand tall. Every time you extend your posture, you deepen your breathing, which means better oxygen intake.[4] Good posture also sends a powerful signal to your body's energy-making mechanisms to "be ready for anything." (See page 85.)

7. Turn down the heat, turn up your energy. When the air is cool, the ambient temperature sends a powerful signal to your Meta-Stat to fire up the body's furnace. In response, your body burns more fat as a means of warming itself to meet the demands of your environment.[5] (See page 94.)

8. Improve hormone balance, hour after hour. In Chapter 2, we saw how hormones play a key role in Meta-Stat function. Research shows that we have a lot more control over our hormones than most of us realize. (See page 97.)

9. Stay calm in an uptight world. If you spend any amount of time with people who are tense, you probably will feel tense yourself. This not only wastes energy and triggers production of fat-storing hormones, it also throws your body chemistry out of whack.[6] Whenever you feel tension creeping up on you, strive for calm. (See page 106.)

10. Stop the stress response. Unlike tension, which usually builds from within, stress is an outside force. When mismanaged, it produces hormones that instantly create fatigue and promote fat storage. To keep your Meta-Stat running optimally, you must learn effective coping techniques to nip stress in the bud. (See page 122.)

11. Ramp up your evening Meta-Stat setting. Your preparation for the evening really starts in late afternoon. How you make this transition will determine how much energy you have when you get home. It will also help overcome your body's natural tendency toward an evening metabolic slump. (See page 136.)

12. Get plenty of good-quality rest. A recent study published in the *International Journal of Obesity* linked deep sleep with lower body fat in nearly 7,000 volunteer participants.[7] Other studies confirm just how vital deep rest is to energy and fat loss.[8] Studies by Eve Van Cauter, PhD, a professor in the department of medicine at the University of Chicago, indicate that even a few nights of poor-quality sleep, or not enough sleep, significantly increase insulin resistance and fat storage.[9] (See page 151.)

THE MSOff SWITCHES

So far, I've emphasized the MSOn Switches, which translate small actions into big results. Unlike other approaches, every switch is within your reach wherever you are throughout the day. You just need to turn it on.

As you might expect, the MSOn Switches have a flip side. As easily as you can turn them on, you can turn them off, reducing metabolism and thermogenesis in the process. When you consciously or unconsciously hit one of the MSOff Switches, you send a signal that increases fat storage and drains energy.

Few people even know when they've activated an MSOff Switch. But they feel the effects over time, in the form of weight gain and fatigue. This is why drastic measures like near-starvation diets never work for weight loss: They flip so many MSOff Switches that the body shifts into preservation mode.

The following list identifies the patterns and behaviors that may be pushing your Meta-Stat from "on" to "off." Pay attention for these as you go about your daily routine; if one sneaks in, take steps to change back to MSOn mode as quickly as possible.

1. Starting the day on the wrong foot. A lack of physical movement, no exposure to bright light, skipping breakfast, and other unhealthy A.M. habits can each increase the body's hibernation-like instincts. This casts a long shadow, since you're more likely to store fat and feel tired all day long.

2. Giving in to inactivity inertia. This is a fat maker extraordinaire. Evolutionarily, we were not designed to sit still very long, vegetating. In fact, sitting for more than 30 minutes at a shot is a surefire way to fuel weight gain and fatigue, as it signals the brain to conserve energy—and therefore fat—rather than burning it. As a result, oxygen intake plummets, blood circulation slows, and hormones become out of whack.

3. Weakening muscle fibers. One of your greatest allies in the fight against fat and fatigue is muscle. But muscle requires regular, intensive stimuli to stay healthy. Some people believe the best way to build muscle is with twice-weekly strength-training workouts. Not true. After each long workout, metabolism falls back to its resting rate. What works is challenging your muscles every day, if just for a minute at a time.

4. Living in the dark. Back when our ancestors were alive, the arrival of winter—with its fewer daylight hours—prompted their bodies to significantly slow metabolism. It was an important survival mechanism when food was scarce. But not today. If you spend most of your waking hours in dim light, you are shutting down a key component of your brain's fat-burning, energy-producing arsenal.

5. Starving yourself of oxygen. Studies show that most people don't get nearly enough oxygen over the course of the day.[10] Part of the reason is poor posture and lack of physical activity: We don't sit in a way that allows us to breathe fully and naturally, and when we're inactive, our brains don't get the signals instructing us to breathe deeply and often. Our bodies have grown accustomed to shallow breathing and oxygen starvation, but that dampens our ability to slim down and energize.

6. Becoming dehydrated. According to research, nearly everyone is slightly dehydrated 24 hours a day. While our bodies have grown accustomed to this lack of vital fluids, as little as 1 to 2 percent dehydration increases cardiovascular strain and accelerates exhaustion.[11] Poor fluid intake—fewer than six glasses a day—causes the body to secrete the hormone aldosterone, prompting tissue to hold on to almost every molecule of water and sodium it can, according to Peter Lindner, MD, in *Fat, Water Retention and You*.[12] Several researchers have suggested that a decrease in water may cause an increase in fat deposits.[13]

7. Maxing out on caffeine. Small servings of caffeinated coffee or tea bump up heart rate and may boost metabolism, at least slightly. But when you overdo, your body reverses the effect in an attempt to resist caffeinism, a condition characterized by high levels of stress hormones as well as physical and mental exhaustion.

8. Overimbibing. Whenever you drink alcohol, your body burns less fat, and more slowly than usual. In a study published in the *New*

England Journal of Medicine, scientists found that two drinks a day reduced the body's ability to burn fat by about one-third.[14] Research also suggests that, in some people, two drinks a day may significantly increase sensitivity to blood sugar. This leads to high levels of insulin, which stimulates the conversion of carbohydrates to fat and increases weight gain.[15]

9. Slumping your way to fat gain. The ability to stand erect on two feet is a uniquely human attribute. But these days, good posture is a rarity. Standing head-forward has become the standard. Unfortunately, it's making us fatter and more tired. You need to stand tall to properly support your body's fat-burning, energy-enhancing powers.

10. Raising body temperature. As discussed in Chapter 1, the human body evolved to produce energy (metabolism) and heat (thermogenesis) as a survival mechanism for being lean and exposed to cool temperatures.[16] When we shiver even slightly, we burn off fat and rev up metabolism. But when we bundle up or hide under layers of covers, the body doesn't need to make its own energy to stay warm. As a result, metabolism—and fat burning—slow down.

11. Living with hormonal imbalance. Hormones get out of kilter for many reasons. When you mishandle stress, have long periods of inactivity, eat the wrong foods or too much, or deprive yourself of sunlight, you negatively alter your hormone balance. Every time you react with a negative emotion such as anger or guilt, your brain triggers a hormonal response that promotes fat storage rather than fat burning.

12. Tensing up. Unlike the deliberate flexing that creates healthy muscle tone, chronic physical tension can be both fattening and tiring. It keeps summoning stress hormones that shift the body's chemistry into fat-making overdrive.[17] It also exhausts your psyche and sours your mood.

13. Giving in to stress. Uncontrolled stress triggers the release of the hormone cortisol, which stimulates the production of the fat-storing enzyme lipoprotein lipase (LPL). Studies also report the stress-related activation of the body's "starvation response," which heightens fat-making processes[18] and fat storage.[19] What's more, stress hormones—including cortisol and epinephrine—appear to increase insulin resistance, which in turn may add to the amount of stored body fat.[20]

14. Skipping meals or snacks. Studies confirm that skipping meals can lower your basal (baseline) metabolic rate.[21] On the other hand, if you eat most of your calories early in the day—at breakfast and lunch, for example—you'll actually stoke your metabolic fire to burn hotter, says Pat Harper, RD, MS, a spokesperson for the American Dietetic Association.[22]

15. Falling into the sugar blahs. This is a killer of a fat maker. To handle even a single teaspoon of sugar or another refined carbohydrate, your body must ramp up its fat-making and fat-storage functions. And a megasize soda has as much as *25 teaspoons* of corn syrup or white sugar. Furthermore, a high sugar intake prevents the brain from producing the vital fats that keep you smart and young.[23]

16. Getting stuck on the fat train. When you eat too much dietary fat, or the wrong kinds of dietary fat, it immediately converts to body fat. So that fat-laden dessert really does head straight for your hips or thighs! Just remember that not all fats are bad; you just need to know which to avoid—namely, the ones that slow metabolism and hinder thermogenesis.

17. Starving for protein. When you don't eat enough high-quality protein throughout the day, your body can react by blocking metabolism and thermogenesis, as if preparing for a long stretch of hibernation. The heat-enhancing, fat-burning effect of protein is 40 percent greater than that of carbohydrates.[24] But if you don't pay attention to the protein content of meals and snacks, you could set the stage for fat storage and fatigue.

18. Accidentally overeating. Evolutionarily speaking, the human body functions best on larger meals and snacks early in the day and very light eating in the late afternoon and evening. The problem with eating even "just a bit too much" in the evening is that your metabolism already has begun to slow down. So the extra calories more easily convert to body fat, and the digestive processes induce sleep when you really should be active.

19. Collapsing when evening comes. Nearly four of every five Americans get no significant physical activity in the evening.[25] As mentioned above, this is the time of day when metabolism slows to a crawl. So if you remain inactive, you effectively turn off your Meta-Stat. A bit of evening relaxation can be wonderful. But if it lasts for more than 30 minutes, uninterrupted by physical activity, both fat storage and fatigue set in.

20. Not getting enough sleep. While you're sleeping, your body is running thousands of crucial metabolic and thermogenic processes to repair and regenerate for the day ahead. But very few of us sleep long enough or, more important, deeply enough, which means these key processes fall behind or fail altogether. Instead of burning excess fat and recharging our batteries all night long, we're waking up even more tired than when we climbed into bed. According to Allan Rechtschaffen, PhD, director of the Sleep Research Laboratory at the University of Chicago, people who are sleep deprived tend to increase their calorie consumption by more than 10 to 15 percent per day.[26]

PART

The MSOn Switches

TWO

The Meta-Stat switches in the pages that follow have evolved not just from my study of the mechanisms behind fat loss and energy but also from the feedback of people who've read my previous books. Like you, they're seeking practical strategies that will improve their health so they feel more fully alive. My readers have been an invaluable source of information on which switches work best and which could use improvement.

All of the switches are consistent with my past recommendations. Here they have been modified or streamlined for the primary purpose of supporting optimal Meta-Stat function.

As we learn more about how the Meta-Stat works, the switches may undergo further transformation. For this book, my goal is to show you how you can take advantage of the latest findings now to burn fat and boost energy. That's what the Meta-Stat switches are all about.

CHAPTER 4

■ ■ ■

M S O n   S w i t c h   # 1

Wake Up on the Right Side of the Bed

How you wake up in the morning sets the tone for the whole day. In terms of your energy and metabolism, this is make-or-break time. Even choices that seem small can have a big impact.

Many people miss this early-morning opportunity. A lack of physical movement, no exposure to bright light, skipping breakfast, and other factors collectively increase the body's hibernation-like instincts. This can result in an increase in fat-storing tendencies and fatigue that lasts all day long.

Early in my study of fat loss and energy production, I determined that many important metabolic processes fire up in the first few minutes of the day. So I recommended switches like this one, to encourage people to start the day on the right foot, metabolically speaking. With further research, I better understand how the switch actually works. It has to do with the Meta-Stat.

> *Success Map Tip:*
> Record your breakfast and your energy level. Describe your morning MSOn Minutes in the space provided.

Within minutes of awakening, you can begin to raise the setting on your Meta-Stat dial with the signals you send it. Six simple keys turn the dial way up, with the message "This is going to be an active, energetic day." Here are the keys.

1. Calm energy instead of tension or rushing

2. Muscle-toning activity within an hour of awakening

3. Exposure to bright light

4. A few bites of a great-tasting breakfast with high-quality protein

5. A focus on self-regulation rather than self-control

6. The MSOn mindset, which establishes the rhythmic use of Meta-Stat signals at regular intervals throughout the day

Let's look at these individually and see how they affect your physical well-being and your mental outlook.

1. CALM ENERGY INSTEAD OF TENSION OR RUSHING

Many people have the misconception that they need to "start the day with a bang." But that's counterproductive. If you jump right up and go into overdrive, you ramp up levels of tension and tiredness, which turn the Meta-Stat backward. Remember, the Meta-Stat obeys a law of ancient wisdom. If you expend a whole lot of energy in the morning, the Meta-Stat will be fooled into thinking you need to conserve energy and protect body fat all day long.

So the key to A.M. success is staying calm—really calm. Stop for a moment to reflect on what this means.

What are your mornings like? Most people feel rushed, even frantic. That's because they set their alarms to get as much sleep as possible, so they don't have much time for lollygagging. As the alarm jangles them awake, they turn on a low-beam light (none of that blinding daylight!). They skip breakfast or simply gulp down a cup or two of coffee, figuring they really don't need to eat a major meal until noon or later. For most people, there's little morning exercise.

If this describes your own morning routine, you should be aware that such habits can backfire. Late awakening, low light, no exercise, little breakfast—all these factors combine to slow your metabolism and therefore fat burning and energy production.[1]

One of the reasons is this: From the moment you get out of bed, your brain cues your body's metabolism to match your current and anticipated physical demands.[2] If your morning ritual takes place in low light, and you're moving in slow motion, your brain gets a low "signal." It has little incentive to push your metabolism much higher than near-hibernation rate.

If you extend this "sleep walk" activity level into the morning—and skip breakfast in the process—you unwittingly fail to turn on this fat-burning switch. You may even stimulate fat-preserving and fat-storing processes instead.[3]

What about the tension factor? Most of us are so accustomed to feeling tense when we waken that we don't even notice the state of our nerves and muscles. If you can manage to leap instead of crawl out of bed, you might think you're full of energy. But it's tense energy, and as soon as it's expended, you'll grow increasingly tired.

The muscles of the body send a signal to the brain indicating tension, but it's more like a freak wave than a tide of energy. The signal is transmitted for a short time, after which the muscles' kinesthetic senses stop sounding the alarm. Energy passes, but the tension stays. We scarcely notice it. That's why, to increase calm energy, it's so vital to tune your senses to become much more aware of tension—and then to release it on the spot, whenever it appears.

2. MUSCLE-TONING ACTIVITY WITHIN AN HOUR OF AWAKENING

According to national surveys, many of us are quite sedentary in the morning hours, and this keeps metabolism sluggish. But it's not difficult to increase your morning metabolism—either before or after breakfast—if you make morning physical activity a part of your routine.[4]

First thing in the morning, you need to do at least some kind of brief, intense exercise. That's because your muscles need to be

One-Touch Relaxation

This pioneering concept, explored by neurosurgeon Vernon H. Mark, MD, of Massachusetts General Hospital, and others,[5] is one of the simplest ways to defuse tense energy and increase calm energy. It helps you stay alert and active all day long.

The principle is quite simple. Using gentle fingertip pressure, you elicit one-touch relaxation from key muscles. Those muscles in turn trigger a "cascade" effect that quickly dissolves tension throughout the body.

Here's how it's done.

- Place your fingertips on your jaw joints just in front of your ears.

- Inhale. As you do so, tense your jaw muscles, bringing the upper and lower jaw together. You'll feel as if you're clenching your teeth for several seconds.

- Exhale. Let your jaw muscles go totally loose, releasing all tension. Drop your lower jaw and relax your tongue until it lies on the bottom of your mouth, with the front of your tongue lightly touching your teeth.

As you're doing this, focus on the contrasting sensations of tensing and relaxing. Then repeat the exercise, but with less force. Tighten your

challenged briefly, and often, to increase their capacity to burn fat and help you feel 100 percent alive. Otherwise, chances are great you'll skip exercise throughout the rest of the day as well.

As I've already emphasized, that doesn't mean leaping out of bed and ratcheting up the tension. In fact, it's best to get out of bed slowly and, for the first half hour or so, gradually increase your activity level. But after that, make sure you do something really active, for an instant boost to your Meta-Stat setting.

My personal favorite morning exercise is pushups. This may sound

jaw muscles about half as much as you did the first time. Again, hold the tension for several seconds before releasing.

You can repeat this a number of times, reducing the tension every time you do so, until it's almost impossible to discern the difference between "tense" and "relaxed." What you're doing is using touch to create a sensory cue for relaxation. You link the sensation of your fingertips pressing your jaw muscles to a highly desirable sensation of releasing tension, so touch becomes a trigger. Your fingertips issue a mental command to relax.

Once you know how to trigger the relaxation response, you can use it in another way, to get some relief from the "shoulds" that add tension to your life. You probably know what the shoulds are—the duties, requirements, and emotional burdens that can make you feel like a bundle of nerves. As you're inhaling and tensing, then exhaling and relaxing, take this opportunity to release those shoulds.

With some practice, you'll be able to simply reach up and use a single touch on your tense jaw to trigger an immediate "wave" of relaxation through that area. You get such an instantaneous payoff because you elicit a powerful calming and energizing response from the brain.[6] This exercise is great first thing in the morning, but you can also use it during the day.

intimidating, but there are many kinds of modified pushups you can do. Instead of trying to lift and lower your whole body, for example, keep your lower legs on the floor and move just your upper body. Or do a standing pushup against a wall. Just plant your feet about 2 feet away from the wall and lean against it with your hands at shoulder level. Bend your elbows to incline your body toward the wall, then push away with your hands.

Whichever kind of pushup you do, try to work up to 20 repetitions. Then, as you become stronger, you can do traditional pushups. To increase the resistance, or "load," on the muscles, you can prop your feet on a stool or the edge of a sofa.

As an alternative to pushups, you can walk up and down a flight of stairs or do some simple, modified knee bends. See Part 3 for dozens of simple options.

Getting started early pays off every day. People who exercise in the morning are much more likely to get in a regular habit than those who wait until later in the day. That conclusion comes from a study by the Southwestern Health Institute in Phoenix.[7] Researchers found that three out of four people who engaged in some morning muscle-toning activity continued the exercise habit 1 year later. The research team compared morning exercisers to people who waited until midday and those who put off their workouts until the evening. The difference was significant. Among the midday group, only one in two kept up the regular exercise habit, and among the evening exercisers, just one in four stayed with the program.

I think this confirms what most of us know intuitively. Toward the middle or end of the day, we're a lot more likely to find reasons not to exercise. We're too busy, too tired—or we just "run out of time."

When is the best time for these brief muscle-toning activities? As I've mentioned, either before or after breakfast is fine. But there's evidence that you're more likely to burn off excess body fat if you exercise in the morning before you eat breakfast. In a study of runners conducted by Anthony Wilcox, PhD, at Kansas State University, two-thirds of the calories burned in prebreakfast workouts were from fat. By contrast, fat calories accounted for slightly less than half of total calories burned in afternoon runs.[8] After a full night's sleep, there is little glycogen (stored carbohydrate) in your muscles to supply energy. Therefore, more fat is used as fuel.[9]

3. EXPOSURE TO BRIGHT LIGHT

The human brain responds to many signals, but few are more powerful than light. "The body has hundreds of biochemical and hormonal rhythms, all keyed to light and dark," suggests Michael Irwin, MD, medical director of the United Nations.

In the late 1980s, a Harvard medical team discovered why the

Brighten Up Your Morning

Here's an experiment that will enable you to experience the immediate effect of bright lighting. In the morning, when you climb out of bed, do you usually turn on a single light? Instead, click on three or four. What do you feel? For many people, the added light instantaneously boosts alertness. Immediately, your physiology shifts away from sleep and toward a new day filled with more energy and higher metabolism.[10]

Although artificial light can be quite intense, real daylight is usually stronger. When you awaken, open all the window shades or curtains. If possible, step outside for a few minutes or go for a brief stroll to flood your eyes with daylight.

human brain seems to be so powerfully affected by exposure to bright light.[11] Professors Richard Kronauer, PhD, and Charles Czeisler, MD, headed the 3-year Harvard study in which they experimented using light with an intensity between 7,000 and 12,000 lux, which is comparable to daylight just after dawn. They discovered a neurological link between the retina of the eye and structures of the brain known as the suprachiasmatic nuclei, which are thought to play a key role in attention focus and energy production.

More recent research offers further evidence to support light's positive influence on the Meta-Stat setting. Scientists have identified a special type of photoreceptor in the eye that helps set the body's circadian rhythms and metabolism to sunlight—even in people who are functionally blind. These photoreceptors are found in the retina's ganglion cells, nerve cells that encode and transmit information from the eye to the brain.[12]

In the morning, it's important to pay your respects to this powerful metabolic signal. How? Spend 5 to 10 minutes in direct sunlight if possible. Or make sure you have bright light in your bedroom, bathroom, exercise room, kitchen—wherever you spend time first thing in the morning. You need that illumination to start your internal Meta-Stat clock on schedule.

On sunny mornings, do you step outside for a breath of fresh air and soak in the brightness? Many of us do this on vacations but not during the rest of the year. Make a point of it.

4. A FEW BITES OF A GREAT-TASTING BREAKFAST WITH HIGH-QUALITY PROTEIN

A study published in the *American Journal of Epidemiology* reported that those who miss breakfast are 4½ times more likely to be obese than those who eat a morning meal.[13] That being the case, why do so many people neglect this critically important daily ritual?

I think we all know the answer. Too often, early mornings are spent rushing around in a state of partial numbness. But if that's been your pattern up to now, you definitely should try to change it. Don't skip breakfast! It's the meal that matters most.[14]

Studies over the past 30 years have consistently shown that breakfast is beneficial in many ways, including:[15]

- Improved weight control

- Increased mental alertness and energy

- A more positive, constructive attitude

- More strength and endurance

- Improved performance at work and in school

- Less irritability and fatigue

In a surprising number of ways, breakfast sends a big message to your Meta-Stat. Here's why. Let's suppose you eat one small serving of a low-fat, high-fiber breakfast—perhaps a bowl of old-fashioned oatmeal with low-fat or fat-free milk, a piece of fruit, or a slice of 100 percent whole grain bread with fat-free cream cheese and all-fruit preserves. Just one small serving—and that, in itself, is enough to switch on your energy and fat-burning power.

On the other hand, when you skip breakfast, you not only keep the body's fat burners in "off" mode, you turn on the fat-making process instead. You lose twice!

Shake Up Breakfast

Protein shakes—combinations of milk or water, low-fat yogurt, whey protein powder, fresh fruit, ice, and other delicious ingredients—can serve as potent snacks and even meal substitutes. Among many scientific studies supporting this is one from the University of Tennessee, which found that people who added three daily servings of yogurt to their diets lost 61 percent more body fat and 81 percent more stomach fat over 12 weeks than people who didn't.

Lots of mornings, our whole family enjoys protein shakes. They're rich in nutrients that help fuel the Meta-Stat for an entire day. Here's the basic recipe. For each serving, you'll need:

- ½ cup unsweetened frozen fruit (your choice of peaches, blueberries, and/or strawberries)

- ¼ cup plain or lightly sweetened fat-free vanilla yogurt or kefir

- ¼ cup fat-free milk, soy milk, or 100 percent fruit juice

- 1 scoop whey, casein, or soy protein powder

Process the ingredients in a blender until smooth. If you are able to use fresh fruit instead of frozen, add several ice cubes before blending to thicken the shake.

Here are a few other favorites. These recipes make two servings; if you want just one, divide the quantities in half.

Strawberry Sunrise: 1 cup frozen strawberries; ½ cup orange juice, fat-free milk, or low-fat soy milk; ½ cup low-fat plain or vanilla yogurt or kefir, 1 banana, 1 scoop protein powder

Blueberry Creamsicle: 1 cup frozen blueberries, ½ cup low-fat plain or vanilla yogurt or kefir, 1 banana, ½ cup orange juice, 1 scoop protein powder

Peaches Praline: 1 cup frozen peach slices, ½ cup low-fat plain or vanilla yogurt or kefir, 2 tablespoons pecans, ½ cup fat-free milk or low-fat soy milk, 1 scoop protein powder

Vanilla Almond: ½ cup low-fat plain or vanilla yogurt or kefir, dash vanilla, 1 banana, 1 tablespoon almond butter or ground almonds, ½ cup fat-free milk or low-fat soy milk, 1 scoop protein powder, ice cubes

"We can't overstress the importance of breakfast," state Peter D. Vash, MD, MPH, an endocrinologist and internist at the UCLA Medical Center, and dietitians Cris Carlin and Victoria Zak. According to this trio of experienced health professionals, breakfast skippers are cheating themselves out of foods that have "thermic potential." That is, you lose an opportunity to burn fat. "When you wake up and get started on a new day," they conclude, "you must have breakfast to turn on your thermic switch, moving your body's rhythm from low ebb to high tide."[16]

Indeed, though breakfast is a morning meal, its ability to reset your Meta-Stat means that you will reap its benefits all day long. According to research at Vanderbilt University, the University of Minnesota, and the University of Health Sciences/Chicago Medical School, eating breakfast—particularly a high-fiber, low-fat breakfast—actually reduces the total number of calories and the total grams of fat eaten over the course of a day.[17] According to research by Sarah F. Leibowitz, PhD, a neurobiologist at Rockefeller University, late afternoon and evening are the times when those who skip breakfast are most likely to pay for it by gorging on high-fat and/or high-sugar foods. This is because of an excessive increase in neuropeptide Y, a brain chemical associated with food cravings.[18]

Other research reports indicate that in general, breakfast eaters are leaner and have lower blood pressure than breakfast skippers.[19] If you get in the breakfast habit, studies show, you'll have an easier time maintaining balanced blood sugar, experience greater energy and strength, and be better able to stick with a healthful, balanced diet.[20]

In one study, moderately overweight women who regularly skipped breakfast were randomly divided into two groups. One group was asked to eat a low-fat breakfast every morning, while the other group was instructed to continue forgoing the morning meal. After 12 weeks, the breakfast eaters lost significantly more weight than the breakfast skippers.[21]

Breakfast eaters who were once breakfast skippers report a measurable improvement in their energy levels during the day. As we now know, this benefit results from a boost to the Meta-Stat setting.

META-STAT STARTER

Creative Breakfasting

There is no reason to have the same breakfast every morning. With the Meta-Stat approach, the key is to expand your taste horizons and test the food options that give *you* the most lasting energy. Here's a sampling of your many healthy options.

Salmon. Although my girls like it at other times of day, they won't touch it at breakfast. I happen to like a few bites of canned salmon, which is very high in protein. (My favorite is from Dave's Albacore, available by mail.)

Fresh fruit. Try a quarter of a cantaloupe, an orange, or a handful of blueberries or strawberries, for example.

Yogurt. Choose fat-free or low-fat varieties.

Whole grain toast. A good choice if it's really whole grain. In our household, favorite toast toppings include:

- ¼ cup low-fat cottage cheese or plain yogurt (no sweetener)

- ½ cup fresh fruit with chopped nuts (for taste and extra nutrients)

- 1 slice reduced-fat Cheddar or Swiss cheese, melted

- Low-fat turkey breast breakfast sausage or turkey breast bacon

- Scrambled egg, Eggbeaters, or tofu

Of course, as with every other meal, you need to make choices. If you have scrambled eggs with sausage, instant microwave oatmeal with whole milk, or white bread with butter and jelly, your blood sugar level could as much as double. That means a sharp increase in fat-forming processes![22]

Protein is certainly beneficial. In fact, Swiss scientists reported that a breakfast high in protein (25 grams or more) can have positive effects on the brain and metabolism all day long.[23] But a good breakfast also supplies a balance of carbohydrates and fiber to rev up hormones and brain neurotransmitters for the day ahead.[24] In fact, the right kind of high-protein, modest-carb, high-fiber, low-fat breakfast helps set the fat-burning rate for your entire day.[25]

When your breakfast contains a moderate amount of metabolism-boosting protein (such as some fat-free milk, low-fat cottage cheese, fat-free yogurt, or fat-free cream cheese), plenty of fiber-rich complex carbohydrates such as whole grains, and a modest amount of good fats, studies suggest that you'll be less likely to overeat or to eat high-fat foods at lunch.[26] Plus, you'll tend to reach for fewer impulsive, high-fat snacks. Eating breakfast can help reduce your appetite for the entire day.

Here are a few quick-and-easy breakfast suggestions to get the right Meta-Stat setting first thing in the morning.

Eat on the way to work. If you're a commuter, you can plan breakfast around foods that are easy to carry with you. Add some frozen berries and a handful of fat-free, whole oats granola to a cup of fat-free plain yogurt. Or choose a fresh whole grain wheat, rye, or pumpernickel bagel and top with a few slices of turkey breast and a thin layer of fat-free or low-fat cream cheese. Voilá—you have breakfast to go!

Eat breakfast even if you think you're not hungry. People who have made a habit of skipping breakfast sometimes tell me, "I'm just not hungry in the morning." If this applies to you, there's a good chance it's because you've learned to override your body's natural rhythms. Once you reestablish your normal, healthy metabolic rate, you'll begin to feel hungry when you get up in the morning. In addition, says C. Wayne Callaway, MD, obesity specialist and former director of the Nutrition and Lipid Clinic at the Mayo Clinic, "you will be hungry at appropriate times throughout the day, and will lose the urge to binge in the evenings."[27]

Have some morning company. Begin a breakfast partnership with your spouse or child or a friend or co-worker. Make the first meal of the day more fun and interesting. If you join your children for breakfast, you get some quality time with them, as well as an opportunity to teach them about healthy breakfast choices. If it's a co-worker, why not meet to eat? On nice days, you can have your breakfast in a nearby park. Or just plan to eat at each other's house on alternate mornings.

5. FOCUS ON SELF-REGULATION RATHER THAN SELF-CONTROL

As we'll discuss in more detail in Chapter 27, the latest neuroscientific research draws a clear distinction between self-control and self-regulation.[28] Self-control rarely works unless everything in your life is going smoothly. The moment stress or a task intervenes, self-control vanishes. You rarely end up following through on your intentions.

With self-regulation, you're able to clearly envision the new you that's taking shape from the fat-burning, energy-boosting practices that you're incorporating into your lifestyle. The image in your mind evokes a positive, meaningful response from you: "I have an attractive, sexy figure" or "I feel the strength and energy that comes from being fit." By conjuring this response every morning, it provides far more motivation over the course of the day, helping to overcome the distractions and temptations that can prevent you from attaining your goal.

This is why the Meta-Stat approach focuses on self-regulation rather than self-control, development rather than performance. When you go the development route, you may set goals, but they are very personal and also very specific. According to researchers, people who grasp their own original goals in distinctive and specific ways are 50 percent more likely to take confident actions to achieve those goals and one-third more likely to feel a sense of control under stressful conditions.[29]

So within a half-hour or so of awakening, make a point of looking ahead to your the day's events and reminding yourself why you need to jump-start your Meta-Stat at regular, consistent intervals. Zero in on specific ways you can stay on track.

6. THE MSON MINDSET

As I've indicated, the Meta-Stat approach is different from any other diet or health regimen in that it is not a once-a-day or once-a-meal solution. Rather, it is a continual self-monitoring, developmental, new-results-driven process. You establish the rhythmic use of Meta-Stat signals and maintain progress by using those signals at regular intervals throughout the day. It requires a different mindset than what you may be accustomed to.

Research indicates that permanent fat loss is more likely when people shift their point of view from first person to third person.[30] In essence, instead of seeing your actions through an "I" lens—"I am going to pause and catch some sunlight" or "I am strengthening my muscles now"—you observe yourself interacting with life and making choices. It's as though you are sitting on your own shoulder, watching what you're doing.

From this perspective, you can much more readily identify and redirect self-defeating behaviors as they're about to occur, instead of looking back at the end of the day and vowing to do better tomorrow. According researchers at Ohio State University, adopting a third-person point of view enables change because it you can readily compare past and present behaviors and make adjustments accordingly.[31]

Each morning, think about where your energy and fat loss signals will come from during the day ahead. Use the third-person perspective to anticipate barriers and identify steps for overcoming them. Then even as unexpected disruptions arise, stimulating your Meta-Stat remains a priority.

CHAPTER 5

■　　■　　■

MSOn Switch #2

Create Activity Momentum

S itting still is getting to be a problem. A big one. The growing tendency—not just in America but around the world—is to sit in front of a computer most of the day and then lounge in front of a TV at night. Computers may be useful, TV entertainment may be enjoyable, but when we're enthralled with these screens, we stop moving. And that's a mistake. Inactivity is an unnatural state for humans.

Whenever you are inactive for more than 60 minutes or so, it's likely that your body is sending a signal to your brain to decrease fat burning and increase fat making. So what happens when you linger over a big meal and then spend hours at your desk or on the sofa? You're more likely to end up feeling tired, and you probably will store more calories from your meal as body fat. It's because you're not heeding your body's innate capacity and need for movement.

The average American spends about 4 to 4½ hours each day watching television. And this doesn't count time watching DVDs or playing video games. Increasing evidence suggests that prolonged television viewing lowers metabolism and puts on the pounds.

The unhealthy relationship between TV and weight seems to become magnified at the 3-hour-a-day mark, suggests Larry A.

> **Success Map Tip:**
> Record your energy level and tally your MSOn Minutes.

Tucker, PhD, professor and director of health promotion at Brigham Young University. In one study, Dr. Tucker and his colleague Glenn M. Friedman, MD, tracked over 6,000 working men whose average age was 40.[1] The doctors discovered that those men who spent more than 3 to 4 hours a day in front of a TV were twice as likely to be obese (with excess body fat accounting for 20 to 30 percent of their total weight) as those who watched TV for an hour or less a day. They also were at greater risk for becoming superobese—that is, with excess body fat comprising at least 31 percent of their total weight. Among frequent TV watchers, the risk of superobesity more than doubled.

This finding mirrors a study of nearly 800 adults, published in the *Journal of the American Dietetic Association.*[2] It concluded that the incidence of obesity was 19.2 percent among those watching at least 4 hours of TV a day, compared with 4.5 percent among those watching an hour or less a day. In effect, the risk of obesity quadrupled!

According to the study, TV had a fattening effect whether or not people snacked heavily while they watched. Even after accounting for excess snacking, the researchers found that frequent viewers still were putting on extra body fat at an accelerated rate. The conclusion: Spending prolonged periods in front of the television seems to produce extra body fat all by itself, perhaps due to lowered metabolism.

ENERGY COMES NATURALLY

Of course, we can't blame our sedentary ways on TV alone. The typical American lifestyle seems to encourage inertia. Driving instead of walking. Sitting instead of standing. Desk jobs instead of physical labor. This has become the predominant pattern for almost half of the US population, including children.

Parents and teachers often give instructions that—however inadvertently—suppress a child's natural energy: "Sit still." "Stop fidgeting." "Stay right where you are." "Don't move." Have you noticed that many children who try to comply simply can't? That's true of adults, too. We need to move. Whether tapping our toes while perched in a chair or drumming a desktop with a pencil eraser, we're compelled to express our energy.

Even when sitting still, we aren't still—at least not for very long. Our energy connects us with the world by moving us into it. Sitting motionless goes against our inherent biological nature. We were born for motion, for activity.

Lucky for all of us, the world is full of interesting things to do. Only a lack of imagination or, more commonly, the suppression of energy stands in the way. Otherwise, each of us would have the attentiveness and vigor to more fully explore our talents and passions. In my view, the restraints on energy deprive us of many opportunities—to be a poet or musician, writer or explorer, astronomer or gardener, inventor or sports enthusiast, community volunteer, independent scholar or scientist, artist or collector.

Even with regular workouts at a gym or health club, you may not have much energy. One reason, as I emphasize throughout this book, is that you must continually activate your energy. Your metabolism relies on the signals you send it. Unless you learn those signals and use them, your overall vigor and vitality noticeably wane and eventually may all but disappear.

When you activate your energy with physical movement at regular intervals throughout the day, you sustain a consistently high metabolism. This produces a wide range of benefits, including:

- Maximum fat burning throughout the body

- Peak energy, with physical vigor and mental drive

- Enhanced ability to handle pressure

- Extraordinary attentiveness to people and tasks

- Increased confidence and ingenuity in facing challenges

- Improved self-regulation of mood

- Deeper sleep and rest

- Exceptional stamina all day long

MOVE AT EVERY OPPORTUNITY

Every one of your bodily systems functions best when activity and motion are integral parts of your daily regimen. Without them, you're apt to gain weight. But apart from that most obvious development, there is hidden damage as well. Muscles atrophy, which interferes with your body's ability to make energy and burn fat. The cardiovascular system suffers. And, to make matters worse, people who sit still for long periods are more likely to feel depressed and anxious than those who engage in regular exercise.[3]

At one time, scientists believed that frequency of physical activity didn't have much of an impact. Duration mattered most. Some research had shown that a single lengthy aerobic session—going for a long run, for example, or pedaling a stationary bicycle for 40 minutes straight—could raise metabolism and keep it high for several days afterward. Better studies show that post-aerobic metabolism returns to near-normal levels within 30 to 60 minutes of a 30-minute exercise session.[4] In other words, the Meta-Stat dampens down. You need to keep restoking it—not just during a formal exercise session but throughout the day, every day.

As I'll discuss in Part 3, your muscles get a lasting benefit from brief intermittent exercise sessions. For now, the important thing to know is that whenever you build new, stronger muscle tissue, the muscle fibers act like a metabolic furnace. That furnace can burn 24 hours a day, improving your overall health and increasing your fat-burning potential. But unless you choose to stay in motion, you can become overwhelmed by sedentary impulses. Sitting still is a fat maker extraordinaire.

Evolutionarily, we were not designed to vegetate. In fact, if a half hour goes by in which you don't move at all, you are actually tiring yourself. Oxygen uptake plummets. Blood circulation slows. Hormones adapt to the inactivity by favoring fat storage. As a half hour of inactivity stretches into an hour or longer, multiple signals are racing to your brain, telling it to conserve energy (and fat) instead of burning it. Your body goes into a sort of mini-hibernation state, just as its ancient programming dictates.

Just think of bears fattening up for a long winter. That's how your biochemistry begins to respond when you sit at a desk or on the sofa, with minutes ticking away. To counteract this effect, you need to slip in some brief, intense activity at regular 30-minute intervals throughout the day.

The trouble is, many of us just don't seem hardwired for movement. According to a study that appeared in *Science,* people who are overweight have an inherent tendency to sit. Those who are lean, by comparison, move around—spending an additional 152 minutes, on average, engaging in basic physical activity such as puttering around the house.[5] "This is not a 'fidget more' story," cautions James Levine, MD, an endocrinologist at the Mayo Clinic. "It's a 'get off your bottom and move' story."[6]

META-STAT STARTER

Motor Skills

Use the "eat-and-move" technique to increase your fat-burning power. Fifteen to 30 minutes after eating a meal or snack, grab some active minutes for calorie-burning benefits.

Here's why it's so important to exercise during that postmeal time frame. If there is no muscular activity to burn off the carbohydrates consumed in low-fat meals or low-fat or fat-free snacks, chemicals in your brain and body respond by quickly converting the carbohydrate for storage as fat.[7] Research indicates that your body's metabolic rate goes up by about 10 percent after a meal or snack as a result of the chemical processes that are activated during digestion. And there's evidence that this 10 percent can be increased—in some cases, doubled[8]—if 5 to 20 minutes of moderate (not vigorous) physical activity such as walking takes place while digestion is in its earliest stages.[9] In fact, you may get up to twice the usual calorie-burning benefits for each active minute within that postmeal period.

By engaging in physical activity within a half hour of eating, you actually pull oxygen into your body, according to Bryant A. Stamford, PhD, exercise physiologist and director of the Health Promotion Center at the University of Louisville. Oxygen is necessary for fat burning and energy production. With short bouts of increased physical activity, Dr. Stamford explains, "food can be made to burn hotter, in a sense, with fewer calories being available for fat storage."[10]

MORE FLEX IN YOUR SCHEDULE

Mark Twain once said, "Exercise is loathsome." Many people today probably would agree with him.

The truth is, you don't need to get out there and do a full-scale formal workout every day. You don't need to join a health club, which is likely to involve even more driving or commuting time. Nor do you need to carve a couple of hours out of your already packed daily schedule.

I know you're busy. And quite possibly, you also feel out of shape. Or your knees, back, arms, hips, or feet hurt. Or, as you're getting older, you have a more "crowded" lifestyle—with responsibilities to your children and your parents and, if you're moving upward in a profession, to your career. With all of these restraints and demands, you're probably wondering where you can find the time for a formal fitness regimen.

The answer: Take the opportunities where you can find them. In Part 3, we'll explore ways to increase the number of "active minutes" in your day—for example, by doing muscle-toning exercises while you stand in line, talk on the phone, or sit in traffic. You have many other opportunities as well, such as taking the stairs instead of the elevator or walking an extra block on your way to work. These may seem like minor adjustments, but they have a major impact in terms of boosting your metabolism and helping to neutralize cravings for high-fat, high-sugar foods.[11]

Do you remember the lightbulb analogy from Chapter 1? With every physical action that makes significant use of major muscle groups, you turn up your Meta-Stat one click, or watt. The light grows brighter, the furnace hotter. There's one important footnote to this observation, however. Just being "busy" doesn't necessarily have the same effect, because we habitually use muscle movements that require little energy. If you're doing busywork at a desk or counter, talking on the phone, or driving around in a car, the small amount of low-energy motion does little to influence your Meta-Stat setting.

HOW SHORT BURSTS WORK

One of the advantages of short but frequent bursts of activity, particularly muscle-toning activity, is that they hinder lipoprotein lipase, a key fat-storing enzyme. So every time you get up and move, it helps reduce excess body fat.[12]

There's another reason that it pays to be active for a few minutes at frequent intervals throughout the day. It involves fat molecules known as free fatty acids, which are extremely small and very mobile.

Free fatty acids are in constant motion. Because they're small, they pass easily through the semipermeable membranes of cells. Sometimes they're being released from fat cells; other times they're being deposited into fat cells. Or they pass into muscle cells, so they're available for energy.

Inside fat cells, free fatty acids link up in threes to form triglycerides. As the fat cells get full, some of these triglycerides spill out into the bloodstream. Once there, they can build up on the walls of coronary arteries, raising the risk of stroke, heart attack, and diabetes.

When you're active, your muscle cells will hang on to their free fatty acids to burn them for fuel. On the other hand, underused or inactive muscle cells have no need for energy, so they send their free fatty acids back into the bloodstream and eventually to fat cells for storage. Over time, this can lead to a spike in triglyceride levels. By engaging in short spurts of physical activity throughout the day, you prevent free fatty acids from finding their way into fat cells.

The action of free fatty acids is similar to that of fat-burning enzymes. These enzymes act as catalysts for metabolizing fat and turning it into fuel in muscle cells. But they function well only when they're called upon regularly.[13] Otherwise, they break down into amino acids (the component units of proteins) and can't do their jobs. This is another reason that long sedentary stretches—such as an entire day or even several days without frequent bouts of physical activity and muscle toning—shift your body's biochemstry toward fat forming and fat storage, and away from fat burning.

BEYOND FAT BURNING

Research indicates that regular physical activity and exercise can produce fat loss even without caloric restriction.[14] In fact, it may be the single most important factor in maintaining fat loss.[15] In one study at the University of California, 90 percent of people who reached and maintained their goal weights engaged in regular exercise, compared with only 34 percent of those who relapsed.[16]

According to Janet Walberg-Rankin, PhD, associate professor of exercise physiology at the Virginia Institute of Technology, you can lose a pound of fat a week just by ratcheting up your activity level a notch or two.[17] As you slowly but steadily burn off excess body fat and improve your overall fitness, you reduce your risk of serious medical conditions such as heart disease, high blood pressure, osteoporosis, and breast and colon cancers. The benefits of physical movement and muscle toning are so profound that, for people who have been very sedentary, even a little exercise can reduce their risk of disease as much as quitting smoking, according to Steven Blair, PED, former president of the American College of Sports Medicine.

The psychological benefits of exercise are equally impressive. Studies have shown that people who are physically active exhibit fewer psychological and physiological overreactions to stressful situations.[18] And research from Harvard Medical School's Institute for Circadian Physiology suggests that every time you get up and move—using

META-STAT STARTER

Something to Chew On

In between regular bouts of physical activity, you might add some embellishments to your daily routine in order to stay in motion. Harvard researchers have discovered that even the simplest movements can have surprising benefits. For example, chewing gum generates enough muscular activity to measurably increase energy.[19] Repetitive jaw movements can spike metabolism upward by as much as 20 percent while you chew.[20]

Chewing gum may not melt away body fat all by itself. But it can increase alertness, which is critical to effective decision making. When you're trying to stoke your Meta-Stat as often as possible throughout the day, every decision matters.

"muscular activity" even briefly—you increase your mental energy and alertness.[21]

The best news of all may be that people who become physically active—even if it's late in life—tend to outlive people who are sedentary. That's the latest word from a panel of experts convened by the Centers for Disease Control and Prevention and the American College of Sports Medicine, who report that "a staggering quarter of a million deaths each year can be attributed to physical inactivity."[22]

Even if you don't want to be more active for your own sake, perhaps you'll want to do it for your children or grandchildren. According to research presented at the National Institutes of Health Conference on Physical Activity and Obesity, when both parents are active, their children are more likely to follow suit. In the same vein, the Framingham Children's Study found that children of two active parents were nearly six times more likely to be active than children of inactive parents.[23]

SHORTCUTS TO FITNESS

When you break up exercise into simple, smaller units, it's easier to do. Still, it can take some getting used to, especially if you have a rather sedentary lifestyle. One idea is to redesign your living environment so that it's less conducive to sitting around. I love sitting around as much as anyone, but I make a conscious effort to avoid doing so for more than a half-hour at a time. On the rare evening when I watch television, I take "activity breaks" during every commercial. I keep a set of resistance bands draped over a nearby chair, so I can grab them for a few simple movements. My family joins in, too. We use a buddy system: If any of us is sitting for more than a half-hour, someone else creates a fun diversion to get all of us out of our chairs for a while.

Another idea is to create a reminder system for yourself. It might be as simple as setting your computer calendar to send a message every 30 minutes, prompting you to get up and move. Not a big deal. If you have reminders and obey them, you'll feel your energy rise. And there will be a hidden benefit as well, as you'll increase fat burning.

As for what you should do every 30 minutes, the possibilities are endless! As a starting point, examine your everyday habits. Where, precisely, in your daily routine can you slip in a few simple muscle-toning or get-moving activities that give you a big fat-burning payoff? Here are some ideas.

12 Instant Muscle Toners

- Slowly open and close one hand, tensing your hand and forearm muscles. Repeat with the other hand.

- With an open hand, slowly rotate your wrist clockwise and then counterclockwise while tensing your hand and forearm muscles. Repeat with the other hand.

- Slowly shrug your shoulders, tensing the muscles. Then drop your shoulders, relaxing completely.

- Make a fist with one hand and slowly do a biceps curl, tensing your hand and arm muscles as you bend your fist toward your shoulder. Slowly return to the starting position. Repeat with the other hand.

- Standing, shift your weight to one leg. Tense your leg muscles and rise upward onto the ball of your weight-bearing foot. Slowly lower your heel. Shift your weight to the other leg and repeat. (If this throws off your balance, use a wall or chair for support.)

- While standing, shift your weight to one leg. Slowly bend and raise the opposite knee. Switch legs and repeat.

- While standing, tense the muscles in both legs. Slowly lower yourself into a knee bend or modified squat. Return to the starting position.

- Press together the palms of both hands so the fingers point outward, away from your chest and parallel to the floor. Tense your arms, chest, and back muscles. Without shifting hand position, apply even pressure of one palm against the other hand, then switch.

- Stand about 18 inches away from a wall with your feet shoulder-width apart. Place your palms flat against the wall, then tense your arm, chest, and back muscles. Do slow pushups, lowering your body toward the wall and then pushing away.

- While sitting, tense one leg and slowly extend your foot away from the chair. Slowly return it to the starting position. Repeat with the other leg,

- Sitting, tense the lower muscles of your right leg. As you do so, flex your toes and extend them as much as possible, like a ballet dancer *en pointe*. Relax, then repeat with the left leg.

- Sitting with your arms at your sides, tense your shoulder muscles and slowly raise both arms, keeping them straight. Bring your hands up to shoulder height, then slowly lower them again.

28 Get-Up-and-Go Actions

- Three or four times a day, climb a flight or more of stairs instead of taking the elevator. (You burn 10 times more calories climbing stairs than you do resting.)

- When you're in a shopping mall, *walk* up the escalators instead of riding.

- At the airport, skip the moving walkway and walk alongside it.

- Tense and flex your arms while you are sitting at a stoplight or stuck in traffic.

- Even if there are empty parking spaces near your workplace or the supermarket, park your car as far away as you can.

- If you're taking a bus or cab, get out an extra block from your destination.

- Stand up and move around while reading letters or talking on the telephone. Research shows that people who are standing burn twice as many calories per minute as those who sit still.[24]

- Move your wastebasket far away from your desk so you need to take a little hike to discard items. (And no shooting baskets!)

- When you need to speak with a co-worker, call ahead to find out if you can stop by his or her office.
- Walk someplace at least 5 minutes from your office to eat your lunch so that afterward, you can enjoy a 5-minute return walk.
- On your lunch hour, plan some errands that are within walking distance.
- Keep moving while standing in line. Do toe raises or gently shift your weight from one leg to the other.
- Walk and talk with your spouse, child, or friend.
- Find a partner for a quick game of Frisbee, table tennis, basketball, soccer, or volleyball.
- Make active dates with friends, involving physical activities you love.
- Sweep your sidewalk and patio, balcony, or deck.
- Rake leaves or weed your garden or flowerbed.
- Jump rope for a minute or two.
- Enroll in a dance class. Or simply put on some of your favorite music and move your feet. (Even tapping your feet burns more calories than sitting still.)
- Plan short bicycle rides.
- Walk your dog instead of just turning him loose in the backyard.
- Take your *neighbor's* dog for a walk.
- Do a 5-minute muscle-toning workout while sitting.
- Sit in a rocking chair and rock as you read or watch TV.
- Stand up and stretch during commercials.
- Walk up and down a flight of stairs at the end of each television show.
- Pedal your stationary cycle or use your indoor rower during a show.
- Stretch in the shower with shoulder shrugs and toe touches.

CHAPTER 6

M S O n   S w i t c h   # 3

Catch Light to Boost Energy

Natural light energizes and sustains us as it helps burn off excess body fat. Increasing evidence suggests that fat loss may be significantly affected by your exposure—or lack of exposure—to sunlight.

This makes intuitive sense if you think about the way our ancestors lived. The duration of daylight sent powerful cues to their metabolism. Shorter days announced the coming of winter and a period of famine or near starvation. Metabolism slowed down as a result.

For our ancestors, burning fewer calories was essential to their survival. They needed to store every available calorie as excess body fat for insulation. This was their primary insurance against cold weather. The human body retains this protective mechanism. As winter approaches and days grow shorter, the body naturally slows the rate at which it burns fat as fuel for energy. During the summer months, the combination of bright sunshine and extended daylight hours signals the Meta-Stat to raise metabolism, burn off excess fat, and prepare for active days.

A brightly lit room has about 500 luxes of light (a lux is the scientific equivalent of the light from a single candle), compared with

> *Success Map Tip:*
> **Under MSOn Minutes, note how you catch the light to boost energy.**

10,000 luxes of light at sunrise and 100,000 at noon on a sunny day. To our metabolism, spending the day indoors is virtually the same as spending the day in darkness. It stimulates the inherent physiological processes associated with sleeping and gaining weight.[1]

Remember that according to scientists, human biology and human metabolism have hardly evolved since ancient times. That's why research finally is showing that light, especially brief bouts of exposure to bright sunshine, is a key to energy and fat loss.

These days, though, most of us limit our time in the sun, instead adapting to relatively dim indoor light levels. We have even less light when we're watching TV or directing our gaze at computer screens. That's too bad, since optimal exposure to light is an effortless way to fire up your Meta-Stat.

THE HORMONE CONNECTION

In understanding how the body responds to various light signals, we need to look at how the hormone leptin plays a role. As discussed in Chapter 2, the body produces leptin in abundance when metabolism is naturally high and fat loss is necessary. Levels of the hormone drop whenever the body slips into fat-conservation mode or makes extra fat in order to protect itself.[2]

Leptin has other effects as well. For example, scientists have discovered that the hormone acts on certain areas of the brain to stimulate production of melanocortin. It's the same antioxidant compound that's manufactured by the skin in response to sun exposure. Research suggests that melanocortin in the skin circulates through the bloodstream, eventually reaching the brain. There it suppresses the appetite centers, which in turn prompts the body to speed metabolism and shed excess body fat.[3] Melanocortin also acts on the thyroid gland to boost hormone output, which further increases metabolism.[4]

Another hormone, agouti, competes with melanocortin. Though agouti is present in the same parts of the brain as melanocortin,[5] it influences the brain in the opposite way. Specifically, it sends a signal to not only slow down fat loss but also to manufacture more fat.[6]

With too much agouti and not enough melanocortin, you become hungry and conserve fat. So there's a little hormonal competition going on, with agouti signaling "Eat more, store fat" as melanocortin urges "Eat less, burn fat."

SOAK UP MORE VITAMIN D

Interestingly, the actions of both hormones on fat cells appear to have some connection to vitamin D, which is synthesized by skin cells in response to sun exposure. Michael Holick, MD, PhD, a professor at Boston University Medical Center and director of its Vitamin D, Skin, and Bone Research Laboratory, has amassed convincing scientific proof that nearly all of us may be deficient in vitamin D. As a result, we aren't getting the full benefits of the nutrient, which we need to thrive.[7]

For example, vitamin D is essential to calcium absorption. Calcium, of course, is necessary to build and maintain bones. A low calcium level has a number of other associated health risks as well. In particular, insufficient calcium triggers the release of calcitrol, the hormone responsible for turning off the mechanisms that break down fat and burn it. Calcitrol also activates the mechanisms that make body fat.[8]

Dr. Holick advocates brief, sensible exposure to sunlight—not just for vitamin D production but also for a number of health reasons. Not that we should spend hours on the beach in unfiltered sunlight. In fact, Dr. Holick says, we don't need much sun at all—no more than 5 to 10 minutes on the face and arms or arms and legs 2 or 3 days a week. He prefers the hours between 11:00 A.M. and 2:00 P.M., because that's when the skin makes the most vitamin D.[9]

As with every other aspect of the Meta-Stat approach, timing is crucial. A few minutes in the sun can elevate metabolism and improve overall health. Longer than that, and sunlight can do more harm than good, increasing your risk of skin conditions from premature wrinkling to skin cancer.

Of course, sunlight is not the only source of vitamin D, but it may be the most abundant and reliable. The typical multivitamin supplies only 400 IU of vitamin D, where most experts recommend 1,000 IU a day, particularly for those who aren't getting enough sunlight. Among foods, fortified dairy products are your best bet.

BECOME A LIGHT HARVESTER

More than you imagine, light is an "on" switch for the brain and senses.[10] It upshifts metabolism and delivers a burst of energy. With that energy, it's easier to stay active and increase your fat-burning power.

So become a light harvester: Seek out bright light as often as you can throughout the day. Heading outdoors for a few minutes of sun exposure is ideal. On cloudy days, you can get similar benefits by soaking up some extra-bright indoor light.

Though we're well past the dark ages, we can shortchange ourselves on light all too easily. And that's unfortunate, especially when something so valuable comes free. As difficult as our ancestors' lives may seem by modern standards, they never had to worry about getting enough light. They were outdoors, hunting and gathering what they needed to survive. Because of their "enlightened" lifestyles, their bodies continuously produced lots of energy and burned off excess fat, so they could meet the physical demands of the active seasons.

These days, we sometimes must hunt for sunlight the way our forebears hunted for wildebeest. It won't come to you. You need to search for it. The alternative is to live and work in dim light. It may seem more convenient, but it effectively shuts down an important component of your body's fat-burning, energy-producing ability.

CHAPTER 7

MSOn Switch #4

Take In More Oxygen

How you breathe is how you live. But since breathing comes naturally, most of us barely pay attention to it. Typically, we get by with short, shallow breaths. And why not? They're enough to keep us going. The trouble is, this pattern of barely breathing limits our access to oxygen, which is a major shortfall.

Oxygen is an essential ingredient in the production of adenosine triphosphate (ATP). As you'll recall from Chapter 1, ATP is essential to fat burning, among numerous other biochemical processes. Fat burning doesn't happen without enough oxygen.[1]

To ensure an adequate oxygen supply, you probably need to break out of the shallow-breathing habit and learn a new technique. Instead of just filling your chest with air, you'll learn to expand your lower ribs, which in turn opens your diaphragm. And every time you do that, you click your Meta-Stat up another notch. Your respiration is not only deeper but also more relaxed. It enables you to optimize your oxygen intake—and as a bonus, you'll stay on top of stress.

> *Success Map Tip:*
> Under MSOn Minutes, note the times when you pause for focused, controlled breathing. Mark the Daily Energy Wave chart before and after each of these breathing breaks.

BREATHE YOURSELF SLIMMER . . .
ALL DAY LONG

Researchers are reporting what I've long suspected—that most people are underoxygenated all day long.[2] If we were fish, of course, we could do some fancy gill work and get all the O_2 we need. But since we humans have evolved beyond that, we now depend on excellent lung work. The fact is, we need to exploit all our powers of respiration if we're going to feel fully alive.

The oxygen molecules in each breath are vital to brain function. They also "feed" mitochondria, the tiny cellular furnaces that generate energy and burn off fat. Depriving the mitochondria of oxygen is like running a car on empty.

Oxygen is the central fuel for metabolism and energy production. When you don't take in enough oxygen with each breath, your metabolism automatically slows down. Your cells are unable to effectively burn off excess body fat or resist turning new calories into stored fat.

Poor posture contributes to oxygen starvation. It's pretty hard to inflate a balloon that's wedged between your hands, but that's essentially the effect you cause when you slump over. The "balloon" is your diaphragm, the ample cavity underneath your lungs that should expand every time you inhale. But if it's being sandwiched by your posture, it just won't work efficiently.

According to research, 9 of every 10 adults have lost the ability to take even a single, full, natural breath.[3] Instead, we breathe just enough to keep the brain's control panel operating. We prevent ourselves from keeling over, and that's about it. But we don't feel deprived because we're so accustomed to the underoxygenated condition.

We need to stand or sit in ways that allow us to breathe most naturally. We also need to be active, because when we're not, we don't get the neurological signals demanding that we breathe deeply and often. Most of us get a whole lot of practice sitting, without much training at all in breathing. The result is a bad case of oxygen robbery. When you grow accustomed to shallow breathing and oxygen starvation, you deprive your body of critical fuel for metabolic processes. No wonder your Meta-Stat becomes sluggish! Without sufficient oxygen, you're choking off air to the engine that drives your whole body.

Master Breather

Tanya Streeter can descend 525 feet underwater with a single breath. No one else can do it better. That's lung power—and courage, which, as Tanya puts it, isn't something you're born with, it's something you train for.[4]

Tanya has trained for a long time, conditioning her lungs to take in more oxygen and sustain her at progressively greater depths. She often trains with a monofin, a single powerful flipper. She says that at 400 feet below the surface, the water pressure feels like ice picks in her ears. "I train in small increments," she notes. "I don't assume that the longer I bear it, the worse it's going to get. It might get easier."

Because Tanya doesn't overdo her training but carefully expands the edges of her capabilities, she has gone where no human has ever gone before. That's one example of the results that come from the power of concentration, commitment, and making one small change at a time.

BREATHE DIFFERENTLY RIGHT NOW!

Evidence shows that breathing power increases through conditioning. The muscles that need the most attention are those in the diaphragm and the ones that lie between the ribs, called the intercostals. Even if you're very athletic or you work out regularly, you probably don't pay much attention to either set of muscles. But if they're neglected and out of condition, they tire easily. Ultimately, that can affect both your performance and your energy level.[5]

Breathing exercises increase oxygen intake and circulation throughout the body. This stimulates metabolism and fat burning, so you're slimming down with literally every breath you take! This exercise helps improve the elasticity of your rib cage[6] and your breathing power. Here's how to do it.

1. Lie on your back on a mat or carpet.

2. Relax your body and flatten your lower back, gently pressing it toward the floor. As you do so, keep your head aligned with your spine. Allow your neck to lengthen as much as possible. Tuck in your chin slightly.

3. Place your hands on either side of your rib cage, with your palms and fingers pressing lightly against your ribs.

4. Inhale slowly and deeply through your nose. To make sure you're using your diaphragm, lift and expand your chest fully as you maximize the inhalation.

5. Exhale slowly through your nose or your nose and mouth.

6. Rest for several moments, breathing normally.

7. Repeat the exercise, again expanding your chest against some light hand pressure, but this time, lift your ribs a little higher.

Some people find this exercise more effective if they use a series of short inhalations to fully expand the chest. Try both techniques to see which works best for you.

DOING WHAT COMES NATURALLY . . . ONLY BETTER

As an All-American swimmer, I've come to truly believe in lung power and its ability to improve fitness and energy. Yet I've observed that most people never fully develop their respiratory capacity. Instead, their lungs languish, slowly atrophying in function from year to year until they can barely accommodate a single breath. This steadily undercuts energy, as well as the ability to lead an active Meta-Stat lifestyle.

For those who may need some assistance to retrain their natural breathing patterns, I recommend a device called the PowerLung. It's a simple-to-use, handheld, dual-action lung muscle strengthener with an adjustable level of resistance to inhalation and exhalation. To me, it's like progressively pursing your lips more tightly to restrict the flow of air into and out of your lungs while you breathe. It delivers measurable results in as little at 90 seconds (10 breaths or so) a day. I keep one PowerLung at my desk and another in my travel bag. To learn more about this device, visit www.powerlung.com.

CHAPTER 8

■   ■   ■

M S O n   S w i t c h   # 5
Seek Ideal Fluid Intake

F eeling sluggish? Low on energy? Not motivated to get up and move, much less exercise?

It could be from a lack of water—or, more precisely, a lack of cool water. One recent medical study showed that sipping 500 milliliters (17 ounces) of ice water can raise metabolism by 30 percent for 90 straight minutes.[1]

More than 75 percent of the human body is water. It is a medium for every enzymatic and chemical reaction, including fat metabolism. It performs a crucial role in fat-burning, fat-forming, and fat-storage processes. Water also is vital to muscle tone and strength, as well as to skin health. Well-hydrated skin looks firm and youthful.

Drinking plenty of water and other fluids helps regulate body temperature and maintain regular bowel movements. It builds resistance to infection by nourishing the mucous lining of the respiratory tract.

Doctors routinely advise anyone with edema or elevated blood pressure to drink plenty of water and other fluids.[2] This may seem counterintuitive, since people with edema are retaining fluids, but the best way

> *Success Map Tip:*
> Note your fluid
> intake throughout
> the day. See how it
> correlates to your
> energy level.

to rid the body of excess fluids is to drink more, according to Kathy Stone, RD, president of Strictly Nutrition. "When an individual senses that he is retaining fluid, then cuts back on his water intake to compensate, the body just responds by retaining more fluid," Stone explains.[3]

As if all these reasons weren't enough to persuade you to keep tabs on your water consumption, here's one more: Water and other fluids have a direct impact on metabolism. Your Meta-Stat depends on water to function at its peak.

Many foods have high water content, so you probably get about 3½ cups of water from meals and snacks during the course of a day. The metabolic process is another source; as your body uses energy, it generates about ½ cup of water as a by-product. But you still need more fluids than food and metabolism can provide.

In general, you should aim for four 8- to 12-ounce glasses of water every day. That's all you need to rev up fat burning and energy boosting. Appetite stays in check, as does fatigue. The benefits of something so simple are amazing.

IT'S A DEHYDRATING WORLD

Research indicates that nearly all of us are chronically dehydrated. Dehydration occurs when you don't take in enough fluids to replace what's lost through perspiration, respiration, urination, and other body processes.

It doesn't take much of a fluid deficit to create problems. For example, as little as 1 to 2 percent dehydration contributes to cardiovascular strain and accelerates exhaustion.[4] At 4 to 5 percent below optimal fluid intake, you could experience a 20 to 30 percent decline in cognitive performance.[5]

Without adequate fluid, the brain appears to go through physical changes that could affect behavior. According to sports medicine researchers Robert Goldman, DO, and Robert M. Hackman, PhD, "Even a slightly dehydrated body can produce a small but critical shrinkage of the brain, thereby impairing neuromuscular coordination, concentration, and thinking."[6] One effect is that you're less likely to pay attention to stimulating your Meta-Stat.

The decline in blood volume that occurs with even slight dehydration impedes the transport of oxygen and nutrients throughout the body, which drains energy levels. The thicker, more concentrated blood not only stresses the heart but also interferes with the elimination of accumulated waste from the body's cells.[7]

Each day, the average person loses at least 2 cups of water through breathing, another 2 cups through invisible perspiration, and 6 cups through urination and bowel movements. That's 10 cups a day, without taking into account lost fluids through perspiration during exercise or hard physical work.[8] When the body becomes this dehydrated, Meta-Stat function plummets.

Our lifestyles contribute to our fluid shortfall as well. Modern, energy-efficient homes and office buildings constantly, imperceptibly wick moisture out of us. So does stress.

"The fatigue, headaches, lack of concentration, and dizziness you may feel at the end of a workday could result simply from not drinking enough water," explains Liz Applegate, PhD, nutritional science lecturer at the University of California, Davis.[9] "It starts every day as soon as you awaken. When you open your eyes in the morning, your body is already facing a water deficit."

Arid Conditions in Low-Carb Land

Have you been following a very low carbohydrate diet? If so, you may need to drink more fluids. The reason: Very low carb diets can cause dehydration.

To help your body process and absorb water, be certain to include complex carbohydrates in each meal and snack. "The only way to avoid extreme water loss is to eat enough complex carbohydrates to produce sufficient glucose for your brain and red blood cells," says C. Wayne Callaway, MD, former director of the Nutrition and Lipid Clinic at the Mayo Clinic. "When your liver is forced to make sugar from stored glycogen or protein, water loss is inevitable."[10]

FLUIDS IN, FAT OUT

We've grown accustomed to getting by with less water and other fluids than our bodies need. But we may not be aware of one of its insidious outcomes—namely, that it causes us to gain fat. There's growing evidence that weight-loss efforts often fail because of a fluid deficit.[11]

As mentioned earlier, you require about four 8- to 12-ounce glasses of water and other fluids every day to stay well hydrated. When you are active throughout the day, as in a Meta-Stat-centered lifestyle, this fluid is vital. It won't cause bloating.

With water deprivation comes increased appetite. What you perceive as hunger may actually be your body's cue to drink more fluids. When you're dehydrated, you're more likely to eat fattening foods, or simply to eat too much.

According to some reports, dehydration also may cause the buildup of fat deposits.[12] An increased fluid intake, on the other hand, enhances the biochemical process that releases fatty acids from fat cells into the bloodstream, where they travel to muscles for use as fuel.

"Water may be one of the simplest, most powerful keys to fat loss," asserts Ellington Darden, PhD, exercise scientist and former director of research for Nautilus Sports/Medical Industries. "If you don't drink enough water, your body's reaction is to retain the water it does have. This hampers kidney function and contributes to the accumulation of waste products. Your liver is then called on to flush out impurities, which minimizes one of its main functions—that is, metabolizing stored fat into usable energy."[13]

A German study found that sipping 2 liters of water a day elevated metabolism and calorie burning by 100 calories per day—about the same increase you'd get from jogging for 15 minutes.[14] While it isn't a substitute for physical activity, water is a superb Meta-Stat booster in its own right.

For fat burning, your best bet is to serve your water on the rocks. You "maximize calorie burn by keeping the water ice cold," Dr. Darden explains. "A gallon of ice cold (40°F) water requires over 200 calories of heat energy to warm it to core body temperature (98.6°F)."[15] A gallon is the equivalent of 128 ounces, or eight 16-ounce glasses.

META-STAT STARTER

Liquids on Standby

In order to meet your body's fluid needs and rev up your Meta-Stat, I recommend keeping a tall container of ice water on hand and taking frequent sips throughout the day. Drink more frequently during bouts of physical activity, as well as at the first sign of symptoms such as dryness in the eyes, nasal passages, or mouth. These could indicate possible dehydration.

Everyone in my family carries a Nissan Thermos Insulated Water Bottle. It's a 16-ounce stainless steel bottle with a handy ergonomic shape, a built-in pop-up straw, and a push-button cap that's easy to open and close with one hand. It's great for keeping water (or another beverage) ice-cold. Fill it from a water cooler, and the water stays chilled for hours. Drinking cold water will probably help burn more calories, since your metabolism will increase to warm it to body temperature.

For more information about the water bottle or to place an order, visit www.thermosonline.com.

Water enables your circulatory system to move hormones into exactly the right locations for incinerating excess body fat. It also helps escort toxic wastes from your system, so your liver can concentrate on fat burning.

A CURE FOR CRAVINGS AND MORE

As you increase your fluid intake, you're likely to notice another benefit: You no longer experience the urge to overindulge in certain foods, especially high-fat ones. The fact is, your body probably has been craving fluids all along. As mentioned earlier, you may be misinterpreting your body's "thirst drive" as hunger. Many people do.

A good way to distinguish between thirst and hunger is to sip a glass of ice water before grabbing something to eat. Then wait 5 to 10 minutes. If you still feel hungry, it probably is genuine hunger. Go ahead and help yourself to a light snack—perhaps four whole-grain crackers topped with thin slices of cheese, a half-dozen almonds with ¼ cup low-fat yogurt or cottage cheese, or half of a low-carb energy bar.

"Drinking generous amounts of water is by far the number one way to head off food cravings and reduce appetite," says George Blackburn, MD, associate professor at Harvard Medical School.[16] Wayne C. Miller, PhD, former director of the Indiana University Weight Loss Clinic, would agree. In clinical studies, Dr. Miller and his colleagues have linked a high daily water intake to successful, lasting weight loss.[17] Of course, it makes sense: Water takes up room in the stomach, creating a sense of fullness and reducing the desire to eat when under stress or by habit.

Increasing your fluid intake doesn't only enhance fat loss. It boosts energy, too. "Because a deficiency of water can alter the concentration of electrolytes such as sodium, potassium, and chloride, water has a profound effect on brain function and energy level," observes neurosurgeon Vernon H. Mark, MD, author of *Brain Power: A Neurosurgeon's Complete Program to Maintain and Enhance Brain Fitness Throughout Your Life*.[18]

If you've been underhydrated for many years, you probably will notice improvements in your appetite, energy level, and overall well-being as soon as you increase your fluid intake. In this respect, it's like adjusting your breathing pattern or practicing relaxation techniques. At first, paying attention to your fluid intake might seem like unnecessary effort. But the payoff comes almost immediately as your Meta-Stat resets to exactly where it should be. Not surprisingly, you'll notice a difference in terms of how you feel. And once hydration becomes a habit, sticking with it is easy.

BEYOND WATER

New research confirms that fluid replacement can take many forms. There's pure water, of course, along with low-carb sports drinks and protein shakes.[19] Even coffee and tea contribute to your fluid intake, as long as you drink them in moderation. It has long been known that the caffeine in coffee, tea, and many soft drinks has a diuretic effect, meaning that it causes fluid loss. But researchers now say that you may be able to consume up to 300 milligrams of caffeine in a 2-hour period before it begins to have a negative effect.[20] That's the equivalent of two cups of coffee or as many as six cups of tea.[21]

Caffeine stimulates the release of fat from fat cells. It also enhances fat burning, as measured by the blood levels of free fatty acids in both lean and obese people.

A cup of tea or coffee also provides enough caffeine to raise metabolism. Caffeine increases the release of fat from fat cells and boosts the consumption of oxygen and fat burning, as measured by the levels of free fatty acids in the blood of both lean and obese people.[22] If you can handle a mild caffeine buzz, coffee and tea offer another option for adding to your fluid intake and stimulating your Meta-Stat.

Drink Smart with Tea

When you're considering your beverage options, be sure not to overlook green tea, whether iced or hot. Recent research at the University of Geneva indicates that green tea may increase metabolism and fat burning by up to 35 percent.[23] According to the research team, green tea or green tea extract "has thermogenic properties and promotes fat oxidation beyond that explained by its caffeine content."[24]

The theory behind these thermogenic properties goes something like this: Whenever your body releases stored fat for energy production, it triggers a corresponding surge in the hormone norepinephrine. But norepinephrine's fat-burning effect wanes quickly. It appears that epigallocatechin gallate, a chemical in green tea, helps keep norepinephrine available in the bloodstream for an extended period, so fat burning lasts longer.

Another study, reported in the *American Journal of Clinical Nutrition,* found that green tea improved energy expenditure (a measure of metabolism) as well as fat oxidation. Initially, the researchers attributed this effect to the caffeine in green tea. Through further investigation, they concluded that other compounds in the tea interact in such a way as to produce the metabolism-boosting, fat-burning benefits.

In fact, based on their findings, the researchers calculated that green tea could boost thermogenesis by 35 to 43 percent. This is significant, in terms of Meta-Stat function.

Fat-Fighting, Energy-Boosting Beverages

In terms of fluid intake, the bare-minimum recommendation is four 8- to 12-ounce glasses a day. At least half of those glasses should be water. For flavor, try squeezing in a slice of lemon, lime, or orange. Or give it a twist of mint, which can stimulate metabolism and alertness.[25]

Try to drink most of your fluids before 5:00 P.M. That way, you're less likely to get up in the middle of the night to urinate.

Here's a short list of beverages that support the Meta-Stat approach by helping to satisfy your body's fluid needs.

- Plain, pure water

- Water with natural lemon, lime, orange, or berry flavoring (unsweetened)

- Water with a dash of pure peppermint flavoring

- Carbonated mineral water, with or without flavoring

- Green tea (my favorite brand is Republic of Tea)

- Naturally flavored decaffeinated black tea, hot or iced (some favorites include Republic of Tea Mango Ceylon, Ginger Peach, Blackberry Sage, Cinnamon Plum, Orange Ginger Mint, Lemon Winter Mint, Carob Cocoa Mint, and Cardamom Cinnamon)

I make a point of sipping green tea—I prefer unsweetened, sometimes with a squeeze of lemon or lime—throughout the day, and especially in the afternoon. That's when the tea's cold temperature and active ingredients combine to boost my metabolism when it would otherwise take a downturn.

Power Up!

I'm a big fan of protein shakes because of their two-for-one benefits. They not only replenish fluids, they also are a lean source of amino acids, the building blocks of protein.

Protein is essential to human life, providing the basic structural components of cells and tissues. It also increases fat burning by trig-

- Decaffeinated coffee, hot or iced

- Decaffeinated coffee with fat-free or low-fat milk or a dash of half-and-half

- Decaffeinated cappuccino with fat-free milk

- Caffeinated tea, hot or iced (no more than six cups per day)

- Caffeinated coffee, hot or iced (no more than two cups per day)

One caveat when making your choices: Be careful not to overdo sweeteners, whether "natural" (such as table sugar, corn syrup, fructose, or sucrose) or artificial (aspartame or saccharine). These can push your appetite and metabolism in the wrong direction.

Whereas fiber-rich complex carbohydrates assist in reducing body fat,[26] large amounts of refined carbohydrates—including sugar and other sweeteners—can contribute to overweight and obesity.[27] Better to use a no-calorie sweetener on occasion than to consume 10 to 12 tablespoons—the amount in a typical soft drink—all at once.

As for alcoholic beverages, they generally don't count toward your daily fluid intake. In fact, some research suggests that two or more alcoholic beverages a day may elevate blood sugar and insulin. This revs up the body's fat-forming processes, resulting in fat gain.[28]

gering the production of glucagons, hormones that enable the body to use fat as fuel instead of storing it. A high-protein meal or snack will burn 40 percent more calories than a high-carbohydrate alternative.[29] It also boosts oxygen consumption by an extra 200 to 300 percent. This indicates a definite spike in metabolic rate.

Feed your body high-quality protein, and it will respond by increasing metabolism and fat burning. By "high-quality," I mean protein that is low in fat and readily absorbable. (I'll talk more about the best protein sources in Chapter 22.) What's great about protein shakes is that you can mix and match lean, nutritious proteins with other ingredients to create your own perfect shake. (I've listed a few of my family's favorites on page 49.)

As much as I like these shakes, I do recommend avoiding certain commercial "smoothies." Some contain over 1,000 calories and 100 grams of fat. Some are high in carbohydrates, in the form of sugar and other sweeteners. If you prefer a commercial product, carefully read labels and choose one that's low in calories, carbohydrates, and fat. If you find a product that meets these criteria, but you don't like the taste, try blending in some fresh fruit.

I suggest purchasing an insulated bottle or a small soft-sided cooler and some freezer packs, so you can carry your protein shakes with you. Then you're ready for a fluid "break" whenever the opportunity arises. The best times to sip a shake are before and after exercise and as an evening snack.

Soup's On!

Soup is a miracle food. It helps replenish vital fluids while controlling appetite and helping to satisfy the body's nutritional needs. Perhaps because I'm a big soup eater myself—vegetable is my favorite—I can't imagine why more people don't order it more often.

I recommend a warm mug of soup as an accompaniment to any meal or by itself. A study at Johns Hopkins University confirmed that soup is superior to other foods in its ability to satisfy. The favorite? Tomato soup. Make yours with fat-free milk and add a dash of cayenne pepper for some extra calorie-burning heat.

CHAPTER 9

■　　■　　■

MSOn Switch #6
Rise Up and Stand Tall

When you sit or recline in a comfortable chair—perhaps in front of the TV—you probably feel the pull of inertia to stay where you are, rather than getting up and moving around. I suppose that seems obvious. What isn't so obvious is why anyone would want to put themselves in that position for long stretches of time. As soon as you "settle in," it's an invitation to munch on food—usually the wrong foods—and a signal to slow your metabolism. Thinking about it rationally, why would we want to even tempt such results?

Using ultrasound scanning, Australian gastroenterologists and other scientists were able to determine that people definitely stay hungrier when they're reclining or slumping than when they're standing or sitting with proper posture. According to research, proper posture stretches appetite sensors in the stomach and turns off false appetite signals.[1] In effect, standing (or sitting) tall can help whittle away those extra pounds.

One of the reasons we're seeing so many potbellies in the United States is that two of every three American adults have weak

> *Success Map Tip:*
> Each time you
> remind yourself to
> stand tall, make
> a note under
> MSOn Minutes.
> Mark your energy
> level, too.

oblique and abdominal muscles. These very muscles are essential for maintaining good posture.[2] What's more, if you slump even slightly, you restrict breathing and circulation, which in turn slows metabolism. In fact, poor posture can diminish vital lung capacity by 30 percent or more.

According to research reports, poor posture contributes to a host of health concerns, from fatigue and poor concentration to digestive disorders and pain syndromes such as headaches and muscle aches.[3] Not surprisingly, poor posture plays a role in 80 percent of all back problems. Compared with sitting or standing straight, slouching exerts 10 to 15 times as much pressure on your lower back.[4] No wonder you feel less inclined to move around, and less inclined to spark your Meta-Stat.

Maintaining proper posture is a choice you make—or don't make— every waking moment. Whether consciously controlled or not, your posture creates its own momentum. Once gravity gets a grip on your tilted head or drooping shoulders, your body feels like a slow wave moving downhill. Slouching gradually becomes slumping, and ease turns into effort. Fortunately, you can turn the tide on poor posture at any point in your life. Why not now?

ARE YOU IN A SLUMP?

Of the nearly 700 muscles in your body, you rely on just four or five to hold your head, neck, shoulders, chest, and back in proper alignment. Yet very few people carry themselves in a relaxed upright position. Poor posture—hunched over, head jutting forward—has become the standard.

Our ability to stand erect, on two feet, distinguishes us humans as a species. It's something we should value. In general, those who sit or stand tall seem to exude greater grace and self-confidence than most. But good posture isn't only about appearance. It's about fat burning and energy production, too. Every time you slump, you contribute to fat gain or fatigue . . . or perhaps both.

So much of modern life prompts us to lean forward in an attempt to see and comprehend with greater clarity. Research shows that all of our neck-contorting pursuits—like watching TV, peering at a computer monitor, or working on an assembly line—induce us to assume an unhealthy posture. "It's extremely difficult to work in a technological society and not develop a 'forward head,'" observes René Cailliet, MD, former head of rehabilitative medicine at the University of Southern California Medical School.[5]

Indeed, any activity that requires you to look down for protracted periods—from reading and sewing to cooking and cleaning—can produce the constant postural stress that contributes to vision problems, tension headaches, and neck and jaw pain.[6] When we get up to walk around, the neck and shoulders don't automatically return to their natural positions.

If you were to spend a lunch hour watching people on a busy street, chances are you'd see that most everyone was still in the same general posture as they were at their desks. The fact that they were up and walking wouldn't make much difference. The head-forward position stresses every part of the body, especially the neck, spine, and shoulders. And that not only takes a toll on energy and alertness, it also interferes with Meta-Stat function.

While slouching isn't healthy, neither is the ramrod-straight posture that many of us associate with sitting or standing tall. You may remember your parents or physical-education instructors telling you to sit up or stand up straight. In response, you'd throw back your shoulders, suck in your stomach, and tuck in your buttocks. That's the military paradigm of proper posture, but you can't hold that position for very long. You're stiffening your muscles, which is tiring—not to mention unnatural.

The truth is, you can't force good posture. Nor is it instinctive or automatic. "We're not born knowing how to do it right," says Wilfred Barlow, MD, medical director of the Alexander Institute in Great Britain. "No reflex system sets up good posture. We have to learn it."[7]

By easing into a relaxed upright posture, your head and spine naturally align. This automatically deepens breathing and frees up circulation.[8] It also alerts your Meta-Stat to fire up the energy-producing furnaces, so it's ready for anything. As a result, you feel more energetic, with greater fat-burning power to boot.

THE MIND-BODY CONNECTION

The benefits of proper posture don't end with the body. How you sit and stand can exert a powerful influence over how you feel emotionally. It makes sense when you consider how slouching restricts breathing and circulation,[9] which in turn inhibits vital blood flow to the brain. Even the simple act of rounding your shoulders forward may reduce the brain's oxygen supply by 30 percent.[10]

Studies indicate that poor posture decreases mental alertness while increasing mental errors.[11] Compared with people who maintain a relaxed upright posture, those who slouch are more likely to experience a sense of helplessness and frustration while completing work tasks and to perceive themselves as under greater stress.[12] More generally, researchers have linked poor posture to more intense feelings of panic and, in some cases, depression.[13]

"Posture is not solely the manifestation of physical balance," writes occupational medicine specialist David Imrie, MD. "It is also an expression of mental balance. Think about the way you stand when you are depressed or tired, with your shoulders rounded and drooping. Your body represents your emotions by giving up the fight against gravity, sagging just as low as you feel."[14]

By lifting and relaxing your body into its natural alignment, you actually help slow or reverse the aging process, functionally as well as cosmetically, according to Dr. Cailliet.[15] With poor posture, on the other hand, you not only appear older, you feel that way, too.[16]

PRACTICE MAKES PERFECT

Honing proper posture means learning to stand and move with grace and vigor. Along with food, water, and oxygen, your body depends on mobility to preserve its natural functions. Over time, a body in motion takes its cues from the patterns that you etch into its memory each time you sit, stand, bend, turn, and walk.

Through the rest of this chapter, you will learn simple techniques for strengthening and controlling the muscles that position and support your body, whether you're at rest or on the move. In this way, you can establish and maintain habits that foster proper, health-promoting posture. As you adjust your body position and move with greater ease, you'll feel more motivated and energized to take advantage of other MSOn Switches.

Centering

Your head weighs between 10 and 15 pounds. To avoid placing undue stress on your neck, shoulders, and spine, it must maintain a comfortable, centered position. It's important for fine-tuning your Meta-Stat setting. The fact is, your metabolism—and your energy

---

META-STAT STARTER

It's All in Your Head

The battle for proper posture is won from the neck up, literally. Sitting or standing tall begins with your head and neck. Once they're in a natural, comfortable position, your shoulders, chest, and back will follow suit and align themselves.

At the crest of your spine is a small muscle called the rectus capitus anterior.[17] It's responsible for flexing and rotating your head. You can tone the rectus capitus anterior with a gentle "head nod" exercise, which you can practice while sitting or standing.

1. After getting comfortable, place your hands on the base of your skull just behind and above your earlobes. Your thumbs should point toward your spine, in the back of your neck.

2. Let your neck lengthen, gently extending upward as if lifted by an imaginary cord attached to the top of your skull.

3. With your neck in this slightly elevated position, nod your head as if in agreement, bringing your forehead a little forward and chin slightly in.

Repeat this exercise about a dozen times a day.

---

level—are influenced by how you hold your head. Here's one way to become more aware of this ideal placement.

1. Sit comfortably on a stool, bench, or chair, with your back unsupported. Breathe naturally.

2. Lengthen your neck and let your head move upward, with your chin slightly in, your shoulders broadening, and your lower back flattening.

3. Gently tilt your head to the left and return to center, finding the most balanced spot you can. Repeat to the right, bringing your head to that balanced, vertical position in the center.

4. Move your head slightly forward, then return it to center. Repeat, moving your head slightly backward.

With this simple, short exercise, you have made a subtle but important discovery. By tilting left and right, then forward and back, you have found the position in which you can hold your head with *the least amount of effort*. Far from feeling unnatural, this position is comfortable, because it creates the least tension in all your muscles.

As you're doing this exercise, you might want to conjure a helpful image in your mind. Envision a 5-pound weight on your head, as though you were carrying a basket. If you lean too far one way or the other, you might drop the weight, so you need to gently push up against the resistance. This image stimulates your senses with signals that help stabilize your head and neck.[18] Your posture will improve automatically.

I recommend performing this exercise several times a day—with your eyes closed, once you learn the steps. If you spend your days at a desk or behind a counter, take just a moment to "find the center" before you resume work. Quickly and consciously, you can determine the position in which you can hold your head with the least strain. It won't be long before this conscious practice translates into a reliable, subconscious habit.

Upward Float

Here's another technique that can train your body in proper posture. I call it simply, "think taller." Whether you're sitting, standing, or walking, allow your head to float upward by extending your neck.

Don't push or strain; simply bring your head over your shoulders and move your chin slightly in. You'll feel the difference—a good indicator that you're stimulating your Meta-Stat. Try it in front of a mirror, and you'll *see* the difference, too. As you'll notice, your head does more than simply perch atop your neck. When comfortably positioned, it almost literally floats there.

In general, try to be more aware of your head position when your whole body is in motion. Whenever possible, your head should lead— not by jutting forward, but by moving upward and away from the rest of your body. Lengthen your body by following the upward direction of your head.[19] This initiates the process of learning a new pattern of moving your body with grace and ease.

Sitting Smart

For optimal Meta-Stat function, your goal is to sit less and move more. If you must sit for long hours at a stretch, make sure you have the right chair. For optimal support and comfort, it ought to fit the length, size, and contours of your body. The height of the seat should precisely match the position of the countertop, desk, or workstation that you're using. Well-positioned armrests also are important. They can relieve about 25 percent of the load on your lower back[20] and provide stability and support when you're changing positions.

If you sit in various chairs during the day, or if another person often sits in your chair, be sure you adjust it each time you return to it. This should become as automatic as adjusting your car seat, steering wheel, and mirrors after someone else has driven your car.

Avoid sitting on your wallet, checkbook, pen, comb, or car keys. A thick back-pocket wallet, in particular, not only throws off your posture but actually can contribute to back pain. The *New England Journal of Medicine* published a study in which a number of male patients experienced complete relief from chronic back pain once they stopped carrying fat wallets in their back pockets.[21]

When you sit, briefly pause and choose the most balanced, comfortable sitting position. First of all, sit squarely. Don't slump. Center your lower back and buttocks far back on the seat. Leaning to one side or sitting off-center shifts the line of gravity, causing tension and impeding circulation.

Let your shoulders and chest come forward. Your thighs should be at right angles to your spine, with the bend in your hip joints, not your lower spine.

Smoothly move your upper body toward the back of the chair, once again "hinging" the movement from your hip joints rather than your lower spine. Whenever possible, place your feet flat on the floor. Another good option is to rest one foot on a chair rung or place it slightly ahead of the other foot on a small stool.[22]

If you must cross your legs, do it at the ankles. Crossing at the knees misaligns the pelvis and can lead to back tension and pain, particularly if you hold the same position for a long time.

Once you're properly seated, balance your neck. With your eyes closed, do the centering exercise described earlier. When you're comfortable, gently tilt your head to the left and return to center, then tilt to the right and return to center. Repeat to the front and back, so you end with your head in the exact center of your body.

Even if you have the most comfortable chair imaginable, make a point to get out of it at frequent intervals throughout the day. Sitting for hours on end is stressful, no matter how ideal your chair or workspace design. Take a break by standing up for at least a minute or two, at least every half hour.

When you read—at your desk, on a train, while flying—bring your reading material up to your field of vision. This reduces neck and shoulder strain from dropping your head. You might want to invest in a bookstand that holds books on a slant near eye level. Also consider buying a small reading light that clips right onto books. Both items are available online and in many bookstores.

Mindful Mobility

Think of walking as a step-by-step technique for releasing tension and improving posture while shifting your Meta-Stat to a higher setting. Hold your head high, with your neck and shoulders relaxed and lower back flat. By concentrating on the actual steps, you can improve not only your posture but also the degree of relaxation you feel as you stroll along.

With each step, let your heel lightly strike the ground. Roll your weight forward across the sole of your foot, gently pushing off with your toes. Many people make the mistake of letting their feet point outward or in. They should point straight ahead. Be careful, too, not to lock your knees, even when you extend your legs. This phenomenon, called hyperextension, can result in knee injury as well as added muscle tension.

As you move forward, practice what's known as a heterolateral walking pattern. In other words, your left arm swings forward in sync with your right leg, and your right arm moves with your left leg. This is a natural gait, and it helps maintain balance.

Of course, not all of your daily walking is at the pace of an afternoon stroll. But there's a cardinal rule for everyday movement: Whenever you reach, turn, or bend, take a step in that direction. This helps concentrate your power while coordinating your body's various moving parts, alleviating strain on the back muscles by utilizing the trunk and legs. As always, lead the movement with your head, following with the rest of your body.

PAY ATTENTION TO TENSION

Stress and pressure are realities of modern life. If we ignore them or pretend they don't exist, they can manifest as physical tension. This tension can influence not only our posture but also our actions and behaviors, as well as our thoughts and moods. It artificially charges the Meta-Stat in a way that produces tense energy instead of calm energy.

Tense energy has become so common that it seems normal. But it isn't inevitable. The key is to develop the appropriate skills and know-how to defuse stress on the spot.

When a muscle stays tense, you become less aware of it as time goes on. With this diminishing awareness, you're more likely to "lock in" tension. So whenever you notice that your body is stiffening or tightening—usually because of stress—take immediate steps to relax. Often this can be as simple as shaking your muscles, shifting your body position, and taking several deep breaths. (For more ideas, see Chapter 13.)

CHAPTER 10

◼ ◼ ◼

Turn Down the Heat, Turn Up Your Energy

For optimal fat burning and energy production, it pays to be cool. When you're in a cool environment, the ambient temperature sends a powerful signal to your Meta-Stat, instructing your body to fire up its inner furnace. It needs to burn fat in order to acclimate to its surroundings.[1]

A warm environment triggers a very different physical reaction. As we perspire, our bodies naturally slow their metabolic rates. It's as though they're prompting us to take a break for rest and recovery, before we become overheated.

> **Success Map Tip:** Compare the graphs of your Daily Energy Wave from a very warm day and a very cool day.

Heating and cooling are basic survival mechanisms that evolved over thousands of years. Among our ancestors, the fittest endured courtesy of finely tuned metabolisms that naturally adjusted to cold and warm environs. They weren't swaddling themselves in clothing and blankets, which contribute to overheating and therefore slow metabolism.[2]

META-STAT STARTER

Chill!

Right now, seek a cooler spot. It could be someplace in the room where you are, perhaps closer to the door or a window. Otherwise, you may need to step outside.

Once you've found your spot, take a deep breath. Let the cool air invigorate you. Every moment of cooler temperature is a signal to increase your metabolism, so you're producing more energy and burning more fat!

According to a study in the *Journal of Physiology,* the cooler your body, the cooler your brain. That's important, because apparently, excessive heat not only saps physical vigor but also undermines brain function. At least up to a point, a cool brain is a healthy brain. And a healthy brain is key to building and sustaining energy, strength, and good health—not to mention enhancing fat burning.[3]

DE-LAYER

Of course, I'm not suggesting that you risk hypothermia in order to stimulate your metabolism. You have many options to cool down and still remain comfortable. For example, shed an extra layer or two of

META-STAT STARTER

Fan the Flames

When you exercise indoors, turn on a small fan and keep the temperature a bit cool. According to some surprising new evidence,[4] mental boredom with exercise may have a link to overheating—and a cool breeze helps solve the problem.

clothing. If you're in the habit of wearing a sweater in your office, try going without one. At home, trade your flannel pj's for cotton.

While we're on the subject of bedtime, researchers stress the importance of a cool night's sleep. When you bundle up at night, with blankets and quilts as an insulating layer, you warm your body too much and slow your metabolism as a result. Try sleeping with one less blanket, even in winter, and forgo the quilt completely.

As your body adjusts to each change, add another one. Gradually, the cooler temperature will seem normal. This will pay off handsomely for your Meta-Stat in terms of stoking your metabolism to higher fat-burning, energy-producing power.

CHAPTER 11

■ ■ ■

M S O n   S w i t c h   # 8

Improve Hormone Balance, Hour after Hour

Throughout human evolution, hormones have played a vital role in ensuring our survival. Now, poor diet, inactivity, lack of sun exposure, and other drawbacks of modern life conspire to undermine optimal hormone levels.[1]

According to endocrinologist Scott Isaacs, MD, author of *Hormonal Power,* anyone who has a high percentage of body fat—even if he or she doesn't appear overweight—likely has some sort of hormonal imbalance. Unfortunately, doctors routinely overlook hormonal disorders as a cause of weight gain.[2]

In Chapter 2, I introduced a number of hormones and their respective effects—positive and negative—on Meta-Stat function. Here we'll explore several key hormones in

> **Success Map Tip:** Review several Success Maps, noting the highest point of the Daily Energy Wave on each. See if this point correlates with a time when you were exercising, eating, or otherwise stimulating your Meta-Stat.

further detail, along with some practical strategies that can support hormone balance and keep your Meta-Stat operating at peak efficiency. The latest research proves that you have much greater control over your hormones than you may realize.

INSULIN: STABILIZE FOR YOUR META-STAT

Have you ever seen a sumo wrestler? They're rather hard to miss. Some of these Japanese bohemoths tip the scale at close to 500 pounds—a real advantage for pushing around an opponent. One of their secrets to fattening up is to skip breakfast.[3] They go straight to practice immediately upon arising, then sit down to a megalunch. Afterward, they sleep for several hours. Metabolism naturally slows after a big meal; a long nap slows it even more.

Though very strong, sumo wrestlers are very obese. They routinely develop serious health problems after they retire. Though relatively few of us Americans desire to take up sumo wrestling, many adopt the eating habits of the sport. Specifically, tend to skip breakfast, then eat a large lunch and possibly a larger dinner. We're so full when we go to bed that we don't feel hungry when we wake up the next morning. And so the cycle continues.

Breakfast is critical to hormonal balance—and to Meta-Stat function—because it prevents the insulin surges that occurs when we feast, then starve, then feast again. Insulin secretion runs with your biological clock. Insulin sensitivity—your body's ability to flawlessly balance blood sugar and keep insulin working in favor of calorie burning and energy production, rather than against it—is highest first thing in the morning. It begins to dip around 6:00 P.M That's why your body is less able to handle carbohydrates, especially simple sugars, during the evening.

To prevent spikes in blood sugar and insulin, then, you need to eat the right foods in the right combinations at the right times of day. The MSOn Eating Plan (Part 4) will provide the framework for building daily menus of meals and snacks that support general hormonal balance. Specific to insulin, here's what you need to know.

Start your day with protein. As Chapter 22 will explain, you should be eating lean protein at meals and snacks throughout the day. But it's

Beware of Ab Fat

Those dimples of fat on the hips or thighs might be unattractive. But they're relatively harmless, compared with fat in the abdominal region.[4]

The fat cells that surround internal organs are more sensitive to hormonal regulation. So a state of hormonal imbalance—too much insulin and cortisol, too little human growth hormone—actually will promote the accumulation of abdominal fat.

To offset this hormonal "hot spot" and start burning abdominal (or visceral) fat, be sure to eat more protein and fewer carbohydrates and to choose only complex carbs. This mix of nutrients can help prevent the hormonal spikes and dips that encourage fat accumulation in the abdominal region.

Also, try to move around at every opportunity—especially in the evening, when metabolism begins dropping off. Strength training, in particular, builds muscle. And the more muscle you have, the more calories and fat you burn.

Finally, pay attention to stress. It triggers the release of cortisol, which can reverse certain positive effects of exercise.[5] It also seems to increase a person's predisposition to abdominal fat.

especially important for breakfast. Research shows that protein not only controls hunger but also supplies energy. And it does so without causing dramatic rises and falls in blood sugar and insulin levels.[6]

Eat starches *before* dinner. Because insulin sensitivity takes a downturn in the evening, your best bet is to get any starchy carbohydrates— whole grain breads, oatmeal, brown rice—earlier in the day. For dinner, choose water-rich carbs such as tomatoes, peppers, spinach, lettuce, and broccoli. The water some calories from fat storage.

Have an evening snack. In many European countries, an afterdinner tradition is to nibble on fresh fruit, savoring each bite. It's a smart idea, because it helps stabilize blood sugar. Then your body won't need to churn out as much insulin to do the job.[7]

On those occasions when you choose an evening snack that's high in refined sugar, be sure to eat it slowly. This reduces the impact on blood sugar and insulin levels, and therefore on Meta-Stat function.

Forgo the sports drink. Unless you're a competitive athlete in training for a high-endurance event, high-glycemic sports drinks probably aren't for you. They can interfere with insulin balance, contributing to fat gain in the process. They're most effective during or after periods of high-intensity physical activity, not before. If you're engaging in more moderate activity, as in the MSOn workout, you may not need sports drinks at all.

LEPTIN AND ADIPONECTIN: THE DYNAMIC DUO OF FAT LOSS

One of the smartest strategies for defusing food cravings and fueling fat burning is to enlist the help of leptin and adiponectin. Working together, these two hormones—which are secreted by fat cells—can reduce fat cell size while increasing fat loss.

In your brain and body, leptin and adiponectin help regulate the intensity of your appetite and influence the speed at which your body burns fat. Levels of both hormones decline whenever your body thinks that you need to conserve existing body fat or make extra fat for survival.[8] You can maximize both hormones naturally, just by heeding this advice.

Eat well. According to research, a diet that's low in fat, moderate in carbohydrates and protein, and rich in plant-based foods helps maintain optimal leptin levels. (Not coincidentally, this is the foundation of the MSOn Eating Plan, which you'll read about in Part 4.) Where high-fat, high-sugar foods suppress leptin production,[9] low-fat foods actually boost leptin levels. They also enhance leptin's effectiveness, helping each molecule of the hormone to attach to cells and improve fat burning.[10]

Fish oil, an excellent source of healthy fats, has a particularly beneficial effect on leptin. When you eat fish, the oil not only improves the efficiency of leptin, it also steps up production of the hormone.[11]

Eat often. Building your meals around a mix of nutritious foods is an important component of having a healthy diet. But you need to pay attention not only to what you eat but also to how often. Whenever you skip meals or snacks, the stomach secretes ghrelin, the hormone that's responsible for triggering a voracious appetite. In other words, when ghrelin is on the scene, you overeat.

The presence of ghrelin causes a decline in leptin, which in turn leads to a slowdown in metabolism. Your body tries to conserve energy by converting any extra calories to fat, as well as "locking down" any fat cells you already have. In the meantime, the excess ghrelin leaves you feeling constantly hungry. You eat more food, but you burn off less fat.

Eating meals and snacks at regular, frequent levels throughout the day helps keep ghrelin in check. Then leptin can do its job of stimulating fat loss. (I'll discuss meal frequency in more detail in Chapter 21.)

Stay physically active. To garner the full power of the "thin hormones," you need to maintain the kind of activity level that I recommend in the MSOn Workout, which you'll find in Part 3. A Harvard study found that regular exercise can dramatically increase leptin levels.[12] Other research has confirmed that adiponectin levels rise as the body burns off fat through regular exercise.[13]

Even brief, 15- to 20-minute cardiovascular workouts or muscle-toning sessions can have a significant effect on leptin, and perhaps on adiponectin, too. It's just another reason to get up and get moving . . . often!

Catch more light. As you may recall from Chapter 2, leptin triggers the production of melanocortin, an antioxidant that supports fat loss by suppressing appetite centers in the brain.[14] Melanocortin levels also rise with sun exposure. In fact, research suggests that the melanocortin secreted by the skin in response to sunlight may circulate through the bloodstream to the brain, where it can influence metabolism.[15]

Remember, too, that as melanocortin suppresses appetite, the hormone agouti stimulates it. Both occur in the same parts of the brain.[16] The key is to maintain proper balance between them—just enough melanocortin, not too much agouti. When levels tip in agouti's favor, you become hungry and burn less fat.

HUMAN GROWTH HORMONE:
THE FOUNTAIN OF YOUTH?

Human growth hormone (HGH) is the body's most potent revitalizer. With optimal HGH levels, you feel younger, stronger, and more energetic. Though the hormone is present in your body through your entire life, it naturally diminishes with age.

HGH is produced by the anterior portion of the pituitary gland. From what scientists have learned about this extraordinarily potent hormone, it appears to be secreted in short spurts, or pulses, throughout the day. About 6 to 12 discrete pulses occur in a typical 24-hour period. The largest occur about an hour after you fall asleep at night. If you go to bed at 11 o'clock, for example, optimal HGH secretion takes place around midnight.

One of the most important functions of HGH is to free up stored fat, which your body burns for energy. Somehow the hormone manages to find its way to every one of the body's 25 to 30 billion fat cells. After attaching to specialized receptors on those cells, it prepares the signal that eventually will induce the cells to release their stored fat. HGH also stimulates the growth of muscle tissue.

A variety of growth hormones simulate the effects of HGH; virtually all are available by prescription. A far better alternative, in my opinion, is to stimulate your body's own HGH production—naturally, without medication. You can do this no matter what your age. Here's how.

Get deep rest at the right time. When you don't get enough sleep, or you don't get good-quality sleep, your body responds by stepping up cortisol production. As discussed in Chapter 2, cortisol helps regulate appetite and metabolism while dampening fat burning and energy production.[17] But cortisol and HGH have an inverse relationship. That is, as cortisol levels rise, HGH levels fall. Your metabolism and fat burning follow suit.

To keep a lid on cortisol production, you need to be sure that you're getting deep, restorative sleep between midnight and 3:00 A.M.—what experts call the critical healing period. This is the window of opportunity in which sleep can have the greatest positive impact on your metabolism and your overall health.

In Chapter 15, I'll say more about creating an ideal sleeping environment. For now, the most important guidelines are these: You need a cool, dark, quiet room in which to sleep, as well as enough time for good-quality sleep. And make a point of waking at approximately the same time every day.

Engage in regular muscle-toning exercises. Every time you intensely work your muscles, you stimulate HGH production. I recommend at least 10 minutes of resistance training either once or twice a day. This is enough to significantly raise HGH levels, not just for the short term but over a 24-hour period.[18]

Build your diet around HGH-friendly foods. Research confirms that all of us require adequate protein intake for optimal HGH production and secretion.[19] Consuming a protein-rich food or beverage after exercise also appears to enhance HGH secretion.[20] Some scientists recommend following a workout with 15 to 25 grams of protein—perhaps in the form of a protein shake or bar, lean turkey or chicken breast, or an egg.[21]

Some foods actually can dampen HGH production. For example, sugary foods such as soft drinks and refined-carbohydrate snacks deplete HGH levels by elevating blood sugar.[22] Fatty foods can have a similar effect when they're eaten in advance of exercise.[23] For this reason, be sure to steer clear of high-fat snacks for at least 60 minutes prior to an intense workout.

TRIIODOTHYRONINE: ESSENTIAL TO METABOLISM

Think of your thyroid gland as the master regulator of your Meta-Stat. It sets the rate at which you burn fat.

Of all the thyroid hormones, triiodothyronine (T3) is by far the most active. A low level of T3 can slow metabolism and cause weight gain.[24] Your body is able to make its own supply of T3 from an enzyme called 5-deiodinanse. To do so, though, it needs selenium. Unfortunately, the vast majority of Americans don't get enough selenium from their diets.[25]

A trace mineral, selenium comes from the soil, and the amount in your diet depends in large part on where your food is grown. Grains, fruits, and vegetables tend to be the best sources, though selenium content can vary greatly even within each food group. To ensure that you're getting enough, you might consider taking a broad-spectrum multivitamin/mineral supplement that contains selenium.

For the best Meta-Stat boost from a healthy thyroid, monitor your consumption of goitrogens, a class of raw foods that can interfere with thyroid function and T3 production. Foods in this group include cabbage, brussels sprouts, turnips, rutabaga, radishes, kohlrabi, kale, and cauliflower. Keep in mind that they cause problems only when eaten raw and in large quantities.

CHOLECYSTOKININ AND GALANIN: FOR AND AGAINST FAT LOSS

In the grand scheme of hormone balance, cholecystokinin (CCK) and galanin seem to be working at cross-purposes. Galanin creates feelings of fatigue, confusion, and vulnerability, along with cravings for high-fat, highly sweetened foods.[26] It also influences the activation of other hormones, virtually ensuring that any excess dietary fat gets stored as body fat.[27]

CCK, on the other hand, works to keep hunger in check.[28] It appears especially sensitive to even small amounts of specialized protein peptides known as glycomacropeptides from high-quality proteins.

To maximize CCK while minimizing galanin, stick with meals and snacks that combine lean proteins with high-fiber complex carbohydrates—perhaps low-fat plain yogurt with sliced fruit or whole grain crackers with cheese. Limit fatty, sugary desserts and soft drinks, especially in the evening, when galanin levels reach their peak. Snack foods such as chips, cookies, and ice cream stimulate galanin production.

CALCITROL: LESS IS BEST

By now you probably have seen news reports about the slimming effects of calcium—namely, stimulating the production of hormones that enhance metabolism and inhibit fat storage.[29] But running low on calcium can raise levels of one particular hormone known as calcitrol. It has a number of effects on the body, the most problematic being the way in which it shuts down some mechanisms that support fat burning while activating others that fuel fat production.[30]

Increasing evidence shows that people who consume low-fat and fat-free dairy products get direct benefits from the increase in dietary calcium. In a recent University of Tennessee study, for example, men who added three servings of yogurt to their daily diets lost 61 percent more body fat and 81 percent more abdominal fat over 12 weeks than men who didn't. Commenting on his findings, the study's author, Michael Zemel, PhD, concluded, "Calcium helps the body burn more fat and limits the amount of new fat your body can make."[31]

CORTISOL: A BY-PRODUCT OF STRESS

The adrenal gland's principal hormone, cortisol plays a major role in the quantity and distribution of body fat.[32] It not only stimulates appetite, it also promotes fat accumulation in the abdominal area.[33]

When cortisol levels rise too high, large amounts of muscle tissue break down, undermining Meta-Stat function in the process. Excess cortisol also stimulates specific receptors that contribute to water retention and bloating.

The most important strategy for stabilizing cortisol levels is to reduce stress as much as possible. At times this might seem easier said than done. But I'll present some can't miss antistress techniques in Chapters 12 and 13. Remember, too, that brief bouts of physical activity—like the everyday movements presented in Chapter 5—can help burn off excess cortisol.

CHAPTER 12

■   ■   ■

M S O n   S w i t c h   # 9

Stay Calm in an Uptight World

When we talk about tension in the context of the Meta-Stat approach, we need to acknowledge that it takes two distinct forms. There's the natural, healthy muscle tension that increases as you build muscle tone, and there's the more general physical and emotional tension that's a by-product of stress, poor posture, and other factors of modern life. The former stimulates metabolism, which leads to optimal energy and fat loss. The latter tilts your biochemistry toward moodiness, fatigue, and an urge to overeat.[1]

If you're not careful, lifestyle tension can sabotage muscle tension. You probably can recall a situation where you skipped a workout because you were on deadline at work or dealing with a crisis at home. Lifestyle tension got the upper hand.

> **Success Map Tip:**
> When you use your MSOn Minutes to loosen up and stay calm, mark your energy level on the Daily Energy Wave.

Over the years, some people have suggested that chronic tension burns calories. It doesn't. Instead, it stimulates production of fattening hormones.[2] This is why stress reduction is so important to fat loss—and, more generally, to optimal Meta-Stat function.

The good news is, you can learn to monitor your tension levels and to replace tense energy with calm energy. This process consists of three steps: awareness, pacing, and releasing. Let's look at each one in turn.

AWARENESS: TREAT TENSION
LIKE A HOT POTATO

Before you can release tension, you need to be aware of it. That isn't always easy, since tension can conceal itself in many different ways. But you must flush it out, because otherwise, it tends to become chronic. Then it's even more of a problem because you may not even notice that you're tense. You just feel "normal."

To increase your awareness of tension, I recommend doing a quick "tension scan." Begin by tensing and relaxing your shoulders. Then shift your attention to other parts of your body in sequence—tensing and relaxing your jaw, neck, back, arms, and so on, down to the tips of your toes. Even your tongue may be carrying excess tension, whether or not you're talking!

PACING: TAKE BREAKS AT REGULAR INTERVALS

Human energy has a powerful connection to the biology of time. Researchers in an intriguing field of scientific exploration known as chronobiology have been mapping the natural rise and fall of energy that we each experience throughout the day.[3] Each rise corresponds to an uptick in your Meta-Stat setting; each fall, a downturn.

Every half hour or so, we have an innate biological need to change our pace, shift our view, revitalize our energy. That's the Meta-Stat asking whether we want to conserve our resources at that moment, or if we want to feel fully alive. Whether or not we realize it, we respond to the Meta-Stat, sending signals to lower or raise energy-producing, fat-burning power.

Overarching and influencing this communication between us and our Meta-Stats are what scientists call the ultradian rhythms, which are regular rises and falls in energy that occur every 90 to 180 minutes. Ultradian rhythms are more frequent than circadian rhythms, which span a 24-hour cycle and encompass waking and sleeping. The current understanding of ultradian rhythms comes from hundreds of biological and behavioral studies in laboratories throughout the world.

Ultradian rhythms are the end product of a complex pattern of messenger-chemical communications that occur among many parts of the body, including the circulatory system and the brain. These messenger chemicals help us regulate our energy levels. Within the ultradian rhythms is a natural downturn. Nature has equipped us with a series of signals that compel us to take a few key minutes to rejuvenate amid the continually shifting challenges and pressures of daily life.

Here's the problem: Few of us heed the opportunity to recharge during the downturn. Instead, we tend to ignore the signals and forge ahead with whatever we're doing. Of course, in the din of modern life, it's becoming harder and harder to hear—and heed—what our messenger chemicals are trying to tell us. Still, we pay a steep price for our negligence, as we accelerate the depletion of our energy reserves.

Our bodies respond to this stressful state with a flood of hormones, including epinephrine and cortisol. We may feel as though we've gotten a "second wind," but it's only an illusion created by the hormonal stimuli. But what happens? We pour ourselves back into the task at hand. Through all the frenetic activity, we deplete those all-important messenger chemicals—the ones that ignite and coordinate memory, perception, and engagement with the world. No wonder we so often feel drained and disoriented by the end of the day!

The Ways of Our Errors

As you can see, it's vital to tune in to your ultradian rhythms and to heed their signals to take brief, rejuvenating pauses every 30 minutes or so throughout the day. Your body will tell you when you need these breaks, but you need to pay attention to it. Here are the cues you should watch for.

- You feel compelled to stretch or move
- You're yawning or sighing
- You're unable to concentrate

- You feel increasing tension or fatigue

- You experience hunger pangs

- You feel anxious or frustrated

- You make errors in judgment

- You slow down when performing basic tasks such as typing or counting

- You can't pay attention, no matter how hard you try[4]

The harder and longer we push ourselves, the more prone we become to missing these signals. That's because the more we're driven by internal and external pressures, the less energy—and therefore the less alertness and awareness—we have. If we don't learn to pace ourselves, we experience countless space-outs and "microsleeps," which occur no matter how hard we try to catch up. In fact, many automobile and airplane accidents are attributed to such brief, preventable moments of inattention.[5]

According to William C. Dement, MD, PhD, professor at Stanford Medical School, "Impaired alertness is one of the greatest potential dangers of contemporary life."[6] When we spend more than 20 or 30 minutes on a single task, our problem-solving time increases by up to 500 percent.[7] So it makes sense for us to pause, take a break, and change focus as often as necessary. But so few people around us stop for even a moment that we believe we shouldn't either.

To observe a more natural rhythm of daily life, notice how many children instinctively pause throughout the day, both at home and at school. Of course, we adults scold them for this behavior, admonishing them to sit still and focus. When they whisper and laugh, we tell them to stop. And if they ask for something to eat or drink, we tell them to wait until mealtime. Yet they're simply responding to their bodies' natural cues, just as we should.

When you think about it, why should anyone—kids or adults—be expected to remain still and feign attention? We may congratulate ourselves for our self-discipline, but what is the cost in terms of our energy?

The Strategic Pause

Among the simplest techniques for establishing a habit of regular, rejuvenating breaks throughout the day is one I call the strategic pause. For only 30 seconds of your time, it produces 30 minutes of elevated metabolism.

The strategic pause consists of six quick steps. Each of them is important, though you can adjust them depending on the situation. Collectively, they'll take just 30 seconds to perform.

1. Breathe.

2. Lift and move.

3. Look.

4. Laugh.

5. Find light.

6. Drink fluids.

1. Breathe: Deepen and relax your breathing. Oxygen is vital to metabolism and energy. According to Sheldon Saul Hendler, MD, PhD, faculty member at the University of California, San Diego, School of Medicine, "There are over 75 trillion cells in your body, and they are all breathing—or should be. It is this inner breathing of the cells that allows us to produce biological energy."[8]

How you monitor your breathing has a great deal to do with how much energy you can generate and sustain all day long. Oxygen interruption—brief, frequent halts in breathing or chronic under-breathing—is a common contributing factor to tension and tiredness. Conversely, every chance you have to deepen your breathing can enhance both calmness and vigor.[9]

Oxygen is essential to the production of the cellular fuel known as adenosine triphosphate (ATP). We need ATP for energy, and for life. As Dr. Hendler observes, "The body and brain are sensitive to even very small reductions in ATP production. This sensitivity is expressed in terms of intermittent fatigue and many other symptoms. . . . Breathing is the first place, not the last, that one should look whenever fatigue or other disordered energy symptoms present themselves."[10]

This is why the strategic pause begins with breathing. With practice, breathing will stay at the forefront of your awareness throughout the day.

Wherever you are and whatever you are doing, notice your breathing as you pull back from the task at hand. Consciously deepen and relax your respiration. This simple action will charge your metabolism and reset your Meta-Stat. You can actually feel the accumulated tension ease as your Meta-Stat edges upward.

2. Lift and move: Rebalance your head and shoulders to stimulate circulation. Poor posture—even a slight slumping of the shoulders—depletes lung capacity by as much as 30 percent.[11] According to René Cailliet, MD, former head of rehabilitative medicine at the University of Southern California School of Medicine, "With poor posture, you not only look old, you function that way as well. In a number of ways you probably don't even suspect, a slightly slumping posture can greatly decrease your vital capacity. . . . "[12]

Another major energy drain is sustained inactivity. The longer we sit still, the less energy we have to get up and get going. Unfortunately, in the quest for innovation and success, we have conditioned ourselves to

META-STAT STARTER

Stand Up Right

According to researchers, the key to proper posture is to frequently check in on the position of your neck. The goal is to keep your chin in and head high. It's a very relaxed feeling of being taller. Imagine a beanbag sitting on top of your head; gently lift your muscles to push it toward the ceiling. Nod your head slightly in a subtle "yes" motion. This stimulates toning of the rectus capitus anterior, a very small but important muscle that's designed to help hold your head effortlessly in place on top of your neck. Next, loosen and realign your shoulders so that they are as relaxed and wide as they can be. This instantly increases oxygen flow to the brain and senses.

remain immobile all day long. It makes no biological sense. It drains energy—and the Meta-Stat—rather than renewing it.

The strategic pause helps change that. Stand up—tall, loose, and at ease—and then stretch or move around. If you spend long stretches of time sitting down, simply standing up every half hour or so may increase energy and alertness by up to 30 percent.[13]

3. Look: Rejuvenate instantly with a visual shift. Most people are surprised when they realize that what they do with their eyes can have a tremendous impact on how much energy they have. Day in and day out, the tiny muscles in the human eye use more energy than any other muscle fibers in the body. Without a brief break every half hour or so, they readily tire, contributing to fatigue, headache, and neck and shoulder tension. In one study of 2,330 people from 15 different regions of the country, 77 percent of VDT (computer terminal) users and 56 percent of everyone else reported problems with eyestrain.[14]

Simply by shifting your focus, you bring about a swift change in the neurons that connect your eyes and brain. Your Meta-Stat resets, and your energy level soars.

As part of the strategic pause, you'll take steps to revitalize your vision. If you've been doing close work, spend a few moments blinking your eyes and looking at more distant objects. Focus on a picture or poster on a wall or a scene outside a nearby window. If you've been scanning faraway scenery, shift your attention to something nearby. These easy actions provide a brief and vital rest for the most active eye muscles, prompting a healthy exchange of fluids in the eyes while delivering oxygen and other vital nutrients.

4. Laugh: Enjoy a quick dose of humor. One of the most common impediments to optimal metabolism and energy production is seriousness. No kidding![15]

Pushing nonstop affects mood. Because we're putting all our physical and mental energy into the task at hand, we miss out on the small pleasures and momentary wonders of life. Without these, we lose perspective.

Among people whom I consider star performers in life and work, one particular characteristic stands out: All of them know how to laugh. In fact, their sense of humor is "on" more than "off"—even when they're under extreme stress. It's one reason they're able to achieve so much with apparently little effort.[16]

You probably wouldn't expect a good joke to kick-start your Meta-Stat, but it can. We have much to learn about the precise nature of the process. We do know that every time a person has a hearty laugh, it triggers a cascade of biochemical events. Energy increases, brain wave activity changes, hormone production rebalances, and the heart responds positively.

During your strategic pause, notice or recall something that tickled your funny bone. Then laugh about it! If you're feeling too overburdened to muster your sense of humor, find someone who can help you do it. A friend or co-worker with a quick wit can bring a smile to your face, even when you feel you can't.

5. Find light: Use brightness to invigorate your senses. More than half of your body's sense receptors are clustered in your eyes.[17] They act as light harvesters, firing neurological impulses in a direct stream to the pineal gland and the higher centers of your brain. This process powerfully influences your biological sleep-wake cycles and, according to research, can produce invigorating antidepressant effects.[18]

The catch is, these sense receptors need stimuli in order to do their job.[19] Yet many of us struggle through our days in dim light.

During each strategic pause, take a few moments to "turn up the lights." Step to a window or click on extra lamp or two. Many people report a strong sense of calmness followed by a surge of energy when exposed to bright sunlight or extra indoor light, even at the intensity level of standard room lamps.[20]

6. Drink fluids: Get an energy boost from every sip. I discussed it at length in Chapter 8, but it bears repeating: Energy production and fat burning depend on hydration. In German studies, sipping a half-liter of water elevated metabolism by 30 percent for 90 minutes straight.[21] When you're fully hydrated, it enhances the physiological processes that release fatty acids from fat cells into the bloodstream, where they travel to muscles for use as energy.

According to some reports,[22] a decline in water consumption may cause an increase in fat deposits throughout the body. The opposite also is true: More water, fewer fat deposits. Adequate hydration has numerous other health benefits as well. It helps regulate body temperature; nourishes skin; and maintains soft, regular bowel movements. When you drink an adequate amount of fluids throughout the day, you enhance your resistance to infection by hydrating the mucous lining of the respiratory tract. Adequate fluid intake also prevents fatigue, urinary infections, kidney stones, high blood pressure, and even fluid retention.[23]

On the other hand, even slight dehydration—not enough to trigger thirst—can measurably diminish your energy. During every strategic pause, be sure to take a few sips of water or another fluid. (For a list of options, see page 82.) By sipping every 30 minutes during the day, you not only improve your overall health and resistance to disease, you also send a regular signal to your Meta-Stat to maintain your energy and alertness. And remember, an ice-cold beverage gives your metabolism a little extra kick.

Essential Breaks

It's an irony of modern life: Because we're constantly on the go, we think we should be getting fit and energized from all the activity. Instead, we're gaining weight and feeling exhausted. In desperation, we push ourselves even harder, using willpower to jam extra activity into our already hectic schedules. This may seem like the solution, but it never is.

Rather than doing more, we ought to be doing less. Introducing short breaks into your daily routine actually accelerates results. You accomplish more over the course of a day. And as a bonus, you boost energy production and fat burning.[24]

When you take longer, 2- to 5-minute breaks at midmorning and midafternoon, you experience natural, powerful biochemical "waves" that generate a continual stream of energy for up to 3 hours.[25] Skip even one of these breaks, and your Meta-Stat dials back.[26]

The essential break includes the following steps.

1. Get some breathing space.

2. Turn on muscle toning.

3. Grab a smart drink and an energizing snack.

4. Find a bit of inspiration.

1. Get some breathing space. By changing your mental pace, you immediately generate a measure of internal restoration and renewal.[27] For this to work, though, you need to disengage from your work—and perhaps even leave the area where you're working, if just for a little while.

"A brief period of time—even a few minutes—away from the normal influx of work and mental information will allow your brain to do some of the filing necessary to sharpen your memory," explains Michael D. Chafetz, PhD, a neuropsychologist and author of *Smart for Life*. "Anything that stops the normal flow and lets your brain redirect is worthwhile."[28]

2. Turn on muscle toning. A formal strength-training workout isn't enough to keep the Meta-Stat functioning optimally. Midmorning, lunchtime, and midafternoon are ideal times to use your muscles to send strong signals to your Meta-Stat to produce more energy and burn more fat.

When you stay active by toning your muscles at regular intervals throughout the day, your muscle cells are better able to burn fatty acids as fuel instead of releasing them back into the bloodstream, where they'd be transported into storage. In this way, toning exercises can help reduce your body's fat stores.

Similarly, fat-burning enzymes—the ones that serve as catalysts for metabolizing fat in muscle cells—function well only if they're called upon regularly.[29] Otherwise, they break down into their component amino acids. This is another way in which long stretches without frequent periods of muscle toning and other moderate activity shift the body's biochemistry toward energy drain and fat forming and away from energy gain and fat burning.

Research conducted at Harvard Medical School's Institute for Circadian Physiology suggests that every time you engage in muscle toning, *even for a minute*, you increase your energy and alertness.[30] So a minute here, a minute there gives you a metabolic boost.

As a bonus, every minute of muscle toning conditions the body and brain to better handle stress. It triggers biochemical processes such as the production of catecholamines, powerful neurotransmitters that enhance energy and responsiveness in stressful situations. Through muscle toning, catecholamines help the body become more resistant and resilient in the face of stress.[31] (For muscle-toning exercises you can do right now, see "Good Moves" on the opposite page.)

3. Grab a smart drink and an energizing snack. Every essential break should include both liquid and solid nourishment. As I mentioned earlier, mild but persistent dehydration can undermine your energy and blunt your fat-burning capacity. You can avoid this simply by keeping water or another no-calorie or very low calorie fluid within reach for a ready sip.

Keep a snack handy, too. Many Americans have given up snacking to help control their weight. It doesn't work. When you go for 4 or 5 hours without eating, it causes a decline in blood sugar, which actually stimulates appetite. Until you eat something, you may need a strong dose of willpower just to get out of your chair, much less do more strenuous physical activity. Low blood sugar contributes to fatigue and tension.[32] If your Meta-Stat were a meter, you'd see the needle going down, down, down.

On the other hand, eating between meals actually increases metabolism through a process that scientists call the thermic effect of food. (The word *thermic* means heat-producing, energy-boosting, calorie-burning.) It also prevents spikes in blood sugar that can trigger overeating.[33]

Research published in the *New England Journal of Medicine*[34] and the *American Journal of Clinical Nutrition*[35] confirms the benefits of divvying up your food intake so you're eating less in one sitting but are eating more often. The combination of moderate-size meals and between-meal snacks helps sustain metabolism, so you feel energized and alert (and you're burning fat, too).[36]

As the day wears on, what you eat takes on greater significance because metabolic activity gradually starts to decline. By mid- to late afternoon, the brain has a strong tendency to crave fatty, sugary foods to compensate for dipping energy levels.[37] This is when planning ahead can make a huge difference. Keep a selection of low-fat, lean protein, complex carbohydrate snacks readily available for your essential breaks. Some suggestions: an apple and a small handful of nuts; low-fat plain yogurt topped with a handful of dried blueberries; or whole grain crackers and a snack pack of tuna. (For more, see page 207).

You also might consider keeping a protein bar in your purse, briefcase, or backpack. Just be careful which kind you choose. Read the nutrition label to make sure it isn't a high-carb candy bar masquerad-

META-STAT STARTER

Good Moves

For on-the-spot muscle toning, try one—or more—of these exercises.

- Right now, grasp this book in your right hand and extend it to the side of your body. Slowly raise the book until it's at shoulder height, tensing the muscles in your hand, arm, and shoulder as you do. Maintaining this tension, slowly lower the book. Change hands and repeat.

- Sit in a chair and breathe smoothly. Tense your abdominal muscles and slowly bend forward into a seated crunch. Slowly return to an upright position.

- While seated, extend one leg in front of the chair. Tense the muscles and slowly rotate your foot at the ankle, clockwise and counterclockwise. Repeat with the other leg.

- For a variation, slowly raise the extended leg until it's straight in front of you, parallel to the floor. Maintaining tension in your leg muscles, slowly lower your foot to the floor. Repeat with the other leg.

- Sit with your feet squarely on the floor and your hands gripping the armrests or the seat of the chair. Slowly rise out of the chair, lifting your buttocks only slightly—about an inch above the seat. Maintaining tension in your lower back and leg muscles, slowly return to the starting position.

---

ing as a protein bar. It should be low to moderate in carbohydrates, with no sugar, fructose, or high-fructose corn syrup.

4. Find a bit of inspiration. On a trip to Ireland, I was out for a walk one evening when an elderly man stopped me to say hello. He asked me if I'd found my "bit of inspiration" here and there throughout the day. "You can't wait to have it all at once," he chided, with a glimmer of lifelong wisdom in his eyes.

Often since then, I've pondered his words. He was right: On a regular basis, we need a dash of inspiration—a thought or feeling that lifts us and drives us to be our best. As neuroscientists are discovering, the mind and heart are great generators of human energy.

So end each essential break by taking a few final moments to savor one of your dreams. Steal a glimpse into your future. Remember someone who had a great influence in shaping you as a person. Recall a genuinely supportive note or comment that you received. Or stop to gaze at a favorite photo of your loved ones, for whom your sustained energy may count the most of all.

RELEASING: TARGET THE TENSION

Contrary to conventional wisdom, tension involves not entire muscles but portions of them. Left unchecked, these so-called trigger points feed on each other. A little tension quickly becomes a lot. Before long, the processes that normally would fuel energy production and fat burning are diverted to address the tension and the corresponding poor circulation in the affected areas of the body.

Many people complain of stiffness and aches as they get older. Chances are these symptoms have nothing to do with aging. Instead, they probably result from chronic, unrelieved tension in the trigger points. According to experts, virtually any of your body's hundreds of muscles can develop trigger points.

Researchers have identified two types of trigger points: active and latent. The active ones can cause debilitating, sometimes incapacitating pain. Latent points cause stiffness and restrict movement, but in general, they are not painful except when pressure is applied to them.

In some cases, the symptoms of a trigger point occur somewhere other than the site of the point itself. For example, a trigger point in the shoulder muscles might contribute to headache or neck stiffness. This phenomenon is known as referred pain.

"Trigger points are extremely common and become a distressing part of nearly everyone's life at one time or another," write Janet G. Travell, MD, and David G. Simons, MD, coauthors of *Myofascial Pain and Dysfunction: The Trigger Point Manual*.[38] (*Myo-* means muscle; *-fascial* refs to a protective tissue that encases the muscles.) One study found latent trigger points in the shoulder muscles of 54 percent of women and 45 percent of men.[39] Another research team determined that people between ages 31 and 50 have the greatest number of trigger points.[40]

"Individuals of either sex and any age can develop trigger points," observe the authors. "It is our impression that the likelihood of developing pain-producing active trigger points increases with age to the most active, middle years. As activity becomes less strenuous in later years, individuals tend to exhibit chiefly the stiffness and restricted motion of latent trigger points."[41]

What causes trigger points? Injuries, certainly. All of us are familiar with the bumps, bruises, and strains that can cause lasting discomfort. But researchers have identified other, more subtle causes as well. These include poor posture, chronically tense muscles, fatigue from overwork, emotional distress, and lack of sleep.

Trigger points vary in irritability from hour to hour and day to day. But once formed, they tend to stay put unless you take steps to treat and release them. The reason is that while most other body tissues heal, muscle tissue adapts to pain. That is, you learn to guard your muscles by limiting their motion.

Beyond causing pain and stiffness, trigger points can restrict circulation and weaken the affected muscles. This can lead to dizziness and loss of coordination.

Self-Care for Trouble Spots

Many, or even most, trigger point problems respond to therapy, researchers say. The trouble is, few health professionals have received proper training to recognize trigger points, much less treat them. The total cost of this oversight "is enormous," according to one medical research team. "When patients mistakenly believe that they must 'live with' trigger point pain because they think it is due to arthritis or a pinched nerve that is inoperable, they restrict activity in order to avoid pain. Such patients must learn that the pain comes from muscles—not from nerve damage, and not from permanent arthritic changes in the bones. Most important, they must know it is responsive to treatment."[42]

Fortunately, in many cases you can learn to locate and relieve trigger

META-STAT STARTER

How to Find Trigger Points

Before you begin pressure therapy, you need to identify the location of your trigger points. When you do this, your muscles should be warm and relaxed. Otherwise, it's difficult to distinguish tense muscles—where trigger points usually occur—from adjoining slack muscles.

Remember, trigger points can affect any of the major muscle groups, including the back of the head, neck, and jaw; the shoulders, arms, hands, and upper back; and the lower back, hips, buttocks, legs, ankles, and feet. If you feel tight or uncomfortable in any of these areas, take a few moments to check for trigger points. It's easy to do. First locate any taut band or cord of muscle fibers. Then press or squeeze the muscle lightly to moderately until you locate the spot that produces maximum tenderness with minimum pressure. That's the trigger point.

In most areas of the body, you can press the muscle against underlying bone using your fingertips or thumb. To identify points in your back, you may need to recruit a partner. Or you can use a tennis ball for a quick diagnostic. Sitting in a firm, solid-backed chair, place the ball behind your back, then move around and press against the ball. It's a crude simulation of finger pressure, but it works.

With practice, you will notice when you're aggravating trigger points—when your muscles are becoming tense from poor posture or an uncomfortable sitting position, for example. Then you can take immediate action to relax the affected area by adjusting your posture and releasing tight muscles. If necessary, apply simple, direct pressure to the trigger points.

Note: For any sudden, severe, or persistent pain, seek medical attention right away.

---

point pain on your own, without medical intervention. My wife, Leslie, and I have used a variety of methods to release trigger points to promote better posture and more energy—literally, on the spot. Over the years, we have shared these techniques with our children. The results have been great.

One simple, drug-free technique to treat pain and other symptoms is a form of pressure-point therapy. Though it's known by many different names, I call it direct pressure therapy (DPT). Its principles have the support of medical and scientific research.[43]

The basic technique is quite simple. Once you have located a trigger point, apply pressure that is gentle enough to create only mild discomfort. Use just the pad of your index finger, reinforcing with the middle finger for extra pressure. Hold for 6 to 10 seconds, then release. Repeat the technique with other points as necessary.

If you're not certain of the precise location of a trigger point, you can use a spiral pattern of pressure to find it. Simply move in a small circle, pressing points as you go. You'll know you've landed on a trigger point when it feels more sensitive than the surrounding area, and it becomes even more sensitive as you press on it. Treat it by applying steady pressure for 6 to 10 seconds, then releasing.

Most trigger points respond well in 6 to 10 seconds. For those that don't, you can try a modified version of DPT that some professionals call direct compression.[44] It involves gradually increasing direct pressure on a trigger point over 30 to 60 seconds. With practice, and with increased awareness of your trigger point locations and tension-holding patterns, you'll be able to determine quite easily which points respond to DPT and which require direct compression.

To preserve the results of either technique, follow up with a few gentle range-of-motion exercises that target the affected area. Also, keep the area warm after treatment.[45]

As it turns out, small things like hidden trigger points can make a big difference in your energy level. Pay attention to what activates the trigger points in your body. Then whenever you notice the first signs of distress, deal with them on the spot. Also, be sure to seek out the cause. Otherwise, tension continues to build, and energy is harder and harder to find.

CHAPTER 13

▪ ▪ ▪

MSOn Switch #10
Stop the Stress Response

Through thousands of years of evolution, the human body has developed an exquisitely sensitive system to help cope with stress. It has been integral to our survival as a species. The Meta-Stat plays a central role in this system—always at the ready to stoke the metabolism for extra energy and fat burning, which the body may require when stressful situations arise.

The trouble is, the stress response wasn't meant to be "on" all the time. Yet that's exactly what's happening in modern life, as assorted stressors bombard us in the normal course of our daily routines. They trigger the release of brain chemicals and hormones that flood the body, setting in motion a cascade of biochemical changes that over time can deplete us—body, mind, and spirit. They also dial down the Meta-Stat.

> **Success Map Tip:**
> Each time you use an MSOn Minute to defuse stress and restore calm, note your energy level on the Daily Energy Wave.

Though we may not be able to control the circumstances that create stress, we can control our response to it. Some people view stress as a challenge to grow and develop. For others, stress becomes distress—increasing heart rate, blood pressure, muscle tension, fatigue, anxiety, and mental distraction. The body simply can't function under these conditions for an extended period. To switch off this response, we must learn first to recognize stress, then to stop it in its tracks—whether by confronting it, sidestepping it, or turning it into something positive.

MORE STRESS, MORE FAT

Each time you experience a stressful situation, your adrenal glands dump epinephrine and cortisol into the bloodstream. These so-called stress hormones prepare you to either take on the situation or to escape from it. Scientists refer to this as the fight-or-flight response.

As part of this response, the body taps its fat stores, releasing fat molecules into the bloodstream. From there the fat molecules travel to the muscles, which can burn fat for energy.[1] But given the nature of modern stressors—deadlines, traffic jams, family disputes—the muscles usually don't need the extra fuel. We're more likely to stew or sulk than to sprint from our troubles. So the fat molecules float around in the bloodstream with no place to go.

Before long, the brain sends out signals for the stress hormones to clean up the fat molecules, which the hormones do. Only instead of returning to the fat cells, most of the fat molecules end up in storage in one place: the abdominal area.[2] Excess abdominal fat is a known risk factor for a variety of health concerns, including heart disease, high blood pressure, and diabetes.[3]

Research from Yale University has shown that overweight women who carry most of their fat in the abdominal region produce more cortisol than those who don't. "We've been able to show that uncontrolled stress in rats not only increases their cortisol production but also seems to favor redistribution of fat to the abdominal region," confirms Marielle Rebuffe-Scrive, PhD, of the psychology department at Yale.[4]

In a separate study, researchers at Wake Forest University determined that stressed male monkeys had more intra-abdominal fat than their nonstressed counterparts.[5] This held true whether the monkeys were active or sedentary. In reviewing their findings, the research team concluded that chronic, stress-induced arousal is a determining factor in abdominal fat distribution.[6]

Defuse Stress in a Single Breath

Right now, take a long, slow, even breath. Hold it for a moment, then exhale, counting backward from 5 as you do. Imagine all the excess tension leaving your body along with the air.

Researchers report that even a single deep breath can ease stress and foster a sense of calm and control.[7] Whenever you notice signs of stress—such as a rapid heartbeat or increased muscle tension—you can restore and sustain relaxation simply by changing the way you're breathing.

In effect, the more stress you experience over the course of a day, the more likely you'll gain weight rather than lose it. What's more, research shows that stress feeds into habits that contribute to overweight and obesity[8]—such as making poor food choices (especially fatty and sugary foods, which you are more likely to crave when under stress[9]), overeating, and skipping workouts. You simply may not be as tuned in to the signals that normally would direct you toward healthy eating. According to some studies, stress can trigger the starvation response, a protective mechanism that inhibits the Meta-Stat and heightens fat making[10] as well as fat storage.[11]

Conversely, the less stress you hold on to, the greater your metabolic power may be.[12] That's because people who are anxious or angry metabolize fat more slowly than others. "Sitting on anger just doesn't work,"[13] observes psychologist Catherine Stoney, PhD, of Brown University. If you can find ways to overcome stress and negative emotions, your Meta-Stat will be self-correcting.

BECOME A STRESS HAWK

To maintain optimal Meta-Stat function, you need to manage stress. It's easier than it may seem. The key is for you to become a stress hawk—that is, to develop the necessary skills to not only detect stress but also to defuse it. Once you master the techniques, they'll become a catalyst to optimal fat burning and energy production, even in the most stressful circumstances.

The beauty of the stress busters in this chapter is their utter simplicity. You can use them virtually anytime, anywhere you need them. They require minimal time and effort, yet they deliver maximum results. And that's critical, according to stress management experts Ronald G. Nathan, PhD, Thomas E. Staats, PhD, and Paul J. Rosch, MD. "The stress response starts in seconds," they note. "Too many stressful minutes can lead to an exhausting day. Instant stress relief is important because it can keep stress—and distress—from accumulating and overwhelming you."[14]

Active Minutes: Move beyond Stress

Research from the University of Pennsylvania School of Medicine shows that physical activity has a direct effect on your ability to handle everyday stress.[15] When you're active, you are less likely to become emotionally upset in stressful situations. As a bonus, you bounce back more quickly, as your Meta-Stat settles into a pattern of modest ebbs and flows rather than severe spikes and dips.

Other research confirms that regular exercise reduces stress and improves mood.[16] In one study at Stanford University, researchers tracked the psychological effects of physical activity in adults ages 50 to 65.[17] Regardless of the activity or the setting (at home or in a group led by a fitness instructor), everyone who engaged in exercise showed reductions in stress and anxiety, with those who worked out most showing the greatest improvement.

Physical activity can have other, long-term benefits for stress management. In studies at the University of Nebraska, health psychologist Richard Dienstbier, PhD, found that regular exercise helps generate changes in the pituitary-adrenal-cortical "arousal system," enhancing the ability to handle stressful situations.[18]

Even brief bouts of muscle toning or cardiovascular exercise—a minute or two at a time throughout the day—train your body to release less cortisol under stress. So instead of storing fat, you keep burning it. In this way, physical activity helps "inoculate" you against the harmful health effects of stress.

Just be careful not to overdo. Studies suggest that while moderate

META-STAT STARTER

Keep a Stress Log

For the next week or so, write down all of the stressors you encounter. What sorts of situations consistently irritate or upset you? Which people? Pick one of the stressors and pay attention to it. How often does it arise? How does it make you feel?

Also make note of any techniques that help overcome these stressors. Pay attention to what works and what doesn't. In this way, you can shape your own arsenal of on-the-spot stress blockers.

physical activity boosts energy, more intense workouts may increase tension in some people. Both lift mood and improve appetite, however.[19]

So when you feel stress creeping up on you, take a short walk around the block. Or, if you have access to gym equipment, put in a brief session on the treadmill, stair climber, or stationary cycle. All will help remove fat from the bloodstream before it goes into storage. Plus, your metabolism will stay at a level where it's producing a steady supply of calm energy rather than an overabundance of tense energy.

Instant Detachment: Get the Monkey Off Your Back

Much of the stress we experience is not of our own making. Rather, it comes from those around us—their tension, their worries, their anger. And it sticks like glue. Unfortunately, you may not even recognize it for what it is or where it came from. You just feel it.

One of the cardinal rules of stress management is this: Understand and accept that you are not responsible for "fixing" everyone else's lives. It doesn't work, anyway! Even children need to do their own problem solving, albeit with some guidance from their parents. Likewise, adults must be willing to handle their own problems and pressures instead of foisting their burden on others.[20]

To withstand the effects of "shared" stress, you need to cultivate inner fitness. By that I mean you create a sanctuary within yourself, a place that's so serene and peaceful that little if anything can disturb you when you're there. With practice, you can retreat to this sanctuary—mentally, if not physically—as you need to.

Your first step is to train yourself to recognize when someone is about to unload his or her stress on you. For example, your antennae should go up when a person says something along the lines of "I don't mean to upset you, but . . . " or "You're not going to want to hear this, but. . . . "

Next, you need to ask yourself these two questions.

1. How fast can I let go? The goal here is to find a way to instantly dissolve the stress that tries to occupy your awareness or grab your heart. The quicker you detach, the more effectively you can interrupt the process before any momentum builds up and you get seriously tense. Remember, stress is fattening and fatiguing. It produces a spike in your metabolism, which results in an unhealthy jolt to your Meta-Stat. Hone your ability to move a half step back from the situation at hand, so you can assess it rather than immediately taking it to heart.

2. How calm can I be? To help answer this question, your task is to instantly create a feeling of deep relaxation. Keep breathing deeply as you release every ounce of unnecessary muscle tension. Concentrate on remaining calm yet alert. Physically remove yourself from the stressful situation if you need to. By detaching mentally and physically, you're able to deter the release of stress hormones.

Humor: Look on the Light Side

Compelling scientific evidence suggests that people who are quick to laugh—especially at themselves—are more energetic and better able to bounce back from stressful situations than those who are not.[21] They also are less likely to experience stress-induced binge eating and to avoid exercise.[22]

In truth, humor has very little to do with telling jokes. Rather, it's about perceiving the absurdities of everyday life and being able to poke fun at the small stuff. From hassles to heartaches to hard times, we benefit from taking ourselves more lightly even when we're facing serious circumstances.

To get the full benefits of humor, most of us could laugh a lot harder and more often than we usually do. Humorous thoughts and, in particular, mirthful laughter work their wonders by initially arousing and distracting the mind, then relaxing us and creating the perception of control in our lives.[23] Here are several ideas for lightening up.

See the humor in the everyday. The healthiest laughter happens naturally, as a response to ordinary events. Seek out the absurdities in what's going on around you and share them with others. Create stories around the funniest things you see or hear to spice up conversation with your partner or family at the end of the day.

Start a personal humor library. What makes you laugh? Whether it's cartoons, television comedies, joke encyclopedias, even letters from an old friend, strive to expand your collection. Leave room on your shelf for books that amuse you. Keep a collection of audiotapes and CDs to play on your morning commute. Pay attention to whatever harmless humor tickles your funny bone—and make a point of surrounding yourself with more of it.

When all else fails, ask "Is it worth dying for?" By slowing your Meta-Stat, an out-of-control stress response has an impact not just on your waistline but also on your general health. For years, researchers have known that mismanaged anger and hostility can raise the risk of high blood pressure and sudden cardiac death—that is, an unexpected fatal heart attack.[24] Some now see a possible link between feelings of anger or helplessness and certain forms of cancer.[25]

Robert S. Eliot, MD, author of *From Stress to Strength,*[26] recommends that during those times when nothing seems to be working, you might ask yourself, "Is it worth dying for?" The answer can bring an instant reframing of whatever situation faces you—and may make letting go of needless tension and anger much easier.

Instant Calming Sequence: Think First, Then Act

Your ability to handle everyday stressors—delays, disruptions, disappointments—is an important predictor not only of your personal effectiveness in meeting major challenges but also of your overall physical and psychological resilience.[27] Remember, if you don't nip stress in the bud, stress hormones can continue to linger in the bloodstream for many hours after the stressor has moved on.[28] With the ebb and flow in these hormones, the fluctuations in the Meta-Stat become more severe.

When you stay calm under stress, you're able to use your inner resources more wisely. As a result, you feel more in control of the situation at hand. One of my favorite techniques for switching off the body's stress response is the instant calming sequence (ICS), which I developed more than a decade ago. Because you perform it while fully alert, with your eyes open, you can use it discreetly in any number of circumstances.

Using the ICS at the onset of a stressful situation creates a sort of gap between the stimulus and your response. You can widen the gap to identify new solutions to the challenge at hand, concentrating on what is within your control rather than what isn't. You're able to think before you take action.

Learning the ICS requires practice, but with time, it will become second nature. The sequence consists of five steps.

1. Continue breathing.

2. Lighten your eyes.

3. Unlock your posture.

4. Acknowledge reality.

5. Mobilize your best.

1. Continue breathing. When we first encounter a stressor, most of us stop breathing for several seconds. This impedes the oxygen supply to the brain, which is very sensitive to even small reductions in oxygen.[29] The shortfall pushes you toward distress as you experience more intense emotions—anxiety, frustration, panic, anger.[30]

Make a point to continue breathing deeply and evenly. It doesn't matter whether you're inhaling or exhaling when you pick up your first cue of a possible stressor. Follow the inhalation or exhalation all the way through to the end, then continue the breathing cycle.

2. Lighten your eyes. The muscles in your face not only show your emotions, they also set your mood. Any tension in your brow or jaw, for example, will spread throughout your body.

At the onset of stress, ease the intensity in your eyes. By this I mean your gaze should be relaxed but awake and aware. Imagine the gaze of someone who is listening to music or enjoying a quiet moment in nature. At the same time, maintain a neutral facial expression—or, even better, relax into a smile. This may not be your instinctive reaction, but it's the right one. Just the change in your external expression can make a big difference in your internal response to a stressful situation.[31]

Positive tension in the facial muscles enhances blood flow to the brain. These muscles also transmit nerve impulses from the face and eyes to the limbic system, which governs your immediate reactions. Lightening the eyes and smiling, even slightly, changes your brain chemistry to support more positive emotions and more constructive actions.

3. Unlock your posture. Here's a little experiment for you. Stand in front of a full-length mirror and assume a slouched posture. Then say something. Does your voice sound natural? Or is it weak or strained? More than likely, it's the latter. Whenever you react to a stressful situation by slumping forward, you worsen any feelings of panic and helplessness.[32]

Now change to an upright, neutral stance. Begin talking again. Do you notice any difference?

Unlocking your posture is one of the easiest ways to overcome what's known as somatic retraction, a common, debilitating response to stress. Somatic retraction is a slightly slouching body position, complete with tightening or collapsing of the chest; rolling forward of the shoulders; and tensing of the neck, abdomen, and back. Merely thinking of a stressful situation can prompt your body to slip into this posture.

By changing your body position and standing upright, you send signals to those areas of the brain that are most likely to react quickly and positively. In this way, you're able to calm down more effectively.

4. Acknowledge reality. Far too often, we become entangled in bemoaning every challenge we face: "Not *another* problem! Why does this always happen to me?" This "woe is me" mindset can set off a biochemical wildfire that ultimately leaves you feeling like a victim, overwhelmed by anxiety and frustration.

A single moment of stress shouldn't disrupt an entire day. With the ICS, you can break this pattern.

Think about some of the mistakes that occur when you allow a molehill to turn into a mountain. One of the easiest ways to fall into an old, negative pattern is to subconsciously link a new problem to a previously stressful situation. If you find yourself saying "Not again!" you may be giving in to an old pattern.

In this step of the ICS, you take a moment to distinguish the current situation from past experiences by identifying its unique features. Pinpoint some ways in which it's different from anything you've dealt with before.[33] Likewise, if someone's behavior is the stressor, focus on what's different now compared with past scenarios. Pause for a split second to empathize. Did this person have a meeting with his or her boss? Did he or she have a long drive home?

By looking for uniqueness in every situation, you bypass the brain's innate, lightning-fast tendency to magnify negative presumptions about people and situations. As you separate the past from the present, you can consider specific solutions to the challenge at hand.

5. **Mobilize your best.** Rather than priming ourselves to go on the defensive against stress, a healthier response is to assume that every challenge presents an opportunity for growth. For this step, I recommend an affirmation: "What's happening is real, and I'm calling upon the best in myself right now," or "I am about to be the person I want to be—the best I can be."

Remember, the ICS is a natural, flowing sequence. You release it rather than forcing it. Practice it throughout the day, using different stress cues and increasingly vivid mental images to speed the ICS response.

If you struggle with any of the steps, practice them one at a time until they become comfortable. If you get partway into the ICS and feel yourself losing control, back up in the sequence and proceed more slowly. Remember, you are training your body and brain to activate the ICS at the first sign of stress or tension.

30-Second Stress Neutralizers

In addition to the above techniques, the following can prove very helpful to instantly turn off your body's stress response whenever you need to.

Learn to breathe through stress. Most of us assume that we take in plenty of oxygen. And we should, since we inhale and exhale about 20,000 times every day. But the fact is, most of us breathe just deeply enough to keep from falling over unconscious. Neuroscientists have reported that although we're staying alive, we aren't supplying our brains with an optimal amount of oxygen.[34]

Part of the problem is that vital lung capacity diminishes by about

5 percent with every decade of life. Mostly, that loss is attributable to a decline in the elasticity of lung tissue.[35] You can compensate for this physiological change, but it requires a combination of proper breathing technique, good posture, and regular aerobic exercise.

You can cultivate deep, or diaphragmatic, breathing simply by increasing your awareness of your breath. For example, sit or stand with proper posture—your head up, your neck long, your chin slightly in, your shoulders broad and loose, your back straight. Place your hands around the sides of your lower ribs, with your thumbs toward the back and your fingertips toward your navel. Slowly inhale through your nose. You should feel your lower ribs move out to the sides as your abdomen expands slightly forward and downward. As you finish inhaling, you should feel your chest expanding comfortably. Then slowly exhale through your mouth, feeling a wave of relaxation flood your abdomen, chest, throat, and face.

Touching the outside of your lower ribs establishes a tactile feedback loop with your brain. As you practice the exercise, you'll become increasingly aware of how you feel when you breathe properly. It will become automatic.

Concentrate on this breathing pattern whenever you feel stress creeping up on you. By breathing properly, you increase the amount of oxygen in the bloodstream, which can counteract the body's stress response.[36] This is how you restore a sense of calm.

Cue relaxation with a mind-escape word. You can use mind-escape words to instantly evoke a sense of calm and peace. Choose a word or short phrase that feels comfortable to you. It could be a sort of mental reminder, like "rest" or "time out." Or it could prompt a particular mental image, such as "beach" or "ocean."

How do you connect a word to an automatic relaxation response? It's simple.

1. Sit in a comfortable place, breathing slowly and deeply.

2. Give yourself permission to let go of all anxious thoughts for a few minutes.

3. Direct your attention to your breathing, focusing on the air as it gently passes in and out of your nostrils and chest.

Deeper Breathing, Healthier Blood

Blood flows constantly through the small capillaries in your lungs. As it does, it becomes enriched with the oxygen that is so vital to your health. But here's the surprising thing: You have vastly more blood flow in your lower lung region than in the upper lungs.[37] So if you're a shallow breather, you probably have underoxygenated blood. This can interfere with fat burning and energy production.[38]

With deep, diaphragmatic breathing, you deliver air to the middle and lower lungs, so oxygen is getting into the region where there's the most blood. No wonder it feels so energizing! Diaphragmatic breathing is of tremendous importance not only for managing stress but also for staying healthy.

4. Begin to notice the sensations of your body—the air or clothing on your skin, the weight of your shoulders and arms, the texture and support of the surface you're sitting on.

5. Vividly imagine yourself thinking, feeling, looking, sounding, and performing at your relaxed best in a specific past circumstance—an occasion where you felt really content with yourself and with life.

6. When the image is at its clearest, think of a word to attach to it. This becomes your mind-escape word.

As you practice, you can further refine your mental image. Are you indoors or out? Is it warm or cool, sunny or rainy? What do you see in all directions around you? What do you hear? Do you smell or taste anything? In what specific ways do you feel connected to nature and to the world around you? The sensations will become stronger as you recognize and acknowledge every aspect of the image.[39]

Whenever you encounter a stressful situation, you can think—or even say aloud—your mind-escape word. In an instant, you'll experience a profound sense of relaxation and control. You can also use your mind-escape word when you anticipate a stress response. For example, before picking up the phone to take an important call, you might think or say your word. You'll feel yourself becoming more calm and confident. It will carry through in your voice.

Shift your attention. According to Frank Ghinassi, PhD, instructor in psychiatry at Harvard Medical School, "Changing your thoughts can give you immediate control over how you respond to stress."[40] What runs through your mind in the initial moments of a stressful situation in large part determines the outcome.

If you were to look back at times when you felt tense or anxious, you probably could recognize how you might have chosen a more effective response had you remained calmer from the start. You would have been able to think more clearly, which might have redirected your course of action.

This is key to rapid stress relief—learning to evoke calm alertness at the onset of a stressful situation. You won't get caught up in impulsive thoughts and feelings that can skew your response. Instead, you're able to focus on what you can control rather than what you can't.

Tune out TV. A 13-year study involving more than 1,200 people and supported by the National Institutes of Mental Health concluded that watching television for long periods—over 2 hours at a stretch—generally worsens mood.[41] And a bad mood impairs your ability to handle stress. In fact, turning to TV to escape a stressful situation actually can backfire, as stress intensifies instead of easing up.

Another study suggests that a television habit could affect your metabolism as well. When researchers at Memphis State University monitored young girls who were watching a TV sitcom, they found that the girls' resting metabolic rates dropped as much as 16 percent below normal.[42] In other words, they burned fewer calories while watching TV than while just sitting.

Whether television has the same impact on adult metabolism remains to be seen. Still, it seems healthiest to limit your TV time. And when you do watch, try to remain active—even if you're just knitting or folding laundry.

Call someone. Taking a few moments to pick up the phone and call a friend or family member is just enough to pull back from a stressful situation. Of course, hearing a friendly, supportive voice at the other end can be tremendously calming as well.

More Easy Stress Stoppers

Whenever you have a spare minute or two, take advantage of these stress-fighting measures.

- Stretch your shoulders and loosen your neck and jaw.

- Take off your shoes and put up your feet.

- Sip some iced or hot tea, concentrating on its flavor.

- Close your eyes and vividly visualize one of your greatest personal blessings.

- Recall your most romantic moment.

- List seven things you've especially enjoyed in the past week or month. (Keep the list.)

- Enjoy nature up close—a flower in bloom, a tree moving in the breeze, sunshine on your face.

"If you look at factors that predict successful, permanent weight loss, social support ranks near the top of the list," says John Foreyt, PhD, coauthor of *Living without Dieting* and director of the Nutrition Research Clinic at Baylor College of Medicine. "I'd go so far as to say it is absolutely critical."[43]

Say a kind word—to yourself. The internal mental chatter known as self-talk goes on pretty much nonstop all day, every day. Unfortunately, it tends to emphasize negative messages over positive ones. And the nagging voices of the subconscious mind have considerable power to harm, especially when they trap you in old, unhealthy habits and behaviors.[44]

When self-talk runs amok, take a moment to stop the negative playback. Tune in to a more positive track—whether it's an affirmation of your good qualities or an acknowledgment of your successes. It becomes a lot easier to manage stress with the right mindset. You need to be on your own side!

CHAPTER 14

■   ■   ■

M S O n   S w i t c h   # 1 1

Ramp Up Your Evening Meta-Stat Setting

According to the body's internal clock—the one that has set itself over the course of human existence—metabolism tends to slow down from late afternoon into the evening. This is precisely the time of day when stress hits extra hard in the form of end-of-day deadlines, rush-hour traffic, after-work errands, and assorted other pressures. It's also when most of us sit down to the largest meal of the day. By then, we're too exhausted for much of anything beyond eating. We'd much prefer to adjourn to a favorite chair or sofa, where we can relax and unwind until bedtime.

In other words, the typical daily routine is taking a downturn just as the body's fat-making and fat-storing processes reach their peaks. Within a matter of hours, we can undo all that we've done to fuel our Meta-Stats throughout the day.

> *Success Map Tip:* Note your evening meals and snacks, fluid intake, and activities.

There is, I'm convinced, a better way.

Just as our metabolic patterns enter a transitional period in late afternoon, so, too, should we downshift from the intensity of the workday. How we approach this transition will determine how much energy we have—for ourselves and our families—through the evening hours.

With regular active minutes to maintain your Meta-Stat, you enhance your ability to maintain a consistent energy level through mid- to late afternoon. You're able to navigate what chronobiologists call the breaking point, the critical period between 3:30 or 4:00 P.M. and 6:00 or 6:30 P.M. when tension and tiredness surge.[1] Once you leave work, however, the inertia of habit sets in—and can drag down your Meta-Stat along with it. You may not feel compelled to be "on" anymore. Nevertheless, you're facing numerous crucial choices that could affect your Meta-Stat for better or worse. Now, even more so than earlier in the day, you need to take steps to boost your Meta-Stat and counteract its innate tendency to cut back its energy-producing, fat-burning power.

GET READY, GET SET FOR DAY'S END

Over the years, I've found a number of simple, practical ways to catch a late-day second wind. You may want to incorporate these strategies into your own postwork routine to help keep your Meta-Stat operating at a consistent level, even as your body clock sends messages to wind down.

Slow Down before Heading Home

After a long day on the job—whether your job is at home or a commute away—"heading home" requires a psychological shift that you must guide with care. It makes sense to allow for a brief "decompression period" before quitting time. Make a plan to devote the final minutes of your workday to the least challenging tasks, such as returning selected phone calls—meaning those that are most likely to be stress free—or straightening up your work area. By slowing your pace in this way, you send signals to your body and mind that will allow you to continue winding down as you head for home.

When you're ready to physically leave your workspace, you can reset your Meta-Stat with a simple visualization exercise. Imagine

META-STAT STARTER

Catch Some Afternoon Light

Look around you right now. How bright is it where you are? Can you see the sun? If so, how much sunlight is reaching the spot where you're reading this? How many indoor lights are on? One or two? How bright are they?

Researchers at Harvard Medical School have discovered that one of the quickest and certainly simplest ways to give a quick boost to the brain's alertness and your overall vigor is to turn up the light. While this is important for everyone, it's critical for those who live and work in northern climes, where there's so much light deprivation during winter months.

Tomorrow, as you wrap your workday, click on a few extra lights or—if possible—step outside for a minute or two of late-day sunlight. From either outdoor or indoor sources, light can lift your late-day energy and mood just when they are primed to fall.[2] It's a simple strategy that can help set your Meta-Stat for the rest of the evening.

yourself already at home, engaging in whatever brings relaxation and pleasure to your after-work hours—whether it's a good meal, the company of family, a brisk walk, or something else. The physical and mental release can be so powerful that in a matter of moments, you feel yourself downshifting into the slower rhythm of home life.[3] With this preparation, both the journey home and the arrival feel less hurried.

Sometime between ending your workday and arriving home, spend a few minutes gazing at something beautiful in nature—a flower, a stand of trees, cloud formations in the sky. I recommend doing this even if you work at home, to help yourself make the transition to being "at home." According to a University of Michigan study led by Rachel Kaplan, PhD, even brief exposure to a natural scene can be a potent antidote to mental fatigue, improving energy levels, mood, and overall health[4]—just what you need to keep your Meta-Stat on high.

Unwind before Unloading

Like my family, yours may be in the habit of spending the first several minutes after arriving home sharing your rendition of "Here's what happened to me today." We don't realize that simply dumping on each other can set the stage for fatigue-driven arguments.[5] What's missing is a brief buffer zone to shake off stress and tension and refocus on making the most of the evening, Meta-Stat-wise.[6]

My advice: Negotiate with your family members to establish a different kind of ritual in which each person expresses in a warm and caring way his or her pleasure to see everyone else. Limit your initial greetings to about 25 words or less, such as "What a hectic day! It's great to be home," or "Things were crazy at work, but I'm really glad to see you!" Then, without ignoring each other, simply postpone any conversation about the day's events until later on. Instead, use the time immediately after arriving home to take a shower, change your clothes, do a few stretches—whatever will give you a brief, relatively

---

META-STAT STARTER

Tone Your Muscles, Loosen Your Thoughts

Why do so many of us finish the workday slumped over, and then stay that way well into the evening? There's no reason for it. In fact, I'm amazed that we don't take a few extra moments to stretch our muscles. We'd feel so much better. By stretching our muscles, we stretch our minds. Likewise, lifting our posture can lift our mood.

Gentle physical movements—such as neck rotations, shoulder shrugs, wrist circles, torso turns, and knee bends—improve blood flow throughout the body, alleviating tension. Pause to ask yourself: Where do I feel tight or tense? Then respond by relaxing these areas—smoothly and slowly, following a circular or front-to-back, side-to-side pattern.

Pay attention to your posture, too, making sure to extend upward rather than slouch forward. It makes a big difference. You'll end your workday with a sense of a fresh start rather than a near collapse.

---

quiet interlude to put both your workday and your home life into proper perspective.

If you have young children at home, you and your partner might consider hiring a babysitter for a half hour or so after you arrive home. Then the two of you can set aside family obligations and go for a stroll, listen to music, or sit on the porch and sip a cup of tea—enjoying each other's company, but not hashing over the day's events. This way, both of you can raise your Meta-Stat a notch or two.

Lighten Up!

Previous MSOn Switches have discussed the Meta-Stat-boosting power of humor. An ample dose of humor is a great way to help your brain shift attention to the evening ahead.[7] There's a good chance you'll have at least one funny story to bring home from work and share with your family. If not, look for the levity in the moment as you go about your after-work routine.

In one study of 50 married couples, humor carried considerable weight in determining the happiness of the unions—as much as 70 percent of all the factors taken into consideration, according to the psychologists who ran the study.[8] Along the same lines, those in happy marriages are more likely to have the necessary skills to create and sustain relationships.

Having a sense of humor doesn't mean being able to deliver a punch line like a professional comedian. It's lightening up even when you feel the weight of the world on your shoulders—and, just as important, helping those around you do the same.

Move and Munch before Dinner

Even though you need to wind down after work, be careful not to come to a complete standstill. Staying active, even for a few minutes at a time, supplies a vital jolt to your Meta-Stat and helps prevent the late-day dip in energy that can lead to sitting around and dozing off. So, too, will eating a snack—preferably something low in fat but high in taste—before dinner.

A number of studies have shown that a predinner snack—with the right nutritional composition—stimulates the production of catecholamines.[9] These neurotransmitters, or messenger chemicals, stimulate the brain to sustain feelings of alertness and energy for up to 3 hours following the meal.

According to William Nagler, MD, a psychiatrist at the UCLA School of Medicine, evidence indicates that low blood sugar and simple hunger-related tension may contribute to negative emotions and arguments late in the day.[10] A predinner snack will head off hunger

---

META-STAT STARTER

Fat-Fighting Bites That Satisfy

It's very important for your predinner snack to be light and delicious. Steer clear of foods that rev up your body's fat-forming, fat-storing processes. Instead, choose foods that do exactly the opposite, easing appetite and delivering a quick surge of fat-burning, energy-boosting metabolism.

Your best bet is to choose a low-fat, high-fiber, lean protein appetizer. Among your options:

- Fresh vegetables with low-fat or fat-free cottage cheese or bean dip

- Whole grain crackers with organic peanut butter or almond butter

- A reduced-fat mozzarella cheese stick with half an apple

- A handful of nuts

- A small protein shake made with frozen fruit and fat-free milk or water

Interestingly, the high-fat, high-carbohydrate foods that most people reach for when they want a snack also tend to be the least satisfying. Rather than the traditional cheese-and-crackers appetizer, for example, you're better off with a cup of soup. In studies, soup reduced calorie intake at a subsequent meal by an extra 25 percent compared with cheese and crackers.

---

while balancing blood sugar levels. As a bonus, you're less likely to overeat during your meal and therefore less likely to store fat.

Reorder Your Evening

If your goal were to gain as much weight as possible as efficiently as possible—and to raise your risk of heart attack in the process[11]—you'd eat your biggest meal of the day in the evening and be sure to load it with fats and refined carbohydrates. As extra insurance, you'd sit and nibble on high-fat, high-carb treats until bedtime.

Of course, no one sets goals like these. Yet most Americans are on the fast track to meeting them because of their eating habits. Beyond expanding waistlines, eating large amounts of high-fat, high-refined-carbohydrate foods late in the day depletes energy and undermines mood—both of which can drive a wedge into family relationships.

The trouble is, the body seems to become more efficient at storing fat in the evening.[12] As mentioned earlier, this is in keeping with the body's internal clock, which slows metabolism starting in mid- to late afternoon—just as evolution has wired it to do. The good news is, you can outfox this natural downturn, delaying it until closer to your bedtime. As a result, you'll stabilize your Meta-Stat to keep burning fat rather than storing it. Plus, you'll feel more energized physically and more alert mentally.

To experience these benefits, you'll need to shake up your evening routine. Here's a six-step strategy that will help.

1. Eat early.

2. Make your meal light but great tasting.

3. Slow down your fork.

4. Start with a few bites of protein-rich food.

5. Save dessert for later.

6. Get up and get moving.

Let's look at each step in turn.

1. Eat early. Simply put, eating late is fattening. In fact, for every hour past 6:00 or 6:30 P.M., you should reduce your calorie intake by

100 calories simply because your body doesn't burn as many calories in the evening. So a 9 o'clock dinner should be about 300 calories lighter than a 6 o'clock dinner—more of a light snack than a meal. No kidding!

According to researchers, one reason the French have a much lower incidence of heart disease than Americans is that the French have their main meal earlier in the day and then follow it with physical activity.[13] They also adhere to the Gallic custom of eating more fruits, vegetables, and fiber-rich whole grains and less meat. But the timing of their main meal is critical.

In observing the daily patterns of French culture, R. Curtis Ellison, MD, a scientist at Boston University School of Medicine, found that most French families consume 57 percent of their daily calories before 2:00 P.M. Then they stay active—usually engaging in physical labor of one kind or another—until evening. By comparison, we Americans take in only 38 percent of our daily calories before 2:00 P.M. And we're much more likely to spend the rest of the day on sedentary tasks, such as watching television.

In a University of Minnesota study in which all the participants followed a 2,000-calorie-a-day diet,[14] those who consumed most of their calories early in the day lost weight—2.3 pounds per week, on average—while those who ate later gained weight. Besides fueling the body's fat-forming and fat-storing processes, eating late may spike blood sugar levels through breakfast and lunch the next day.[15] That is, if you even eat breakfast. Research shows that people who have dinner late in the evening are more likely to skip breakfast the following morning.[16]

For maximum benefit to your Meta-Stat, plan your evening meal as early as you can. Ideally, you should be eating before 5:30 or 6:00 P.M.; 6:30 or 7:00 P.M. is okay, at least on occasion. If you regularly eat after 7:00 P.M., make a point to trim your calorie intake and to build your meals around fresh fruits and vegetables, whole grains, and lean proteins.

On weekends, try eating your main meal at midday. Otherwise, aim for earlier than 5:30 or 6:00 P.M.

2. Make your meal light but great tasting. View your dinner not as a mountain climber's feast but as another in an ongoing series of vital

META-STAT STARTER

Keep It on the Record

Surveys show that most of us are amazingly unaware of what and how much we eat from 5:00 P.M. on into the evening. According to Albert F. Smith, PhD, a cognitive psychologist who studies memory at the State University of New York at Binghamton, everyone has trouble keeping track of their food intakes.[17] There is a solution, suggests Kelly D. Brownell, PhD, codirector of the Eating and Weight Disorders Clinic at Yale University.[18] "The first, and perhaps most important, lifestyle behavior is to keep records," he says.

A study published in the *Journal of the American Dietetic Association* confirms the link between recordkeeping and successful fat loss. Those who most accurately documented their food consumption lost the most weight, on average.[19]

signals to your Meta-Stat. Research shows that if you want to burn excess fat during the evening hours, you may need to rethink dinner in a way that's almost the exact opposite of what you're probably accustomed to. Specifically, you should limit your evening meal to about 600 calories—and make sure those calories come from satisfying, low-fat, complex carbohydrate and lean protein sources.

If this doesn't seem like much, remember that you'll be eating snacks before and after your evening meal as well, so you definitely won't go hungry. (You'll learn more in the presentation of the MSOn Eating Plan in Part 4.)

3. Slow down your fork. People who are overweight almost always eat too fast, racing right past their bodies' fullness signals. Savoring each bite not only saves calories, it also enhances enjoyment of the meal. Many cultures make an event of mealtime by focusing on the food and getting the most from every morsel. Eating this way helps balance the body's hormones, since they aren't overreacting to a massive intake of food in a relatively short timeframe. The slower pace also allows satiety—the "I'm full" signal—to kick in, with help from the hormone cholecystokinin (CCK).

4. Start with a few bites of protein-rich food. Think about it: One of the main reasons for eating dinner is to give you the energy to enjoy your evening. Yet the high-fat, high-carbohydrate fare that usually begins the evening meal has the opposite effect. From the first few bites of oil-drenched salad, Cheddar-smothered nachos, or butter-laden garlic bread, a full dose of dietary fat plunges you into an extended period of physical and mental fatigue.[20] We may perceive it as "relaxation," but in reality, our bodies are preparing for accelerated fat storage. What's more, all those fat calories can leave us feeling too tired for physical activity, including sex. (According to one recent nationwide survey, nearly half of all respondents who complained of being too tired for sex or "having a headache" were men![21])

Perhaps the simplest strategy for turning dinner into a more energizing experience is to forgo the high-fat appetizers and begin your meal with a lean protein. Unlike high-fat or high-carbohydrate foods, lean protein offers a real boost to your Meta-Stat. Among your lean protein picks:

- A small serving of bean or lentil salad

- Fat-free or low-fat plain yogurt

- Cottage cheese with several slices of fresh fruit

- A small glass of fat-free milk

META-STAT STARTER

Spice Up Your Meal

When Japanese researchers served soup seasoned with hot pepper to a group of volunteers, they found that the pepper diminished appetite, as well as fat intake. Hot-pepper pills had the same effect, which led the researchers to conclude that effect is brought on by a change in metabolism, not the heat sensation in the mouth.[22] These findings echo those of British researchers, who determined that the capsicum in hot peppers enhances fat burning.[23]

For a Satisfying Mealtime Experience

Once you sit down to your evening meal, follow these tips to eat less and enjoy more.

Set your meal to music. Studies suggest that people eat less and eat more slowly when they listen to soft, slow music. The kind of music is definitely important. "Rock-and-rollers practically inhale food,"[24] observes Maria Simonson, PhD, ScD, director of the Health, Weight, and Stress Program at Johns Hopkins University Medical Institutions. But if you choose slow, soothing music as the accompaniment, you are less likely to race through your meal or unconsciously reach for second helpings.

Volume also matters, according to research from the University of Ulster in northern Ireland. The louder the music, the higher the intake of food.[25] And, of course, the more you eat, the more your Meta-Stat fluctuates. Other studies report that up-tempo and/or loud music increases the rate of eating, the amount of food, and/or the preference for refined carbohydrates and fat.[26]

Slow your pace. According to researchers, people who are overweight are more likely to eat fast.[27] When you eat fast, you eat more—and the extra food is more likely to be stored as body fat.[28]

In a study[29] by Theresa Spiegel, PhD, and her colleagues at the University of Pennsylvania, those participants who extended their mealtimes by an average of 4 minutes burned more body fat than those who ate more quickly. In addition, the people who paused for 15 minutes before taking second helpings felt fuller and more satisfied without needing to eat any more. Do some experimenting to find the pace that works best for you.

You also might try a cup of soup, which research has shown to reduce cravings and total calorie intake.[30] In a study at Johns Hopkins University, soup fared much better than other foods in terms of its ability to satisfy. The favorite: tomato soup (make it with 1 percent or fat-free milk).

5. Save dessert for later. Clearly, one of the hurdles in retooling your evening meal is to keep from going over the 500- to 700-calorie maximum. If you exceed that, you're venturing into an overeating—and fat-forming—zone. One solution, of course, is to get up from the table without having dessert.

But what if you love dessert? Try postponing it instead. With a bit of practice, you'll become accustomed to saving this treat for later, mainly because you're giving your taste buds something to look forward to.

How much later? An hour and a half or 2 hours after dinner should be fine. By then you'll have gotten in a bit of physical activity (which I'll discuss next), and you'll be engaging in some enjoyable personal or family pursuit. In the meantime, your digestive system has processed and absorbed most of your meal's nutrients.

In general, stick with desserts that are low in fat and refined carbohydrates, moderate in complex carbohydrates (the fiber-rich kind), and higher in protein. Once a week, you can have any treat you wish, regardless of calories or fat. The catch: You can take just three bites of it. Chew each bite slowly, savoring every moment that it's in your mouth. As you'll discover, it's not the quantity that makes you feel good, it's the taste sensation. (If keeping leftovers of your favorite dessert is too much temptation, divide it into three-bite servings, put one serving in the refrigerator, and freeze the rest in a sealed container.)

All of the flavor-packed desserts beginning on page 361 meet the energy-boosting, fat-fighting requirements of the Meta-Stat program. You also might try the following options.

- Low-fat or fat-free plain cottage cheese with fresh fruit

- Low-fat or fat-free plain yogurt with fresh fruit

- Low-fat cheese (Jarlsberg lite Swiss, reduced-fat mozzarella, or reduced-fat Cheddar) with fresh fruit

- Fresh, unsweetened fruit

- Dried blueberries, strawberries, or cranberries

6. Get up and get moving. What you do—or don't do—in the 30 minutes after eating your evening meal sends powerful signals to your Meta-Stat and sets the stage for a night of restless wakefulness or deep sleep. In this crucial half hour, the last thing you want to do is park

yourself in front of the television, particularly for hours at a time. This posture promotes fat storage and fatigue rather than fat burning and a pleasant rush of positive energy.

On the other hand, exercising after eating could increase calorie burning by 30 to 50 percent[31] for a period of at least 3 hours following the meal. "Eating stimulates your sympathetic nervous system," explains Bryant A. Stamford, PhD, exercise physiologist and director of the Health Promotion Center at the University of Louisville. "Exercise after eating seems to give a double boost, so it burns more calories."[32]

This is consistent with the research of J. Mark Davis, PhD, and his colleagues in the department of exercise sciences at the University of South Carolina. They measured and compared energy expenditures among women who followed each of four programs—exercise only, meal only, exercise then meal, or meal then exercise—for 3-hour periods.[33] According to the study findings, the meal-then-exercise program increased energy expenditure by an average of 30 percent over the other programs. The researchers concluded that exercising after eating can lead to "exercise-induced postprandial thermogenesis"—in other words, fat burning.

As physiologist Melanie Roffers, PhD, puts it, "Exercising at this time of the day elevates the metabolic rate just as it's winding down."[34] Light evening activity also may alleviate late-night cravings for high-fat foods.[35] If a craving does hit, you may be better able to choose a non-fattening alternative and bypass the tendency to binge.[36]

To turn up your Meta-Stat a notch or two—and to kick fat-burning and energy production into high gear for the rest of the evening—I recommend the following routine.

- Excuse yourself from the table. Make a point *not* to sit and talk for more than 15 to 30 minutes after finishing your meal. Staying at the table is an invitation to munch on leftovers or to nibble at dessert. In fact, just the act of sitting ramps up fat storage and fatigue. Push back your chair and get up. Just standing boosts your energy level on the spot.

• Engage in 5 to 10 minutes of cardiovascular activity. It could be a formal workout, or it could be routine household chores like washing the dishes (by hand) and taking out the trash. According to some research, getting active right after supper—even at low intensity—provides a fat-burning metabolic boost that can last all night.

According to studies at the Cooper Institute for Aerobics Research in Dallas[37], the most effective postmeal cardiovascular activity may be slow, sustained walking. In fact—assuming the same duration, distance, and intensity—you may burn 15 percent more calories walking after a meal than you would walking on an empty stomach.[38] Other studies suggest that brief muscle toning or resistance training could have an even more potent metabolic effect.[39]

There are other immediate benefits as well. For example, walking can help dissipate harmful stress chemicals,[40] so you feel calmer and more resilient under pressure. In addition, a postmeal walk can measurably deepen sleep, as shown in the research of Peter Hauri, PhD, director of the Mayo Clinic Insomnia Program.[41]

• Perform some muscle-toning exercises. I've said it numerous times, but it bears repeating: Muscles rule the Meta-Stat. If you sit around for more than an hour, especially in the evening, your metabolism will slip into fat-storing, fatigue-producing mode. Use your postmeal time to squeeze in a series of easy muscle-toning moves, such as neck rotations, wrist rotations, and leg raises and extensions. (For complete lists of exercises, with instructions, see Part 3.) Whether your moves are overt or covert, the key is tone, tone, tone.

It's best to plan your postmeal activity for approximately the same time each evening because, according to researchers, you're more likely to keep doing it night after night if you consider it part of your routine. "Your body responds very nicely to habit," explains Frederick C. Hagerman, PhD, professor of biological sciences at Ohio University and physiological consultant to U.S. Olympic teams. "Do your best to keep your evening exercise scheduled at consistent times."[42]

WHAT'S YOUR PLEASURE?

One of my favorite pictures of Albert Einstein shows him at middle age, wearing a business suit and riding a bicycle. He is just rounding a street corner. From the photo, it's obvious that he wasn't especially adept as a cyclist. Nevertheless, he's smiling broadly, feeling the glide of the wheels and the wind in his face. He may have been going nowhere, but clearly, he was enjoying every moment of it.

Cycling was one of Einstein's customary early-evening enjoyments.

When was the last time you felt this way? I believe that such active moments, with built-in relaxation and fun, are what renewed and ignited Einstein's creative genius. We can, and should, learn from his example.

CHAPTER 15

M S O n   S w i t c h   # 1 2

Get Plenty of Good-Quality Rest

I t doesn't take a battery of medical tests to prove that you're tired. Your eyelids tell the story. If they're starting to droop, you know precisely what you need—and it probably involves a pillow and a mattress.

Of course, you can resort to a number of artificial methods—from a cup of caffeine-laden coffee to a splash of ice-cold water—to try to stay awake. But if you're sleep-deprived, there's only one real solution to your fatigue. It's spelled s-l-e-e-p.

Sleep has restorative powers. With the right amount of quality sleep, you'll be at your best, physically and mentally. That much may be obvious. But a good night's sleep has other, lesser-known benefits as well. For example, your hormones behave differently when you're well rested. Fat burning improves, too. And both have a direct impact on your Meta-Stat.

One study published in the *International Journal of Obesity* linked a good night's sleep with lower body fat in nearly 7,000 volunteer

> **Success Map Tip:**
> Pay special attention to your evening consumption of food and fluids and note your preparations for bedtime. Compare a Success Map after a night when you slept well to a night when you slept poorly. What were the differences in your routines?

participants.[1] Other research has confirmed the vital role of sleep in energy production and fat loss.[2]

The trouble is, most of us aren't getting the sleep our bodies require. This disrupts the natural renewal processes in millions of the body's cells. When you have "shallow sleep," you essentially turn nighttime into a fat-storing extravaganza. Studies by Eve Van Cauter, PhD, of the University of Chicago vividly demonstrate how a few nights of poor-quality or insufficient sleep significantly increase insulin resistance and fat storage.[3]

To ensure sound sleep, you need to turn on one final MSOn Switch at the end of the day. I'll reveal how a bit later in the chapter. First, let's delve a little deeper into the profound impact of sleep on your Meta-Stat.

THE CRITICAL HEALING PERIOD

It begins the moment you nod off. Thousands of crucial metabolic and thermogenic processes kick in, all designed to continue running while you're sound asleep. Nutrients and hormones revive your metabolism, which slows to what's known as your sleeping metabolic rate. Muscle fibers gain muscle tone, thereby increasing their metabolic capacity.[4] Circulation removes impurities from the body. All this occurs during the "critical healing period" from approximately midnight to 3:00 A.M.

Unfortunately, very few of us get enough sleep—or, more critically, enough *high-quality* sleep—for these processes to run as they should. In fact, nearly 7 of every 10 adult Americans fail to get enough high-quality sleep every single night.[5] Those who get less than 6 hours of sleep per night over six consecutive nights lose up to 30 percent of their insulin response. This makes fat gain much more likely.[6]

Chronic sleep deprivation affects health in other ways. For example, when you're tired, you're much more likely to fill up on high-fat, high–refined-carbohydrate foods in an attempt to feel more energized.[7] One small but provocative body of research has demonstrated that both laboratory animals and humans lacking in good-quality sleep not only end up with increased appetites, they're more likely to overindulge in high-fat foods.[8] These findings may prove important to weight-control efforts because "people eat more when they are tired," observes Donald Bliwise, PhD, director of the Sleep Disorders Center at Emory University Medical School.

In fact, according to Allan Rechtschaffen, PhD, director of the Sleep Research Laboratory at the University of Chicago, sleep-deprived people tend to increase their calorie consumption by more than 10 to 15 percent per day.[9] Just one night of sleep deprivation causes an increase in the hormone cortisol, which contributes to muscle atrophy as well as fat storage, according to studies at the National University of Singapore.[10]

Inadequate or poor-quality sleep has other hormonal effects, too. For example, researchers at the University of Chicago have found that partial sleep deprivation—an hour or two of lost sleep every few nights—alters the levels of leptin and ghrelin, hormones that regulate hunger and fat gain. Study participants showed a 24 percent increase in appetite, with cravings for sweets, salty foods such as nuts and chips, and starchy foods such as bread and pasta.[11]

At the National Institute of Mental Health, scientists who tracked nearly 500 adults over 13 years determined that those who gained the most fat had lost the most sleep.[12] And a study from Columbia University concluded that the rate of obesity is 23 percent higher among people who get just 6 hours of sleep per night, compared with those who average 7 to 8 hours per night.[13]

As nights of subpar sleep add up, your alertness goes down. As a result, you're more likely to inadvertently turn on a number of fat-making switches in the brain and body.[14]

SEVEN SECRETS TO SUPERLATIVE SHUTEYE

Some sleep researchers have suggested that we need an average of 12 hours of rest every night. The trouble with this thinking is, a long night of poor-quality sleep is worse than a shorter period of high-quality sleep. In fact, more recent studies indicate that people who sleep about 7 hours a night live the longest.[15]

META-STAT STARTER

Restore the Good to "Good Night"

Exactly how did you fall asleep last night and the night before? Were you sitting on the sofa watching TV? Reading? Paying bills? When you fall asleep with lights on, or in an awkward position, you sabotage the overall quality of your slumber.

Now look ahead to this evening. What simple change could you make that would ensure a good night's sleep?

Perhaps you could head to your bedroom 15 minutes earlier. Turn off the TV before the late-night news comes on. Take an extra minute to tense and then relax the muscles in your jaw, neck, shoulders, arms, hands, thighs, and feet before climbing into bed.

Even a small change in your sleep habits can make a big difference in your energy level. It can also help shift your metabolism from fat storage to fat burning and keep it there all through the night.

So how much sleep do you need? Enough for your body to adequately rest and recover. "Recovery ability pertains to the chemical reactions that are necessary for your body to produce efficient fat loss and muscle building," explains Ellington Darden, PhD, former director of research for Nautilus Sports/Medical Industries and author of numerous studies on fat-burning metabolism. "An optimal recovery ability is dependent on adequate deep rest."[16]

With this in mind, the following seven strategies can help improve your sleep quality and quantity starting tonight—and maximize sleep's potential as a fat-fighting, energy-restoring ally.[17]

1. Get warmed up 3 to 5 hours before bedtime. Deep sleep requires a warmup—literally. Research has shown that a brief period of post-dinner physical activity within 3 hours of bedtime can significantly improve sleep quality.

Numerous studies have established a connection between physical fitness and sleep quality.[18] It isn't just the exercise that's beneficial; it's also the corresponding rise in body temperature.[19] This passive body heating, as it's known, has been shown to measurably deepen sleep.[20]

"If you can increase your body temperature [with exercise, for example] about 3 to 6 hours before going to bed, the temperature will drop most as you are ready to go to sleep," explain Peter Hauri, PhD, director of the Mayo Clinic Insomnia Program, and Shirley Linde, PhD. "The biological 'trough' deepens, and sleep becomes deeper, with fewer awakenings."[21]

Passive body heating need not come from exercise, notes James A. Horne, PhD, a sleep scientist at Loughborough University in Great Britain. Dr. Horne has discovered a similar beneficial effect from taking a hot bath or shower within 3 hours of bedtime.[22]

2. Shed new light on the day. One of my mom's favorite stories is of President Teddy Roosevelt, who would take visitors out on the White House lawn each evening. There he would point to the stars, naming the various constellations. Even as his guests shivered in the cold, Roosevelt would continue roaming the grounds, looking in all directions to catch glimpses of the night sky. At last, he would turn to his guests and say, "There, now I feel small enough. Let's go get some sleep!"

Each of us needs to use a bit of our evening energy to gain proper perspective on the day's events and to regain our bearings before we fall asleep. The truth is, stress and sleep don't mix. For this same reason, you and your partner should make a pact to check your troubles— whether professional or personal—at the bedroom door. They prime you to stay awake. Over time, they "train" your body in what some researchers describe as a learned association with sleeplessness.[23]

Reserve your bedroom as a comfortable, relaxing haven for sleep or for a warm, loving sexual relationship. Nothing else.

3. Choose the right bed. This really matters. Poor-quality sleep often begins with a bed that over- or undersupports the body.

Take notice of what happens when you climb into bed. Do you feel instantly comfortable and relaxed? Does your bed support you? If not, consider how you might change it to make it more inviting. For example, you might purchase a top cushion that fits between the mattress and sheets. Many department stores and online retailers carry them. You'd be surprised at what a difference they make.

Or perhaps you need to invest in a new bed. There are more options than ever, so be sure to shop around to find the one that's best for you.

4. Be cool. A cool bedroom temperature promotes the decline in body temperature that's vital to deep sleep. "Your body will burn significantly more calories each night if [your room is] cool," Dr. Darden explains. "I'm convinced that most people bury themselves under too many covers. . . . This prevents their normal thermostats from kicking in and supplying natural body heat (and burning off fat to provide that heat).

"If you tend to sleep with too many covers, try to eliminate one or two," Dr. Darden advises. "Wean yourself from cranking up the temperature on an electric blanket or using flannel sheets during the winter months. During the summer, try sleeping with only a single sheet on top of you. Soon you'll be burning several hundred more calories each night."[24]

By the way, warm feet are fine. If you get cold feet, wear warm socks to bed rather than piling on the covers. Swiss researchers found that the combination of a cool room temperature and a cool body with warm feet helped speed the onset of sleep.[25]

5. Avoid going to bed hungry. Interestingly, some scientific evidence suggests that crash dieting and low-calorie diets disrupt body temperature. If you're on such a diet, you may be jeopardizing the all-important restorative phase of sleep known as slow-wave sleep, according to a study in the *American Journal of Clinical Nutrition.*[26]

In terms of your metabolism, not eating anything before bedtime may be nearly as bad as stuffing yourself with high-fat snacks. The combination of an early dinner and no midevening snack may cause a drop in blood sugar that interferes with the sleep process. On the other hand, delaying dessert and eating it or another light snack between 8:00 and 9:00 P.M., as I recommend, increases your chances of truly restful slumber.

In general, it's a good idea to avoid coffee, tea, and other caffeinated beverages within 4 or 5 hours of bedtime. The same rule applies for chocolate, which contains more than enough tyramine to impair sleep. An amino acid, tyramine triggers the release of norepinephrine, a brain stimulant that can keep you awake.[27]

Beyond that, feel free to experiment to find out how various foods influence the quality of your sleep. Here are a few options to start.

Cottage cheese. Try a half cup of low-fat cottage cheese, which is one of the best sources of casein. This protein reduces nighttime catabolism, the process by which the body breaks down muscle tissue instead of burning excess fat during sleep cycles.[28] Eating dairy products before bedtime may help retain healthy muscle tissue as well as naturally increase your daytime metabolism.

Warm milk or cool yogurt. The American Society for Nutritional Sciences recently published a series of articles in the *Journal of Nutrition* discussing the various potential benefits of dairy products for fat loss.[29] The results are promising. If you opt for yogurt, choose a low-carbohydrate variety. This way, you won't get a huge dose of simple sugars that throw fat storage into high gear.

Turkey. Turkey contains tryptophan, the amino acid that converts to the sleep-enhancing neurotransmitter serotonin. A few bites of turkey may bring about deeper, more restful slumber.

6. Sleep deeper—with no clock in sight. It's not enough to simply reach a level of deep, metabolism-enhancing sleep. You need to sustain it through the night. According to research from the Mayo Clinic Sleep Disorders Center, perhaps the simplest strategy to ensure a good night's sleep is to hide your clock. "For most people, the bedroom should be a time-free environment," Dr. Hauri says. "Set the alarm if you must, but put the clock where it can be heard and not seen. Then you won't wake up again and again during the night and keep looking at the clock. People sleep better without time pressure."[30]

7. Rise and shine at the same time every morning. One widely celebrated American habit is sleeping in on weekends. Unfortunately, it confuses the body's internal clock, creating a jet lag–like sleep disturbance known as free-running.[31] When free-running sets in, it tends to lower your energy rather than raise it. Beyond leaving you feeling worn out and less alert, too much sleep can impair your ability to doze off the next night.[32]

Even if your night's sleep has been poor or cut short, you still should get up at about the same time as usual. This helps keep your internal clock in sync through all seven days of the week.[33]

If you do decide to sleep in, it's a good idea to limit your extra time in bed to an hour at most. When you awaken, give yourself a minute or two to allow your body to gradually adjust. Lie in bed, blink your eyes, move your arms and legs. Then open the curtains to expose yourself to daylight as soon as you can. Even better, start your day by walking in the sunlight or sitting near a bright window. These actions help stabilize your body's sleep-wake rhythm.[34] They also have a significant influence on your energy and performance all day long.

PART

The MSOn Workout

THREE

Along with the MSOn Eating Plan in Part 4, the MSOn Workout provides the foundation for the Meta-Stat program. The workout requires a bit more time and effort than the MSOn switches, though it should easily fit into your daily routine. On any given day, you'll spend no more than 20 minutes on "concentrated" exercise.

The MSOn Workout has five components.

- 20 minutes of aerobic activity 3 days a week
- Muscle tone-ups any time throughout each day
- Core strength training (abs and legs) twice a week
- Upper-body strength training (chest, back, shoulders, and arms) twice a week
- Balance and flexibility 4 days a week

Collectively, these support optimal Meta-Stat function. They also enhance the effectiveness of the MSOn Switches, so your body is burning fat and generating energy around the clock.

You can track your workout sessions using the Meta-Stat Success Map on page 246. Remember, too, to find ways to elevate your activity level throughout the day, as discussed in Chapter 5. These brief bouts of movement remind your body how it feels when it's active, so concentrated exercise comes naturally. In effect, you're reacquainting your body with its evolutionary tendency to move. And that's good for energy and fat loss.

(*Note:* If you have a preexisting medical condition, or if you've been sedentary, please check with your doctor before beginning any exercise program.)

CHAPTER 16

■ ■ ■

A Cardio Kick for Your
Meta-Stat

If you walk, jog, bicycle, or swim, you're engaging in an aerobic activity. This form of exercise is terrific for cardiovascular function. While it doesn't build muscle, it does burn calories and therefore fat. That's why it's so important to your Meta-Stat.

I recommend aiming for at least 20 minutes of sustained aerobic activity at least 3 days a week. To qualify as aerobic, an activity should increase your heart and respiration rates. A leisurely lunchtime stroll might provide a much-needed relaxation break, and it certainly will count toward your day's "active minutes." But it won't stimulate your Meta-Stat as a brisk walk would.

CARDIO 5 × 10S FOR GET-UP-AND-GO POWER

Canadian researchers report that intervals of high-intensity physical activity are necessary to burn body fat. In fact, their findings suggest that spurts of intense exercise are nearly *900 percent* more effective than the slow-and-steady approach in reducing fat.[1]

You can experience the difference yourself, using aerobic exercise equipment such as a stationary cycle, stairclimber, elliptical stepper, or treadmill. First, warm up by going at about half-speed, or 50 percent of your perceived maximum effort, for at least 3 minutes. After that, begin a sequence where you go close to all out for 5 seconds, then slow to your warmup speed for 10 seconds, then follow with another

Local Motion

Right now, you can experience for yourself the energizing effect of active minutes. The following exercise sequence produces immediate rewards, though it requires only minimal effort.

Find a flight of stairs where you can smoothly and steadily walk up and down a total of four times. Hold on to the handrail, if necessary. In the absence of stairs, head outside and walk the length of a block—up and back—twice. Make sure your stride is brisk and smooth.

Though not as intense as a full aerobic workout, either option will increase your metabolism as well as improve your circulation and oxygen intake. That's what you need to activate your Meta-Stat.

5-second spurt near maximum. Repeat the fast-slow-fast cycle as many times as you can, up to a maximum of about 10 minutes. Once you have a sense of the timeframe, you can count to yourself instead of watching a clock. Finish with a cooldown, gradually slowing your pace for several minutes or more.

This 5 × 10 pattern is easy to track and parallels the ideal aerobic formula identified by a team of Australian researchers. They found that adults who engage in 6 seconds of intense aerobic activity followed by 9 seconds at warmup speed burned 300 percent more fat than those who went all out for 24 seconds followed by 36 seconds at warmup speed.

I suggest doing the 5 × 10 workout three times a week to start. Over time, you can add intervals until you're exercising for a total of 20 minutes, including a 5-minute warmup and a 5-minute cooldown.

With the 5 × 10s, you take your Meta-Stat to a whole new level. Your metabolism improves, as does your energy. Don't be surprised if you feel more alert and alive after this workout.

GET MORE OUT OF EVERY CARDIO MINUTE

Research is confirming that various types of aerobic exercise equipment can significantly boost your Meta-Stat. It also provides an edge, in the sense that you'll burn more fat and produce more energy than you would without equipment. But just as with strength training, proper form and technique are essential. Otherwise, you may not be getting an optimal workout—or, worse, you could increase your risk of injury. Here's what you need to know.

Treadmill. With the treadmill, the more intense and smooth the workout, the less time it will take and the better your results will be. Hold your head level. Too much bobbing is tiring and hampers results. The same is true for a pounding, jarring stride. When you walk or run, you should feel almost as though you're floating. Avoid too many long, flat walks or runs, instead varying speeds and inclines. You'll rev up fat burning this way—and the effects will last throughout the day. Start with a 1 or 2 percent incline and gradually work up to a 10 percent incline over the course of several weeks.

Stairclimber. You'll get the best results from a stairclimber, in terms of burning fat and toning muscle, if you work out at a slow pace but with greater resistance. Avoid stiffly holding the handrails; it diminishes energy production while elevating tension and fatigue. Instead, rest your hands on the rails only when you need to for balance. Your body should be upright and leaning slightly forward as you climb, much as it is when you're navigating an actual flight of stairs.

Elliptical trainer. Unlike the treadmill, the goal with the elliptical trainer is *not* to float. The biggest time waster and results blocker is too little resistance. You don't want your own momentum moving you forward. You should feel as though you're smoothly and forcefully pushing down on each stride, staying balanced and relaxed as you go. Try doing intervals, going all out for 90 seconds, then following with a recovery period of 2 or 3 minutes.

Stationary cycle. Before beginning your workout, take a moment to set the seat at exactly the right height. It must fit your leg length and your most comfortable stride, in which your leg movement feels strong and smooth as you pedal. If the seat is too low, pedaling will exhaust your legs and potentially injure your knees. Too high, and it will strain your hips as they rock from side to side—very inefficient form that hampers results.

CHAPTER 17

Anytime Muscle Tone-Ups

Consider this chapter your primer for on-the-spot muscle toning. You'll learn a series of simple exercises, each of which sends signals to your Meta-Stat to step up your metabolism for fat burning and energy production. The remainder of the MSOn Workout will present other, more formal resistance-training options, but activating the Meta-Stat begins here!

Even with simple movements like these, you can push your muscles a bit harder each time. I always pay attention to my intensity, and I won't give myself full credit for my workout unless I work just a little harder than before. I recommend that you set the same criteria for yourself. If you don't, you're likely to hit a plateau—and eventually, you may even notice declines in muscle tone and strength.

Before I get too far into a discussion of the muscle tone-ups, let's look more closely at the importance of muscle and resistance training to optimal Meta-Stat function.

MUSCLE MATTERS

Your body has 684 muscles, each one responsive to strengthening and toning. Every day—in fact, every waking hour—your muscles get a little stronger or a little weaker. None of them stays the same.

Unfortunately, more and more people are losing muscle tone rather than gaining it. By age 74, nearly half of all men and two-thirds of all women can't lift a gallon of milk, which weighs just 8 pounds.[1] That's a shame, because muscle is the body's primary fat burner and energy booster.

Not that muscle naturally begins to atrophy after a certain age. In fact, in an ideal world, no one would lose a single muscle fiber ever. But with muscle, the adage "use it or lose it" certainly applies. You need to work it in order to keep it in peak condition for optimal metabolic performance.

Muscle is highly efficient at burning calories for energy—far more efficient than fat. For each pound of muscle, you automatically use an extra 75 calories a day—and that's just to maintain your body's normal processes. By comparison, a pound of fat uses just 2 calories a day. Put another way, muscle is 37½ times more metabolically active than fat.

Research suggests that muscle is responsible for 50 to 90 percent of the body's calorie-burning capacity—even during sleep.[2] "To effectively wage war against body fat, you need to be a good calorie-burning machine 24 hours a day," explains Bryant A. Stamford, PhD, exercise physiologist and director of the Health Promotion Center at the University of Louisville. "Having adequate muscle tissue is the only way to do that."[3]

META-STAT STARTER

Get a Better Grip on Life

There's no time like the present to start preserving and strengthening your muscles. Think for a moment: Which major muscle groups do you use every day? Your abs? Back? Thighs? Arms? Shoulders?

This book will double nicely as a resistance device to work your shoulder muscles. Hold it in your right hand, with your arm at your side. Without bending your elbow, slowly raise the book out to the side at shoulder height, then slowly lower it. Repeat several times with your right arm, then switch to your left.

By strengthening and toning your muscles, you raise your resting metabolic rate,[4] the one that keeps your body running smoothly even when you're sedentary. Research from the University of Wisconsin–La Crosse has shown that muscle-toning activity can boost metabolism and fat burning for a full 2 days after a workout. It works in part by raising muscle temperature, which triggers the release of uncoupling proteins, chemicals that elevate metabolic rate.[5]

In the past, many experts did not view muscle toning as an effective means of burning calories. They advised people who wanted to lose weight to engage in aerobic activity—walking, running, or cycling—rather than resistance exercise. Recent research from the University of Colorado shows that 70 minutes of muscle toning burns as many calories during the subsequent 24-hour period as running for 50 minutes at 70 percent of perceived maximum effort.[6] Strong, well-toned muscles also help maintain healthy circulation, which ensures delivery of oxygen and vital nutrients to the farthest reaches of your body, which needs them to melt away stubborn layers of body fat.[7]

YOUR ANTIAGING DEVICE

Even if you've neglected muscle toning over the years, you can make up for lost time. It's never too late to get stronger and stay stronger—and to raise your Meta-Stat setting as you do. After age 40, resistance exercises may be most effective for building muscle and preventing weight gain, according to research from William Evans, PhD, director of the Nutrition, Metabolism, and Exercise Laboratory at the Univeristy of Arkansas for Medical Sciences.[8]

"There's a myth that we lose the ability to respond to exercise as we age, that we can't get stronger or make our muscles bigger," observes Dr. Evans, former director of the Human Physiology Laboratory at the Jean Mayer USDA Human Nutrition Research Center on Aging at Tufts University. "That's not true. We can make 65-year-olds stronger than they've ever been in their lives. We can make a 90-year-old stronger than a 50-year-old. Our oldest exerciser is 100 years old. We can triple muscle strength in old people."[9]

According to studies published in the *Journal of the American*

Medical Association,[10] few of us should lose much if any muscle tone before age 90. But if you're like most sedentary adults, you began losing muscle—up to a pound a year—in your midtwenties! Even if you're physically active, you may have experienced a decline in your lean muscle mass, especially if you build your workouts around aerobic activities such as walking, jogging, and cycling. These types of activities are great for cardiovascular fitness, but they aren't the best for muscle tone.

In one study involving 72 men and women, conducted by Wayne L. Westcott, PhD, consultant to the YMCA of the United States, the American Council on Exercise, and the National Academy of Sports Medicine, those who engaged in aerobic-only workouts lost an average of 3 pounds of fat *plus* ½ pound of muscle over the course of 8 weeks.[11] In the group that combined aerobic activity with resistance training, people lost an average of 10 pounds of fat while gaining 2 pounds of muscle. Several follow-up studies produced similar results.[12]

When you lose muscle, it lowers your resting metabolic rate. As a result, your body needs fewer calories to function. Any excess calories, especially those from dietary fat, end up as body fat.

The good news is, even if you're showing signs of muscle atrophy, you can start reversing the process within a few weeks by performing

---

META-STAT STARTER

Get Psyched to Succeed . . . Anywhere, Anytime

Press the fingertips of your left hand against your right upper arm as you tense your arm muscles. Next, place your fingertips against your abdomen as you tense your ab muscles. Do you feel firm, toned muscles in these areas? Or do you detect some degree of looseness and flab?

Strong, taut muscles not only sustain metabolism, they also create a fit, trim appearance. But you need to be proactive about preventing muscle atrophy, primarily through resistance training. Otherwise, muscle fibers will waste away, and you'll pay the price in low metabolism—not to mention unattractive sagging.[13]

---

simple toning exercises. As you regain muscle strength and tone, you'll notice improvements in your energy level and your fat-burning capacity.

The key is resistance training, which is really muscle strengthening. With resistance training, you not only increase energy and metabolism, you also burn more fat, especially in the abdominal area. And the effects are relatively long term. In fact, with rather short but intense bouts of resistance training, you can measurably increase your metabolism for 2 *full days* following a workout.[14]

Research suggests that women, including older women, get even better results than men from resistance training.[15] Which brings us to an important point: Muscle toning is just as important for women as for men, according to Barbara Drinkwater, PhD, past president of the American College of Sports Medicine.[16] One recent study, published in the *Archives of Internal Medicine*, found that resistance exercises reduced "bad" LDL cholesterol and strengthened bones in premenopausal women.[17]

THREE KEYS TO YOUR MUSCLE-TONING SUCCESS

For both genders, the basic principle of resistance training is simple: Stress your muscles by making them work against resistance, and they'll grow stronger to meet the challenge. You can stress your muscles in various ways. For the MSOn Workout, I recommend a combination of brief, on-the-spot exercises and more comprehensive resistance-training sessions. You'll get the best results by adhering to these three principles.

1. Create a high intensity of muscle load.

2. Progressively increase the intensity from day to day.

3. Engage your muscles throughout the day, not just in formal workouts.

Perhaps what most distinguishes the MSOn Workout from other resistance-training regimens is that it asks you to shift your focus from total number of repetitions to each movement within each exercise.

Slow Doesn't Equal Success

Lately there has been lots of talk about superslow lifting improving the results of resistance training. Lifting this way produces really long workouts, but not much else.

At the University of Alabama, researchers monitored two groups through a 29-minute strengthening workout. One group performed each exercise by counting 5 seconds for exertion, then 10 seconds for release. The other cycled between 1 second for exertion and 2 seconds for release. The "fast" lifters burned 71 percent more calories and lifted 250 percent more weight than the "slow" lifters.

A simple rule for better results: Move through the exertion phase as smoothly and quickly as possible, maintaining good posture and correct form. Then switch for the release phase, moving slowly and with greater control.

The more muscle tension you generate, the more strength you will build and the higher your Meta-Stat will naturally go. In this way, you'll get far better results in far less time. Research proves that even brief spurts of intense activity elevate post-workout metabolism for more than moderate activity.[18]

For a quick demonstration, make a fist with one hand. Squeeze tighter and tighter, generating all the tension you can. You will feel it flowing from your fist up your arm and into your shoulder, chest, and back. During any exercise, you can significantly enhance its effectiveness by creating tension instead of just holding on.

Building muscle strength and tone does require regular incremental increases in resistance. There's just no way to keep doing the same exercise at the same level of resistance without reaching a point of diminishing returns. You need to find the maximum level of resistance that you can handle, and then gradually work past it. Add extra weight or resistance, intensify the tension, dig deep for concentration. Notice how your muscle fibers respond.

As you challenge yourself in your workout, remember that you're learning more about your own untapped potential. In the process, you're enhancing your body's natural fat-burning, energy-boosting power.

META-STAT STARTER

Practice Peak Focus

Concentrate all of your attention on a single muscle—say, your biceps. Flex your arm and increase the tension in the muscle fibers. With your opposite hand, touch your muscle as you hold the tension. This provides tactile feedback. With touch, you form a connection between the brain and the muscle. The combination of movement and feedback can significantly improve the results of any exercise.[19]

This demonstrates the power of peak focus. When you can harness that power and direct it into your life, you not only improve muscle strength and tone, you can apply it in myriad other ways as well.

For the muscle tone-ups, I recommend combining peak focus with peak intensity. Intensity is a measure of your ability to harness your attention and put the spotlight of action directly onto the right muscles. This is key to muscle toning, especially for the abs and lower back.

Forget aiming for hundreds of repetitions. Perform a dozen repetitions with peak focus and peak intensity, and you're done.

STRENGTH TRAINING ON THE SPOT

Like many other people, you might assume that resistance training requires high-tech equipment and endless hours in the gym. The truth is, it doesn't. If you select a core group of exercises and then practice each one with peak resistance and smooth, well-controlled movements, you will quickly feel and see the results.

The beauty of the muscle tone-ups is that you can perform them almost anytime, anywhere. They're perfect for turning spare time into active minutes. For example, you could perform the toe raises (see page 175) while standing in line at the bank or post office. All you're doing is rising up on the balls of your feet, then lowering your heels to the floor. Anyone standing nearby probably wouldn't notice what you're doing, yet you're creating enough of a muscle load to produce results.

In general, I tend to vary my muscle tone-ups throughout the day, according to the muscle groups they involve. If I'm sitting at my desk, I can do exercises that target my neck, shoulders, forearms, hands, thighs, and lower legs. If I'm standing in the kitchen, I hang on to the countertop for modified knee bends or toe raises. A minute or two of muscle toning here and there throughout the day adds up.

Dynamic Resistance and Dynamic Visualized Tension

Simply moving your muscles through their full range of motion while maintaining maximum tension is enough to stimulate muscle fiber growth and therefore metabolic rate. You can enhance this effect through dynamic resistance (DR) and dynamic visualized tension (DVT), techniques that call for targeted movement with or without mental concentration.

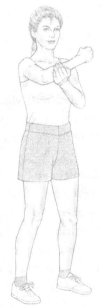

In dynamic resistance exercises, one muscle group provides resistance for another while allowing for a full range of motion. As an example, do a lateral raise with DR. Bend your right arm at the elbow, then use your left hand to grip the elbow from behind. Tense both arms as you slowly raise your right elbow, as shown, maintaining resistance with your left hand. It isn't quite enough resistance to stop the motion of the right arm, but almost. Repeat with the left arm, using the right hand to provide resistance.

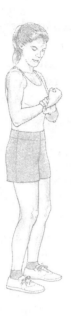

Next try a biceps curl with DR. Make your right hand into a fist, with the palm facing upward. Grasp your right wrist with your left hand. With maximum tension in both arms, slowly bend your right elbow so that your fist moves toward your shoulder. Next, place your left hand under your right wrist to provide resistance as you slowly lower your right arm to the starting position. Repeat with your left arm.

In dynamic visualized tension exercises, you focus your full attention on the muscle group that you're working, maintaining slow range of motion and maximum tension. Again, let's use the biceps curl as an example.

Do a curl with your right hand, raising your fist toward your right shoulder and then lowering. Repeat the exercise—this time very slowly, concentrating on the movement with laserlike precision. Think about awakening every muscle fiber in your right arm. Maintain the tension as you slowly lower your arm to the starting position. Repeat with your left arm.

You can apply DR and DVT to virtually any exercise, including pushups, pullups, and crunches. Both techniques enhance strengthening and toning, so you're getting better results with fewer repetitions.

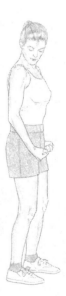

Muscle Tone-Ups for the Upper Body

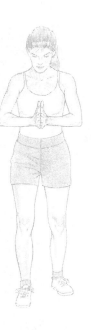

The large muscles in the shoulders, upper arms, chest, and upper back often show significant improvement with muscle tone-ups. You can spark your Meta-Stat and increase metabolism in just a half minute or so. In addition to the two preceding exercises, try the following.

Chest cross with DVT. Stand in a balanced position, with one leg slightly in front of the other. Position your arms as shown, with palms facing each other and touching. Next, with full focus, slowly move your arms out to the sides, tensing your chest and upper-body muscles as much as you can. Slowly return to the starting position, maintaining maximum muscle tension all the way.

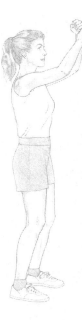

Rope pull with DVT. Stand in a comfortable position, with your knees slightly bent. Extend your arms upward, with your left fist on top of your right at forehead height, as shown. Engage the full power of your concentration as you imagine going hand-over-hand up a rope. Push downward with your left hand against the resistance of your right hand, tensing all of the muscles in your chest, upper back, and upper arms. Slowly move your hands down in front of you, as if advancing up the rope. Repeat, this time starting with your right hand on top of your left.

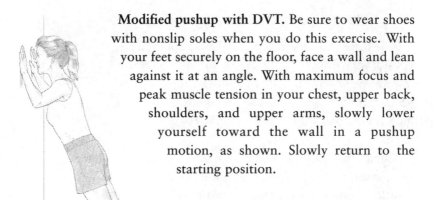

Modified pushup with DVT. Be sure to wear shoes with nonslip soles when you do this exercise. With your feet securely on the floor, face a wall and lean against it at an angle. With maximum focus and peak muscle tension in your chest, upper back, shoulders, and upper arms, slowly lower yourself toward the wall in a pushup motion, as shown. Slowly return to the starting position.

Two-arm lateral raise with DVT. Unlike the lateral raise with DR, this exercise uses visualization to work both arms and shoulders at the same time. Stand in a comfortable position, with your feet shoulder width apart. Make fists with both hands, creating maximum muscle tension all the way up your arms to your shoulders. Slowly raise your arms out to the sides as shown. When you reach the top, imagine that you are holding two watering cans and pouring water from both at the same time. Slowly return to the starting position.

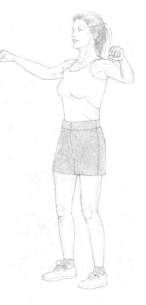

One-arm extension with DVT. This exercise targets the triceps in the back of the upper arm, as well as other muscles in the arm, shoulder, and upper back. Stand comfortably, with your feet shoulder-width apart. Place the fingertips of your left hand on the right side of your upper chest as shown. This provides a centering point for balance. Make a fist with your right hand, tensing the muscles in your right arm and shoulder. Slowly extend your right arm out to the side until it's fully extended. Return to the starting position, then switch arms and repeat.

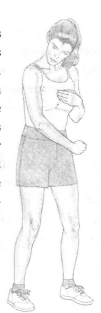

Muscle Tone-Ups for the Lower Body

The following exercises target the muscles in your abdomen, hips, lower back, and legs. We'll start with one of the simplest.

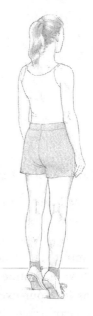

Toe raise with DVT. When you do toe raises, your body weight provides resistance. Stand with one foot slightly in front of the other. Slowly rise as high as possible on the balls of your feet, then slowly lower until you're flat-footed again. If you have a countertop or another secure object to hang on to, you might try this exercise on one leg for added resistance and strengthening power.

Step ahead with DVT. Stand with your feet shoulder width apart. Keeping your spine erect, smoothly step forward with your right leg, as shown. Maintain tension in all of your leg muscles and keep mental focus throughout the movement. Slowly shift forward until your right knee is directly above your toes and your left knee is beneath your hips. Slowly return to the starting position. Repeat with your left leg. For additional muscle toning, add weight—for example, by wearing a backpack containing a few books.

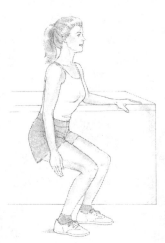

Modified knee bend with DVT. Place one hand on a desk or countertop for support and stand with your feet shoulder width apart. Tense your buttock and thigh muscles as much as you can, then slowly bend your knees until your thighs are almost parallel to the floor, as shown. (Imagine that you're sitting in a chair.) Slowly return to the starting position, maintaining muscle tension as you do. End the movement by rising on the balls of your feet, then lowering.

Create Your Own Muscle Tone-Ups

The beauty of muscle tone-ups is how easily you can modify or add to them to suit your own preferences. You can change your routine as often as you wish, so don't become a slave to habit. Be creative! For example, if you do your resistance training at a fitness center, tinker with your routine to see if you can come up with DR or DVT variations for your exercises. Then you can do them whenever you want. Keep exploring—and see the results!

CHAPTER 18

■ ■ ■

Lower-Body Strength:
Abs and Legs

A trim, toned abdomen may be the most recognizable, and desirable, symbol of fitness. When strong and taut, the abdominal muscles flatten your waist, support your internal organs, and stabilize your lower back at its most vulnerable point—the lumbosacral angle of the pelvis.[1] They power your every move, whether you're bending, lifting, stretching, twisting, or reaching.

The abdominal muscles also help maintain balance, in every sense of the word. As researchers explore the complex connections between physical, mental, and emotional health, they are finding that abdominal strength can help people prepare for and navigate life's changes and challenges.[2] In one large-scale Canadian study that tracked various health markers among 8,116 participants, those with weaker abs had a higher death rate, even after the research team adjusted the results for age, weight, and body fat.[3]

Of course, the Meta-Stat couldn't do its job without the support of the abdominal muscles. Just consider all of the metabolism-related processes that occur in the "core" of your body—including circulation, respiration, and digestion. These processes benefit from the fitness of your abdominal muscles. Whenever your work your abs, your Meta-Stat gets an on-the-spot boost, clicking your body's fat-burning, energy-producing power to a higher level.

META-STAT STARTER

Lean-Back Tone-Ups

Here is a quick muscle tone-up that will provide an instant boost to your core strength. And you don't need to leave your chair to do it!

Sit up straight, with your buttocks near the front edge of your chair and your hands on your waist. Lean back slightly as you tense your abdominal muscles. Slowly rotate to the right, then to the left. Return to the starting position.

WHITTLE YOUR WAISTLINE

In the quest for the "ideal" abdomen, many people build their workouts around crunches, perhaps the best-known abdominal exercises. Unfortunately, crunches won't produce the desired effect, no matter how many you do—not even 5,000 repetitions a month![4] On the other hand, repeated crunches can cause or aggravate lower-back pain by pulling on the front of the lower spine.[5] The back sways inward as the lower abdomen pushes out, creating a potbellied appearance.

In terms of abdominal fitness, less can be more. "You don't need to do hundreds of crunches or other exercises to see an effect," says Wayne L. Westcott, PhD, consultant to the YMCA of the United States. "The abdominal muscles are small. Slow, controlled movement for up to 10 repetitions per exercise is all you need."[6]

As discussed in Chapter 17, the most effective way to tone muscles—and to boost your Meta-Stat is to increase *resistance*, not repetitions. This certainly holds true for the abdominal muscles. You need to strengthen each muscle fiber, and you can't do that by lifting and lowering your upper body over and over again. Instead, slow your pace and practice dynamic visualized tension (DVT), in which you consciously create resistance through the power of concentration. (For a refresher on DVT technique, see page 172.)

Depending on the type of exercise, you can also add resistance by using a medicine ball, a weighted backpack, or another weight that you

can hold safely and securely. When an exercise calls for lifting your feet off the ground, you might try wearing ankle weights to enhance the strengthening effects.

Take your time with your exercises; try not to rush through. "In my opinion," says Ellington Darden, PhD, former director of research at Nautilus Sports/Medical Industries and author of *Living Longer Stronger*, "at least 90 percent of the people who do toning exercises perform their repetitions in a manner that could be described as fast, jerky, and explosive. Research proves that slow, smooth lifting and lowering on each repetition is much more productive, as well as safer."[7]

Proper form is critical. For the abdominal muscles, in particular, the best predictor of an exercise's effectiveness is how well you perform each and every repetition. You should be able to feel the contraction in your midsection, and you should be able to maintain that squeezing sensation through the entire movement.

To pace yourself properly, use a 3-second count during the "lifting" phase of the exercise, followed by a 5-second count during the "lowering" phase—when most of the benefits may occur. When in doubt, opt for slow movements over fast. Also follow these guidelines, which can enhance the effectiveness of your abdominal workout.

- Read the instructions for each exercise.
- Use smooth, controlled movements.
- Take care not to hold your breath or clench your teeth.
- Count the number of repetitions. Lifting and lowering to the starting position is one repetition (rep).
- Concentrate. The most effective muscle-toning exercises are mental as well as physical. The more you focus your attention on the muscle groups you're working, the more your brain activates those muscles. Results improve dramatically.
- Anticipate some minor soreness. Whenever you tax underused muscles, you're going to feel it. This is natural. The soreness should subside within a few days.

I recommend performing all of the exercises in this chapter, in sequence, 2 days a week. You can alternate with the upper-body routine

META-STAT STARTER

10-Second Midsection Strengthener

For years, fitness experts have been using this technique, called the abdominal vacuum, to trim and tone the midsection. It will introduce you to a whole new way of breathing.

Begin with a normal breathing cycle, inhaling and exhaling. As you exhale, forcibly blow as much air from your lungs as you can. This will push key lower abdominal muscles inward and upward. Touch your abdomen so you can feel the contracted muscles. This tactile feedback increases your brain's receptivity to muscle activation.

The entire exercise takes only about 10 seconds. I recommend repeating it two or three times before each meal and snack. Don't worry if you don't notice a big change at first. It may take a few tries before these lower abdominal muscles "wake up" and start working again.

in Chapter 19 so your muscles get a day (or two) of rest between workouts. Once you become accustomed to the exercises, you can use them whenever you feel your Meta-Stat setting begin to slip. They immediately reset your Meta-Stat to where it should be.

Targeted Toners

The transverse abdominis (TVA) and the pyramidalis may be the two most overlooked and underworked muscles in the body. Located in the lower abdomen, they play major roles in flattening the lower abs and stabilizing the lower back.

The first four exercises target these two muscles. Practice all of them for immediate, lasting results.

TVA ab tightener. Besides the TVA and pyramidalis, this exercise also works the oblique muscles (in your midsection) and lower-back muscles.[8] The instructions are for a seated position, but you can also perform this exercise while standing.

Sit up straight, lifting your chest and pulling in your stomach. Smoothly exhale (try to force all of the air out of your lungs) as you tighten your abs and squeeze your buttocks all at the same time. You should feel as though you're rising up an inch or two. Release, then repeat. Aim for 3 to 5 repetitions.

Transpyramid toner. This exercise, sometimes called voluntary contraction, is very effective for the lower abdominal region.[9] Fitness expert Lawrence E. Lamb, MD, describes it as "the most important exercise to flatten your abdomen."[10]

To begin, sit or stand in a comfortable position. Place your hands on your hips, with your thumbs pointing toward your back and your fingers spread across your abdomen. Your index fingers should point to your navel. Relax your shoulders. If standing, slightly bend your knees.

Take a deep breath. As you exhale, notice which direction your lower abdomen moves. If you're engaging the TVA and pyramidalis muscles, as you should be, you'll feel your abdomen pulling inward toward your spine. Next, inhale and notice how your belly "pops" outward against your fingers.

To make a clear distinction between the two movements, exaggerate both of them—pushing outward on the inhalation, pulling inward on the exhalation. As you complete an exhalation, use your lower abdominal muscles to pull inward even more. Then consciously release your abdomen on the next inhalation. Work up to 4 or 5 repetitions.

Exhalation towel roll-up. One reason I don't recommend a traditional crunch is that it doesn't work the abs through their full range of motion. You can get better results from a similar exercise with the help of a towel.

Fold a medium-size bath towel in half lengthwise, then roll it up. (Once you're comfortable with the exercise, you can switch to a larger bath towel or a beach towel.) Lie on the floor with your knees bent and your feet flat. Place the towel under your lower back. The curve created by the towel helps increase the abdominal stretch as well as range of motion.

Place your hands on your abdomen. Alternatively, you could cross them on your upper chest or entwine your fingers behind your head. Tense your lower abdominal muscles, then exhale as you raise your shoulder blades off the floor, crunching your rib cage toward your pelvis as shown. By pulling your lower abdomen inward, you engage your TVA muscle. Pause for several seconds before slowly returning to the starting position.

Work up to 4 repetitions, adding resistance when you're comfortable with the exercise. For example, you might hold several books or a hand weight across your chest.

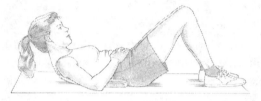

Elbow-to-knee curl-up. When biomechanics researchers at San Diego State University used electronic measurements to compare various pieces of gym equipment, they found the Icarian crunch machine to be most effective at working the abdominal muscles. What if you don't have access to one of these machines? Researchers suggest including the bicycle crunch—what I call the elbow-to-knee curl-up—in your abdominal workout.[11] It targets the rectus abdominis muscle 150 percent better than traditional crunches.

Lie on your back with your hands behind your head. Bring your left knee toward your right elbow, then return to the starting position. Repeat, this time bringing your right knee toward your left elbow. Continue alternating sides using a pedaling motion, as shown. When one leg is bent, the other can be extended slightly. Work up to 4 or 5 repetitions per side.

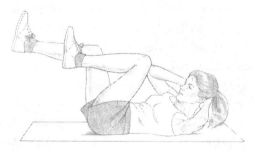

More Ab Strengtheners

In addition to the preceding exercises, I recommend the following for a trim, toned abdomen.

Twisting exhalation roll-up. Both this exercise and the reverse trunk rotation that follows are great for firming up the muscles around the waistline. For extra support, you can place a rolled-up towel behind your lower back.

To begin, lie on your back, cradling your head in your hands. Slowly raise your head and shoulders, but keep your shoulder blades flat on the floor. Imagine your abdomen sinking into your lower back. Focus on this sensation and maintain it throughout the roll-up.

Gently exhale as you slowly bring your left shoulder and rib cage toward your right knee, as shown. Keep your elbow and back relaxed, so the twist is gentle and comes from your waist rather than your arm or neck.

Return to the starting position, then repeat, this time bringing your right shoulder toward your left knee. Work up to 4 repetitions per side.

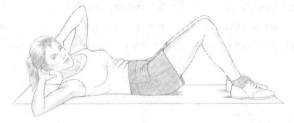

Reverse trunk rotation. This exercise not only improves abdominal fitness but also is great for posture.[12] It requires a full range of motion that builds strength and flexibility in the waist and lower back—ideal for preventing back pain and injury.

Begin by lying on your back, with your arms extended out to the sides and perpendicular to your body. Bend your knees and pull your heels toward your buttocks. Maintain this leg-trunk angle as you slowly lower your knees to the right side. Your right knee and ankle should be flat on the floor, as should your arms and shoulders.

META-STAT STARTER

Return your legs to the starting position. Repeat the exercise, this time lowering your legs to the left side. Work up to 4 repetitions.

As you get comfortable with this exercise, gradually work on extending your legs until they're perpendicular to the floor. If you're struggling to maintain good form through the base movement, try bending your knees more before lowering them to the side.[13]

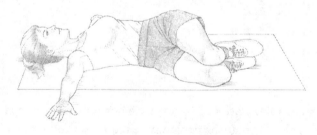

NEXT, THE LEGS

We've been focusing most of our attention on the abdominal muscles, but the leg muscles are just as important to lower-body strength. To a significant extent, your ability to stay fit and active depends on leg power.

Modified knee bend. I first introduced this exercise as a muscle tone-up in Chapter 17. For a refresher: Using a desk or countertop for support, stand with your feet flat on the floor and shoulder width apart. Tense your buttock and thigh muscles, then slowly bend your knees and lower your buttocks until your thighs are parallel to the floor, as shown. Slowly return to the starting position. End by rising on the balls of your feet, then lowering your heels to the floor.

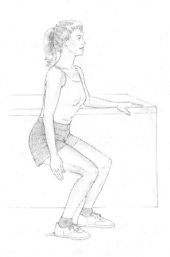

Once you're comfortable with this exercise, you might try adding resistance, such as a backpack filled with books. Work up to 4 repetitions.

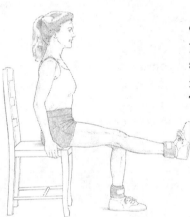

Seated leg extension. For this exercise, you'll need ankle weights, which you can buy in most sporting goods stores. Choose a pair that feels comfortable and is adjustable for poundage. They should fit around your lower legs just above the ankles.

Sit straight on the edge of a chair, with both feet planted firmly on the floor. Concentrate on tensing your buttock and thigh muscles, then raise your right knee slightly so your foot is off the floor. Maintaining concentration and muscle tension, extend your lower leg so that it's parallel to the floor, as shown. Slowly return to the starting position, then switch legs. Perform up to 4 slow repetitions.

Standing side leg raise. This exercise works the sides of your legs. To perform it safely, lean against a doorframe, desk, or countertop for support.

Stand straight with your feet firmly on the floor. Concentrate on your outside leg, tensing all the muscles from your hips to your toes. Slowly

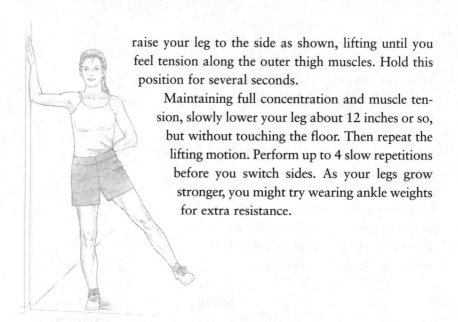

raise your leg to the side as shown, lifting until you feel tension along the outer thigh muscles. Hold this position for several seconds.

Maintaining full concentration and muscle tension, slowly lower your leg about 12 inches or so, but without touching the floor. Then repeat the lifting motion. Perform up to 4 slow repetitions before you switch sides. As your legs grow stronger, you might try wearing ankle weights for extra resistance.

Hip raise. This exercise will help tone your buttock muscles. Lie on your back with your arms extended out to the sides, palms facing down. Bend your knees, keeping your feet flat on the floor. Concentrate on your buttocks, hips, and thighs, generating maximum muscle tension in these areas.

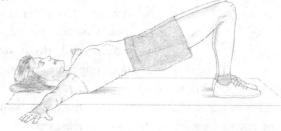

Slowly raise your hips off the floor. Your head, shoulders, arms, and hands should remain stationary. Arch your lower back slightly. Maintaining full concentration and muscle tension, slowly return to the starting position. Perform up to 4 slow repetitions.

Standing calf raise. This exercise targets your lower leg muscles. To do it, you should find stairs with a railing. As an alternative, you can use a solid block of wood as a step and hold onto a desk or countertop for support.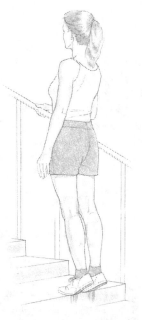

Grasping the railing for balance, stand with the balls of your feet on the edge of the stair. Your toes should point straight ahead.

Concentrate on your lower legs, tensing all the muscles there. Bending your knees slightly, allow your heels to drop as far below the stair as comfortably possible. They need not touch the floor.

Continuing the motion, slowly rise as high as you can on the balls of your feet, making sure your ankles don't roll outward. Then return to the starting position, maintaining your concentration and muscle tension all the way through. Perform up to 4 slow repetitions.

To more fully engage your lower leg muscles, you can perform this exercise with your legs straight rather than with knees slightly bent. Or bend your knees on the downward motion (as your heels drop below the stair) and straighten on the upward motion. For more intensity, try working one leg at a time.

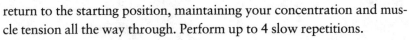

CHAPTER 19

Upper-Body Strength: Chest, Back, Shoulders, and Arms

U pper-body strength is a reliable indicator of overall fitness. When your chest, upper back, shoulders, and arms have exceptional muscle tone, chances are you feel vital and energetic.

But the benefits of upper-body strength go much farther. By improving muscle tone in your chest, back, shoulders, and arms, you increase metabolic efficiency. So your Meta-Stat climbs to an even higher setting.

But to maintain that muscle tone—and to keep stoking your Meta-Stat to burn excess fat—you must include specific toning exercises in your weekly workout regimen. As long as you keep raising the level of resistance, you'll see results!

THE SUPER SEVEN

To get the most from your upper-body workouts, pay special attention to these seven guidelines.

1. Warm up. Precede every resistance-training session with a series of smooth, comfortable motions to increase blood flow and loosen up your muscles and joints.

2. Know your 1-repetition maximum. Your 1-repetition maximum—1RM for short—is the most weight that you can lift in a single movement or muscle contraction. It should be heavy enough that you would be unable to lift it again without resting for a while.

When working your upper-body muscles, you want to approach but not exceed your 1RM, advise Irwin H. Rosenberg, MD, of the Jean Mayer USDA Human Nutrition Research Center on Aging at Tufts University, and former colleague William J. Evans, PhD, now director of the Nutrition, Metabolism, and Exercise Laboratory at the University of Arkansas for Medical Sciences. "In our studies at Tufts, we exercise our subjects at 80 percent of their 1RM," they write. "We recognize that to build strength appreciably, a person must work out at that level."[1]

Once you know your 1RM, be certain to keep checking it every 2 to 4 weeks. As you get stronger, your 1RM will change, and you'll need to adjust your resistance level accordingly.

3. Listen to your body. You can expect slight soreness after your workout, especially if you're just beginning to exercise. But if you feel any pain during a particular movement, stop immediately. Continue only if the pain subsides, and then only after reducing the amount of weight you're lifting. Consult your physician with any questions.

4. Stay centered. During each exercise, use good posture and smooth, controlled movements. Avoid arching your back or twisting and turning in ways that aren't called for in the exercise. Also, be careful not to hold your breath, as this may cause a rise in blood pressure. Breathe evenly and steadily.

5. Use peak focus to reach full intensity. How effective your upper-body workout is depends a great deal on how sharp and focused your mind is. Make every effort to tune out distractions, so each moment of muscle toning produces optimal results. Exercise better, exercise less!

When possible, touch with your free hand the muscle that you're working. This creates a tactile feedback loop with your brain, which in turn increases the number of muscle fibers that you're able to strengthen and tone.

6. Keep passing your peak. As you get stronger, progressively increase the resistance you use. You need to keep challenging your muscles in order for them to grow.

7. Cool down. After your workout, avoid coming to a sudden stop or sitting still. Keep moving as you shift from "exercise mode" to your normal routine. Allow your heart rate and circulation to gradually return to preworkout status.

SMOOTH, BUT NOT TOO SLOW

Almost all of the upcoming exercises call for additional weight. I mention dumbbells, but you can also use variable-resistance elastic bands or even plastic milk jugs partially filled with water. The extra weight increases the resistance level, which in turn stimulates metabolism and builds muscle tone.

If you go with dumbbells, you need to choose your starting weight. I suggest experimenting until you find the heaviest dumbbell that you can use safely and effectively. When you can easily perform twice as many repetitions as recommended, you should increase the weight. Just be sure to do it gradually so you don't overstrain your muscles.

Every toning exercise has two parts. First is the *concentric* motion, which is when the muscle shortens or contracts (during the lifting phase of a biceps curl, for example). The second, *eccentric* motion, occurs as the muscle lengthens (the lowering phase of a curl). For building muscle, the eccentric motion is key.

"Without the eccentric component in an exercise, you don't get much muscle growth," says Maria Fiatarone Singh, MD, a visiting scientist at the Human Nutrition Research Center on Aging at Tufts.[2] Through magnetic resonance imaging, researchers at the University of Southern California determined that smooth, rapid eccentric motions lasting just 2 seconds activated significantly more muscle fibers than slow eccentric motions lasting more than 10 seconds.[3]

Thus, when performing upper-body exercises, pay particular attention to the eccentric motion, maintaining resistance all the way through. This not only strengthens and tones the muscle, it also helps prevent injury.

I suggest performing the following routine twice a week, alternating with the core strength exercises in Chapter 18. This way, your upper-body muscles can recuperate between workouts.

Toning Your Chest, Upper Back, Shoulders, and Arms

Start with the following exercises.

Modified pushup. This update of a classic exercise strengthens muscles in the chest, back, shoulders, and arms. To begin, lie facedown on the floor, with your knees together and your hands on either side of your chest near the front of each shoulder.

Slowly raise your upper body off the floor, supporting your weight with your arms and keeping your knees in contact with the floor. Keep your back as flat as you can. Concentrate on your chest, upper back, shoulder, and arm muscles, tensing them as much as you can. Maintaining concentration and muscle tension, lower your upper body to the starting position. Perform as many slow repetitions as you can.

Keeping your hands beneath your shoulders as you raise your upper body will maximize the strengthening effect of this exercise for your back and upper arms. If you'd rather focus on your chest muscles, position your hands so they're farther than shoulder width apart. You can add resistance by wearing a weighted backpack or by shifting your body weight onto one arm, then the other. Move smoothly and be creative!

Chest and shoulder raise. For this exercise, you'll need some extra weight—a dumbbell if you have one, or a plastic milk jug partially filled with water. Start at the resistance level you can comfortably handle, knowing you will add resistance in the weeks ahead.

Sit in a chair, holding the weight at your left side. Concentrate on your chest, shoulder, and upper-arm muscles, tensing them as much as you can.

Keeping your elbow straight, slowly raise the weight until it's above and slightly to the front of your head, as shown. Maintaining concentration and muscle tension, slowly return to the starting position. Perform as many slow repetitions as you can, then change hands.

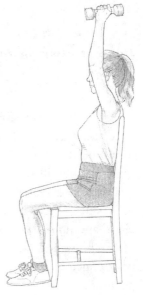

Chest cross. You'll need 2-pound dumbbells for this exercise as well. Begin by lying on your back, with your knees bent and your feet and lower back firmly against the floor. Holding a dumbbell in each hand, extend your arms to either side of your shoulders so they're perpendicular to your body.

Concentrate on your chest, shoulders, and arms, tensing all of the muscles. With your elbows slightly bent, slowly raise the dumbbells in an arc, bringing your hands toward each other, as shown. The weights should touch above the center of your chest. Then slowly lower the dumbbells in an arc, returning to the starting position. Perform as many slow repetitions as you can.

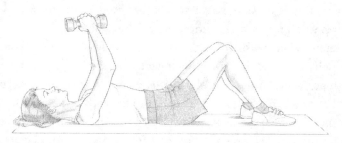

Concentrating on Your Upper Arms

The following two exercises will help strengthen and tone your upper arms.

Arm curl. This is a variation of the biceps curl with dynamic resistance and dynamic visualized tension, which I discussed in Chapter 17. You'll need 2-pound dumbbells or, as an alternative, two plastic milk jugs partially filled with water.

Begin in a seated position, holding a dumbbell in each hand by your sides, palms facing up. Concentrate on your arms, shoulders, chest, and upper back, tensing these muscles as much as you can. Bend your elbows and raise your arms toward your shoulders. Maintaining your concentration and muscle tension, slowly return to the starting position.

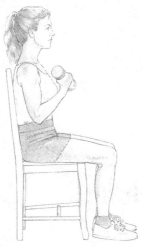

You can alternate your left and right arms rather than lifting the dumbbells simultaneously, if you wish. For another variation, try lifting the dumbbells with your palms facing down rather than up. Perform as many slow repetitions as you can.

Upper-arm extension. This exercise strengthens the triceps muscles, located at the backs of the upper arms. You'll need a 2-pound dumbbell to start. When performing this exercise, you may want to lean on a chair seat or flat bench to support and stabilize your body.

Concentrate on your arms, shoulders, chest, and upper back, tensing these muscles as tightly as you can. With the dumbbell in your left hand, bend forward at the hips until your torso is parallel to the floor. Your left arm should be bent at a 90-degree angle, with your upper arm against your torso and parallel to the floor.

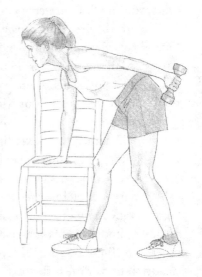

Slowly straighten your arm behind you, lifting it slightly higher than the starting position. Slowly return to the starting position. Perform as many slow repetitions as you can, then switch hands.

CHAPTER 20

■　■　■

Balance and Flexibility

The previous chapters explain the importance of aerobic activity and resistance training to raising your Meta-Stat. There's one more component that we need to discuss, and it may be the most important of all. I'm referring, of course, to balance and flexibility.

Though they're not as visible as trim, toned muscles, balance and flexibility are what allow you to move with grace and ease. Even the strongest, fittest body can falter with a rigid neck, a stiff back, or a weakened spine. This drains your energy—and with it, your motivation to keep activating your Meta-Stat throughout the day.

What's more, physical balance and flexibility tend to translate into emotional balance and flexibility. With just a few stretches a week, you can feel more vital and resilient, with a greater zest for life.

The key with stretches is to do them regularly. The MSOn Workout calls for four stretching sessions per week, though every day is even better. I tack them on to my resistance-training routine, stretching after my lower-body toners on Mondays and Thursdays and my upper-body toners on Tuesday and Fridays. This helps keep my Meta-Stat in a steady state, with few fluctuations to drain my energy.

I've highlighted a handful of basic stretches here. You're welcome to expand your repertoire and explore new favorites. Just try not to add so many that they complicate your workout. Then you're more likely to stop doing them—and that's a mistake!

NECK FLEXIBILITY

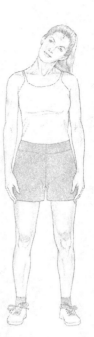

Few things make us feel older or less fit than a stiff neck. Often, neck problems are a by-product of a sedentary lifestyle, as we live and work in pretty much the same positions all day, every day. This limits the neck's range of motion. Here's how to loosen up.

Neck rotation. This safe, simple stretch helps maintain your neck's flexibility. It also contributes to better balance and posture.

Stand comfortably, with your arms at your sides. Drop your chin toward your chest, then slowly rotate your head to the left until your ear is over your shoulder. Return your chin to your chest, then repeat to the right side. Once you feel comfortable with this stretch, you can add some resistance in the form of light muscle tension.

BACK STRENGTH

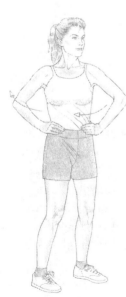

Both back strength and posture determine how much your abdomen protrudes, as well as whether or not you can engage in activities without fatigue or injury. The stretches here, each one recommended by an expert who specializes in back care, may help build your back muscles.[1]

A word of caution: It's best to perform these stretches after you've warmed up—with toning exercises or a short walk, for example. If you have a history of back problems or are currently experiencing back pain, be sure to consult your physician before engaging in any exercise program.

Torso rotation. Stand with your hands on your hips and your feet about shoulder width apart. Your posture should be upright but relaxed. Gently and smoothly rotate your torso first to the right, then to the left. Your head should remain centered on your neck and facing forward.

Back arch. Lie facedown on the floor. Gently rise onto your elbows so that you're leaning on your forearms, as shown. Relax into this stretch for 5 or 6 seconds.

Next, gently push up on your hands as far as you comfortably can. At the height of the stretch, your back is extended as much as possible and your arms are as straight as possible. Relax and hold this position for 5 to 20 seconds. Return to the starting position.

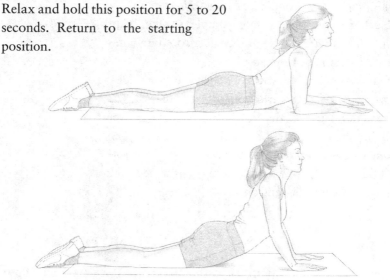

Single knee-to-chest lift. This stretch helps loosen and strengthen the muscles and connective tissues that support the back and hips. Lie on your back with both knees bent and your feet flat on the floor. Using both hands, grasp one knee and slowly and gently pull it toward your chest, as shown. Hold for a slow count of 5, then release your knee and slowly return to the starting position. Repeat with the other leg.

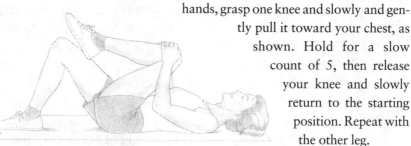

Seated lower-back stretch. Sit with your knees and feet about shoulder width apart. Slowly bend forward toward the floor, as shown. Reach as far as you comfortably can without bouncing, grasping your ankles if you can. Hold this stretch for a slow count of 5, then return to the starting position.

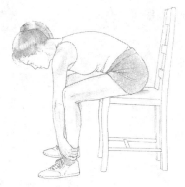

Pelvic tilt. This relaxing stretch helps strengthen the front spinal structures while loosening the back ones. Lie on your back with your knees bent and your arms stretched out to the sides, perpendicular to your body. Gently press your lower back into the floor, as shown. Hold for a few seconds, then release.

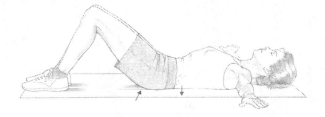

PART

The MSOn Eating Plan

FOUR

If you're accustomed to restrictive diets that limit what you eat, the MSOn Eating Plan just might surprise you. It isn't about avoiding the "wrong" foods. Rather, it emphasizes eating the right foods, in the right amounts and combinations, at the right times of day.

In fact, once you learn to properly balance your protein, carbohydrate, and fat intakes, you may discover that you can eat more than you imagined—and still burn fat and generate energy. Your Meta-Stat uses food to fuel metabolism and thermogenesis. If it doesn't get what it needs, it can't function at its peak. That means you store fat rather than burning it and deplete energy rather than generating it.

In the chapters ahead, you'll learn how to build your diet around just the right mix of quality proteins, moderate carbohydrates, and healthy fats. And you'll discover how to pace your meals and snacks to support your Meta-Stat and prevent overeating.

Remember to track your meals and snacks, as well as your fluid intake, using the Meta-Stat Success Map on page 246. With this information, you can see how certain food choices and eating patterns affect your energy level and your fat-burning capacity.

CHAPTER 21

■ ■ ■

Rethinking Mealtimes

We're so accustomed to experts telling us to eat less that we feel guilty when we eat often. Well, guilt may be fattening—it produces stress hormones that slow metabolism and increase fat gain—but eating often is not. Frequent meals and snacks are key to energy balance and fat-burning power. They crank up your Meta-Stat and keep it at a healthy level.

Infrequent megameals, no matter how nutritious they may be, overwhelm your metabolism. Eating this way can be just as bad as skipping meals. So many dieters think, "I'll save calories if I just don't eat." In reality, they're turning down their resting metabolic rates,[1] since their bodies shift into conservation mode. Instead of burning fat, their bodies store it—an evolutionary response to protect against starvation in the absence of an adequate food supply.

Scientists at Georgia State University pioneered a technique to measure hour-by-hour energy balance—that is, how many calories you are burning versus how many calories you are taking in. The researchers discovered that people who kept their hourly surplus or deficit within 300 to 500 calories at all times were significantly more successful at losing fat and adding lean, toned muscle tissue. People with the largest energy imbalances—whose surpluses or shortfalls exceeded 500 calories from hour to hour—were the heaviest. These are precisely the sorts of calorie fluctuations that occur when you follow the typical three-meals-and-no-snacks eating pattern.

To keep your Meta-Stat on an even keel, you need to pay attention not just to *what* you eat but also to *when* you eat. This is why the MSOn Eating Plan emphasizes smaller but more frequent meals and snacks spread over the course of the day. Actually, if you get most of your calories early in the day—at breakfast and lunch, for example—you'll stoke your internal metabolic fire to burn hotter, according to Pat Harper, RD, MS, a spokesperson for the American Dietetic Association.[2]

Recent studies confirm that for fat loss and energy production, eating small but frequent meals is superior to the usual three large meals a day because it improves the rate of thermogenesis and subsequent calorie burning.[3] In fact, even when people ate the same number of calories over the course of a day, those who ate every few hours showed a significantly higher thermic or metabolism-boosting effect than those who ate two or three times a day.[4]

TURN OFF THE FAT MAKERS

The average human body has 25 to 30 billion fat cells, which serve as storehouses for fat molecules that accumulate both from food and from the body's own fat-making processes. Typically, these cells congregate on the abdomen, hips, and thighs, as well as in layers beneath the skin.

Eating a few large meals a day, as most of us do, can overwhelm the body's existing fat cells. They trigger a hormonal signal that the body interprets as a "no vacancy" sign. In response, the body begins producing new fat cells to accommodate the excess fat molecules. This is how we gain weight.

What's more, eating a few large meals a day causes sharp fluctuations in blood sugar levels, another factor in the "battle of the bulge." With the initial upward spike in blood sugar, the body releases a larger than normal amount of the hormone insulin, which is responsible for escorting blood sugar from the bloodstream into cells. The presence of so much insulin inhibits lypolysis, the process by which the body

META-STAT STARTER

Eat and Move

Follow each meal or snack with a few minutes of easy activity, such as walking around your work area or performing a few muscle tone-ups. Medical research confirms the alertness-boosting, fat-burning effects of these opportune "active minutes."[5]

releases fat from storage for use as energy. After all, the body doesn't need fat when it has all that blood sugar as a readily available fuel source. Instead, fat stays put in its cells.[6]

As insulin does its job, blood sugar begins to drop to a normal level. This not only saps your energy,[7] it also triggers appetite. So by the time you sit down to your next meal, you're more likely to stuff yourself. And you're more likely to eat fatty, sugary foods, which the body naturally tends to crave in the mid- to late afternoon.[8] In effect, you're feeding the cycle by which the body accumulates fat—and you're doing so at precisely the time of day when metabolism gradually falls off.

For successful fat loss, it's vitally important to break the habit of eating too much food in too few sittings. This takes some effort; after all, you probably have been following the "three square meals" ritual since you were a kid. But as you shift toward a pattern of smaller meals and snacks at more frequent intervals, you will notice almost immediate improvement in your energy level—the result of more stable blood sugar. In fact, you may feel so much better that you'll wonder why you haven't been eating this way all along!

3 + 4 = SUCCESS

The MSOn Eating Plan builds on the principle of less food more often. You may eat a smaller amount at each sitting, but I guarantee that you'll never feel deprived. That's because you'll be enjoying not the customary three meals but *seven* meals and snacks on a daily basis. Just remember the formula 3 + 4. That's three light meals and four healthy snacks, spread between 2 and 3 hours apart from morning to night.

Eating small but frequent meals and snacks appears to have numerous health benefits, according to a study that appeared in the *New England Journal of Medicine*. For the study, researchers assigned 14 men of average weight to one of two groups. Both groups consumed the same number of calories per day, in the same proportions of protein, carbohydrate, and fat. But one group divided its calories among three large meals, while the other ate seven smaller meals.

In just 2 weeks, the men following the "minimeal" eating plan showed measurable improvement in several key health markers. For example:[9]

- Their blood cholesterol levels fell by 15 percent.

- Their cortisol levels dropped by more than 17 percent. (Cortisol is the pesky fat-storing hormone that the body churns out when under stress.)

- Their insulin levels declined by nearly 28 percent.

The positive effect on insulin is especially noteworthy because it suggests that blood sugar levels were remaining relatively constant. In other words, small but frequent meals help prevent the blood sugar fluctuations that contribute to overeating[10] as well as to fat storage.[11]

Other research published in the *New England Journal of Medicine*[12] and the *American Journal of Clinical Nutrition*[13] confirm that meal size and frequency play a pivotal role in metabolism and fat burning. Meal composition is important, too. The right combination of lean protein, complex carbohydrate, and healthy fat can trigger a process that's known as the thermic effect of food. In other words, it actually increases metabolism. It also may reduce the urge to overeat, especially at night.[14]

"Many, if not most, people are better off with low-fat, moderate-carbohydrate, high-protein snacks at midmorning and especially at midafternoon," says Richard N. Podell, MD, director of the Overlook Center for Weight Management in New York City. "For one thing, eating at these times helps handle the midafternoon blood sugar dip. Also,

Food for Thought

Eating small but frequent meals has a positive effect on cognitive function—and not just by stabilizing blood sugar, though that's important.[15] The simple act of taking a break from your daily routine to eat helps build what's known as vital memory. "A brief period—even just a few minutes—away from the normal influx of information will allow your brain to do some of the filing necessary to sharpen your memory," explains neuropsychologist Michael D. Chafetz, PhD, author of *Smart for Life.* "Anything that stops the normal flow and lets your brain redirect is worthwhile."[16]

There is growing evidence that pulling back at regular intervals throughout the day can enhance performance and productivity. "Laboratory experiments have shown that if you work too long at mental tasks, your problem-solving time can increase by 500 percent," notes Donald Norfolk, MD, in *Executive Stress.*[17] On the other hand, "introducing rest breaks actually speeds up work, and this more than compensates for any time lost during pauses and breaks," according to Etienne Grandjean, MD, an expert on work productivity and director of the department of ergonomics at the Swiss Federal Institute of Technology.[18]

a midafternoon snack helps steady your blood sugar level, so you won't become ravenous by dinner."[19]

EAT TO RAISE YOUR META-STAT

The MSOn Eating Plan allows you to determine the ideal mix of nutrients for optimal metabolic function. In general, people do best with meals and snacks that consist of 20 to 35 percent lean protein, 40 to 60 percent complex carbohydrate, and 20 to 25 percent healthy fat. This ratio promotes steady, sustained energy production and fat burning.

Through the next several chapters, we'll explore the MSOn Eating Plan from the perspective of each core nutrient—protein, carbohydrate, and fat. For now, let's review the general guidelines for meal size and frequency.

Eat every 2 to 3 hours. Going for more than 3 hours without a meal or snack will cause a dip in blood sugar and energy. You're more likely to overeat and more likely to gain fat.

Limit each meal to about 600 calories and each snack to about 300 calories. The effectiveness of the MSOn Eating Plan is contingent upon portion control. If you increase meal frequency without proportionately reducing meal size, you'll boost fat storage rather than fat burning. The MSOn Eating Plan has a degree of built-in portion control, since by eating more often, you'll feel less hungry over the course of the day. Still, it's very easy to pass the point of satiety, especially if you eat fast or without awareness.[20] You need to pay attention to your body's hunger cues. (I'll talk more about calorie intake in Chapter 25.)

Keep a stash of favorite snacks. Research suggest that adults make 20 to 30 food choices a day, on average.[21] The healthiest choices need to be as accessible as possible. Otherwise, you may end up at the nearest vending machine or minimart, buying a meal or snack that supplies an entire day's worth of calories—not to mention fat—at once.

The key to making healthy choices is to plan ahead. In my family, we stock the car with snack-size bags of unsalted soy nuts, a few protein bars, and a few bottles of water. Then we always have nutritious snacks on hand for whenever we might need them, whether we're sitting in traffic or running errands. Stash a few favorite snacks in your desk, your purse or briefcase, your gym bag—anyplace that's handy, so nutritious foods are ready when you are.

Steer clear of synthetic sweeteners and fake fats. Studies suggest that these manufactured additives may reinforce your taste for sugary, fatty, greasy foods.[22] In particular, "excess use of artificial sweeteners may impede weight loss by increasing hunger," cautions John A. McDougall, MD, founder and director of the McDougall Program at St. Helena Hospital in California.[23] That's because artificial sweeteners reduce serotonin, a feel-good brain chemical, while elevating insulin.

Go easy on dried fruit. It certainly seems like a healthy snack. The trouble with dried fruit is that it's far less filling than fresh, so you can easily eat too much. And it contains so much sugar—even though it's the natural kind—it actually can stimulate the body's fat-storing process.[24]

Energy-Boosting, Fat-Burning Snacks

All of the following snack options comply with the guidelines of the MSOn Eating Plan, supplying a maximum of 300 calories and a mix of lean protein, complex carbohydrate, and healthy fat. The list is meant only as a starting point. Feel free to sample a variety of nutritionally balanced snacks to build your own repertoire. Seek out foods that give you lasting energy-boosting, fat-burning power—the hallmark of the Meta-Stat approach.

- 1 slice 100 percent whole grain bread or two whole grain crackers topped with one of the following: low-fat cream cheese; a very light smear of natural peanut butter or almond butter; ½ slice reduced-fat Cheddar or Jarlsberg lite Swiss cheese; 1 slice organic turkey breast and Dijon mustard; 1 slice organic chicken breast and fresh salsa; 1 rounded tablespoon canned salmon or tuna (in spring water) and salsa

- 1 rounded tablespoon from a foil-pack serving of tuna (with no water or oil, so you can eat it right from the pack) and a few whole grain crackers

- ½ cup low-fat or fat-free plain yogurt or cottage cheese topped with a handful of fresh blueberries or raspberries or 2 tablespoons whole oat granola

- Grape-Nuts cereal

- A reduced-fat mozzarella cheese stick and a small handful of dried blueberries

- A piece of fresh fruit (apple, peach, cantaloupe) topped with a very light smear of natural peanut butter or almond butter

- A very small handful of nuts or seeds, such as peanuts, walnuts, pumpkin seeds, soy nuts, or sunflower seeds

- ½ cup fresh vegetable juice, lightly salted (such as Bolthouse Farms), and one reduced-fat mozzarella cheese stick

- Half of a low-carb, low-fat, high-protein bar made with whey protein

- ½ cup fresh-cut, mixed raw vegetable pieces and a very small handful of nuts or a reduced-fat cheese stick

An added problem, according to Dr. McDougall, is that "fruit sugar causes significant increases in blood fats (triglycerides) in some people. It also stimulates insulin production, which stuffs these fats into fat cells."[25]

Choose fresh whole fruit over dried or even fruit juice. Whole fruit contains fiber, which slows the breakdown and absorption of the fruit sugar into the bloodstream. Blood sugar won't spike upward, and neither will insulin production. Even fruit juice can be a problem if you consume lots of it. "Processing fruit into juice or sauce disrupts and/or removes fiber," Dr. McDougall explains.

Get out of the fast lane. Now that you're going to be eating more often throughout the day, take the opportunity to turn your meals and snacks into breaks from your daily routine. This should be obvious, yet if you're like most people, you probably race through your mealtimes in order to get back to "more important" things—whether it's typing a report or getting to the bank before it closes.

The fact is, few things are more important than eating. It nourishes the body as well as the soul. Since ancient times, people have used the daily repast to take a pause in their lives, whether for conversation or personal reflection. These breaks are among the simplest and healthiest of human pleasures, and they're more important than ever, given the frenzied pace of the modern world.

Use the minutes of your meal or snack to stop whatever else you may be doing. Listen to music (classical is best), gaze out the window, or head outside and find a spot where you can eat in relative peace and quiet. You'll feel and perform better the rest of the day.

MENUS FOR MSON EATING

My wife Leslie and I have created the following menus to whet your interest in and appetite for the MSOn Eating Plan. Please keep in mind that they're suggestions, not requirements. Too many diets prescribe foods and portions. The MSOn Eating Plan isn't a diet. It's a focused, strategic eating style that's tailored to your size and activity level.

The MSOn Eating Plan builds on the principles of biochemical individuality. A concept pioneered by biochemist Roger Williams, PhD, it means that each of us is unique in how we digest and absorb various foods, and how we respond to them. You need to pay attention to your own body when deciding what or how much to eat in any meal or snack.

For this reason, our menus don't specify portion sizes. The ideal portion for you is the one that meets your body's energy needs and satisfies your appetite without supplying any extra calories. You shouldn't be stuffing yourself.

Use these menus as a starting point for changing about what, when, and why you eat. Then create your own, personalized plan. The only caveat is that you follow the 3 + 4 formula—3 meals plus 4 snacks per day.

For those meals and snacks in italic, you can find recipes beginning on page 269. Store any leftovers for another day.

DAY 1

Breakfast: Muesli
Midmorning snack: *Peanut Butter Burst* (page 376); small banana
Lunch: *Roasted Chicken Salad with Mango and Pistachios* (page 299), served with several whole grain crackers
Midafternoon snack: Edamame (fresh soybeans) or a small handful of roasted soy nuts or walnuts; part-skim cheese stick
Predinner snack: Small cup (6 to 8 ounces) tomato soup made with fat-free milk and served with 2 low-fat whole grain crackers
Dinner: *Italian Insalata Mista* (page 293); *Roasted Salmon in Parchment with Lemon and Dill* (page 341); *Broccoli and White Bean Puree* (page 354) or steamed broccoli with lemon; *Blueberry Walnut Biscotti* (page 361) or 1 slice whole grain bread
Evening snack: *Chocolate-Raspberry Tapioca Parfait* (page 363)

DAY 2

Breakfast: *Strawberry Sunrise Shake* (page 47); 1 slice whole grain toast with a very light smear of peanut butter, all-fruit spread, or light cream cheese
Midmorning snack: A small handful of unsalted almonds; a piece of fresh fruit (apple, orange, plum, or peach)
Lunch: *Seafood Chowder* (page 312); mixed green salad with low-fat, sugar-free dressing
Midafternoon snack: Low-fat cottage cheese served with several low-fat whole grain crackers

Predinner snack: Small serving edamame (fresh soybeans) or small handful roasted soy nuts
Dinner: *Beet and Apple Salad with Cheese and Walnuts* (page 287); *Roasted Chicken Breasts with Lentil Ragout* (page 330); *Garlic Green Beans* (page 349) or steamed green beans with lemon; *Smashed Orange-Ginger Sweet Potatoes* (page 359)
Evening snack: *Ricotta Cheesecake Cup* (page 374)

DAY 3

Breakfast: Scrambled eggs or Egg Beaters with part skim cheese and salsa, served over 1 slice whole grain toast; small glass of orange or tomato juice
Midmorning snack: Low-fat, sugar-free yogurt
Lunch: *Greek Chopped Salad* (page 289), served with several whole grain crackers
Midafternoon snack: Small portion of fresh fruit; small handful of unsalted walnuts
Predinner snack: Small cup (6 to 8 ounces) minestrone soup served with 2 low-fat whole grain crackers
Dinner: *Seafood and White Bean Chili* (page 309); *Multigrain Cloverleaf Roll* (page 280) or 1 slice whole grain bread; assorted raw vegetable plate with low-fat dip
Evening snack: *Oatmeal Chocolate Chip Cookie* (page 366)

DAY 4

Breakfast: Plain low-fat yogurt, topped with low-fat granola and mixed berries
Midmorning snack: 1 whole grain toasted pita topped with a very light smear of peanut butter, all-fruit spread, or light cream cheese
Lunch: *Black Bean Soup with Lime* (page 304); mixed greens with fresh tomatoes and low-fat, sugar-free dressing
Midafternoon snack: Several whole grain crackers topped with *Roasted Garlic Hummus* (page 271)
Predinner snack: Small portion fresh fruit (such as half an apple) served with 1 tablespoon low-fat plain yogurt or small handful unsalted almonds or walnuts
Dinner: *Asian Cashew Shrimp with Brown Rice* (page 337); *Jicama Slaw* (page 294)
Evening snack: *Light Pumpkin Cheesecake* (page 368)

CHAPTER 22

■   ■   ■

Protein Principles

During the low-fat movement of the 1990s, protein suffered the same persecution as fat, in large part because the two tend to occur in tandem in foods. If fat was bad, the theory went, then protein had to be bad as well.

Eventually, this thinking began to shift, as carbohydrates became the bad guys in the battle of the bulge. We were free to eat as much protein as we wanted, in any form we pleased.

Between the two extremes is a healthier, more balanced view of protein, which finally is gaining ground among experts and laypeople alike. It acknowledges the vital role of protein in human life. Quite simply, we need it not just to sustain optimal Meta-Stat function, but to survive.

What matters most with protein—as with carbohydrate and fat—is the type and quantity in our diets. Protein gets its structure from long chains of amino acids. Our bodies are able to produce some of the amino acids, but the rest come from foods. We need to be sure that we're getting enough of these essential amino acids by choosing high-quality protein sources. And we need to eat them on a regular basis, since our bodies have a very limited capacity for storing extra protein. As with eating generally, the timing of protein sources is critical. If you eat a large amount at once, then deprive yourself for hours, your

Meta-Stat setting bounces between high and low. That's precisely what you don't want.

To get the maximum benefit from protein, you need to know which kinds are most absorbable, which foods provide them, and how to incorporate those foods into your diet at regular intervals. Because the amino acids from proteins remain in the bloodstream for only about 4 hours after eating, it makes sense to include protein sources in most if not all of your meals and snacks.

FAT BURNER EXTRAORDINAIRE

When we don't eat enough high-quality protein throughout the day, our bodies may respond by slowing metabolism, as if preparing for a long stretch of hibernation. On the other hand, an optimal protein intake instantly increases fat burning, or thermogenesis. In fact, a protein-rich meal or snack can burn 40 percent more calories than a high-carbohydrate alternative.[1] It boosts oxygen consumption by 200 to 300 percent, an indicator of a much higher metabolic rate.

META-STAT STARTER

Cool Down, Then Eat Up

Some experts recommend eating 15 to 25 grams of protein immediately following an intense strength-training workout. This is when muscles are absorbing more protein for faster recovery. By eating protein right after exercising, it gives an extra boost to metabolism, too.[2]

In a small study at Vanderbilt University, 10 healthy adults engaged in 60 minutes of moderate-intensity exercise.[3] Then half of the group consumed a protein-carbohydrate supplement immediately following the workout, while the rest waited for 3 hours. The researchers found that muscles synthesized protein 3 times faster, and replenished their glycogen stores 3.5 times faster, in those who got the supplement right away.

What's the best post-workout protein source? Good choices include a protein shake, a protein bar, lean turkey or chicken breast, low-fat soy milk, or low-fat dairy products.[4]

Recent research has shown that high-protein, moderate-carbohydrate, low-fat meals produce a greater and longer-lasting sense of fullness than high-fat meals.[5] A chief reason is that protein breaks down more slowly than fat and even more slowly than carbohydrate.

In Australian studies, people who followed high-protein diets showed significantly greater reductions in total fat and abdominal fat than people who followed low-protein diets.[6] "High-protein" wasn't so high at all—just 30 percent of calories, compared with 15 percent of calories in the low-protein group.

Protein also triggers the production of glucagon, the hormone that enables the body to use fat as fuel instead of storing it. It's essential for building new muscle tissue, as well as for boosting energy. According to studies by Judith Wurtman, PhD, a research scientist at MIT, protein tends to change neurotransmitter balance in favor of alertness[7]—a sign that your Meta-Stat is ramping up. You can test by eating a protein snack when you need an extra burst of energy and mental sharpness—before heading into an important meeting, for example.

Researchers have asserted that natural protein supports the production and secretion of human growth hormone (HGH).[8] In particular, consuming a protein-rich food or beverage right after exercise may elevate secretion of the hormone.[9] In both women and men, HGH appears to enhance fat burning and energy production.

EAT MORE PROTEIN, BUT WISELY

As people have reintroduced protein to their diets, the general tendency has been to not cut back on anything else. Big mistake. The extra calories can overwhelm the body's metabolic adaptability and turn to body fat. Look for places to save calories—by cutting back on high-fat chips and other munchies, for example. And be sure to choose lean, high-quality protein sources.

Actually, if you're getting an adequate amount of complex carbohydrate in your diet, you don't need to eat as much protein. With enough slow-burning complex carbs at its disposal, the body won't tap muscle and organ tissue for protein to use as fuel, so more dietary protein is available for other purposes.[10]

So just how much protein do you need? In its 2002 nutritional guidelines, the National Academy of Sciences proposed that an optimal protein intake—the amount necessary to protect against chronic degenerative disease—could be as high as 35 percent of calories. The low end of the healthy range is 20 percent of calories. So if you typically eat 2,000 calories a day, between 400 and 700 of those calories should come from protein.

The more active you are, and the more muscle mass you have, the more protein your body requires. Studies have shown that men and women who exercise at high intensity on a regular basis need about 1 gram of protein per pound of body weight per day, if not more.[11] That's lean, high-quality protein, not the kind that's laden with fat.

To determine your optimal daily protein intake, follow these steps.

1. Estimate your ideal healthy weight. The operative word here is "healthy." Chances are, you already have some idea of how much you should weigh. But if you're like most people, your goal weight may be influenced by factors beyond health—such as the images of celebrities and supermodels in popular magazines.

Truth be told, some more objective measures may be no more reliable. For many years, physicians and other health professionals relied on the Metropolitan Life Insurance height/weight tables to determine ideal weights for their patients. Published in 1959, the tables provided a graphic representation of which policyholders had the lowest mortality rates. Because they lived the longest, their height/weight measures were seen as healthiest.

Over time, the tables came under fire for failing to account for other variables, such as age, ethnicity, body type, and body fat percentage. In response, MetLife issued revised tables in 1983. The primary change was to add 10 percent to the ideal weight for each height.

The National Institutes of Health cautions against using either version of the MetLife tables as the sole indicator of your ideal weight.[12] After reviewing 25 major studies on weight and longevity, a Harvard research team concluded that the research used as the basis for the height/weight tables underestimated the health risks of being overweight. Any assumptions based on the tables contain inherent biases that allow ideal weights to creep upward.[13]

Your best bet may be to discuss your ideal weight with your physician or a dietitian. Keep in mind, too, that as you trim fat and build muscle tone, you probably will look much thinner than the number on your scale may indicate. That's because muscle is heavier than fat.

2. Determine your daily calorie limit. Write your approximate ideal weight in the appropriate space below. Do the math, and you'll get a good estimate of your optimal daily calorie intake.

If You Are . . .	And You Want to Weigh . . .	Multiply by . . .	For Your Daily Calorie Limit
A sedentary woman	_____ lbs.	12	_____
A sedentary man	_____ lbs.	14	_____
A moderately active woman	_____ lbs.	15	_____
A moderately active man	_____ lbs.	17	_____
A very active woman	_____ lbs.	18	_____
A very active man	_____ lbs.	20	_____

3. Calculate the amount of protein you need. Multiply your daily calories by 0.25 if you're very inactive, 0.30 if you're relatively active, or 0.35 if you're very active. Divide this figure by 4—the number of calories in 1 gram of protein—to arrive at your daily protein budget.

SEEK QUALITY AND VARIETY

Once you know your optimal daily protein intake, you can assess whether you're getting enough—and, just as important, whether you're getting the right kind. Of course, the leaner the protein source, the healthier. Try not to load up on high-fat proteins like bacon and sausage. True, some diets allow such foods in nearly unlimited quantities. While they may help shed fat, we don't fully understand their long-term impact on health. Your best bet is to go lean. Here are some recommendations.

Shop for wild salmon and other seafood. In the Cooper household, wild salmon is a family favorite. I even have it for breakfast on occasion, with fresh fruit as an accompaniment.

Wild salmon is not only high in protein, it also contains an abundance of omega-3 and omega-6 fatty acids. These "good fats" are essential to energy production and fat loss.

Other smart choices in the fish and seafood category include Alaskan halibut, tuna, trout, sea bass, striped bass, farm-raised tilapia, mahi mahi, herring, sardines, Dungeness crab, shrimp, oysters, clams, and farm-raised mussels and scallops. The oil from all these species enhances the efficiency of the hormone leptin, which reduces fat cell size and enhances fat loss.[14] For this and other reasons, a growing number of experts recommend eating fish two to four times a week.

Choose skinless turkey and chicken breast. Lean animal protein isn't all that easy to come by. Much of the red meat and pork that's available in supermarkets supplies too much "bad" saturated fat and few if any good fats. The sole exceptions are turkey and chicken. By removing the skin, you vastly reduce the proportion of saturated fat to lean protein.

A typical 3-ounce serving of skinless turkey breast supplies 0.2 gram of saturated fat. By comparison, a same-size serving of ham contains 5.5 grams of saturated fat; 3 ounces of flank steak has nearly 5 grams.

Stick with organic poultry as much as possible. It limits your exposure to harmful growth additives, among other contaminants.

Enjoy an egg on occasion. After years of avoiding eggs, many people are welcoming this longtime dietary staple back into their diets. And for good reason: Eggs are an ideal protein source because they contain no saturated fat. They not only have little effect on total cholesterol, they might raise beneficial HDL cholesterol.

If you like eggs, feel free to enjoy one several times a week, whether for breakfast or as part of another meal. With eggs as with poultry, I suggest scouting around for organic, which have measurably higher levels of beneficial omega-3 fatty acids.

Tap the slimming power of dairy. There's mounting evidence that people who regularly consume fat-free and low-fat dairy products as part of a balanced diet are less likely to be overweight. Beyond their protein content, dairy products are among the best dietary sources of calcium. This mineral triggers the production of hormones that elevate metabolism and prevent fat storage.[15]

In a study led by Michael Zemel, PhD, at the University of Tennessee, men who added three servings of yogurt to their daily diets lost 61 percent more body fat and 81 percent more abdominal fat over the course of 12 weeks than men who didn't eat yogurt. Calcium seems to be key. According to Dr. Zemel, the mineral helps the body burn existing fat while limiting the manufacture of new fat.[16] Choose fat-free or low-fat plain yogurt and add your own fresh fruit for sweetness. That way, you'll avoid the fattening natural and artificial sweeteners in flavored yogurt.

Another healthy option in the dairy aisle is cottage cheese. Researchers in Denmark report that people who replaced 20 percent of their carbohydrate calories with high-protein foods such as cottage cheese experienced measurable increases in energy—and the effect lasted all day long. The cottage cheese eaters also burned 5 percent more calories.[17]

In limited quantities, low-fat cheese is an acceptable protein source, but be cautious with cheese dips and spreads, as well as small mountains of sliced cheese and crackers. Eating too much of these "finger foods" is all too easy. A healthier alternative is reduced-fat mozzarella sticks. They go anywhere, and they taste good.

Give soy a taste drive. Soy is something of a rarity in that it's one of the few plant sources of complete protein. It's also rich in vitamins, minerals, disease-fighting phytonutrients, and soluble fiber.

In my family, roasted soy nuts are a popular snack. Each ¼-cup serving supplies 15 grams of protein. One-half cup of tofu contains 18 to 20 grams. You also might try soy milk, tempeh, and edamame (soybeans that are harvested before they ripen).

Go crazy for nuts. Nuts have something of a bad reputation nutrition-wise. While some varieties are high in fat, most contain unsaturated fats that help reduce bad LDL cholesterol while raising good HDL cholesterol. Several long-term, large-scale studies have produced evidence to conclude that people who eat nuts at least twice a week as part of a balanced diet are at 30 to 50 percent lower risk for heart attack and heart disease.[18]

What's more, nuts—specifically, almonds—appear to aid weight loss, according to a study from Purdue University.[19] The mechanism is unclear, but researchers speculate that the protein in nuts may help burn more calories during the digestive process. Nuts also promote satiety, or a feeling of fullness, so you eat less.

With nuts, the key is portion control. You can't eat them one handful after another. As long as you choose low-sodium varieties and keep the serving size in check, you'll be fine.

An ounce of peanuts, pistachios, almonds, or walnuts supplies 8 grams of protein—the equivalent of the protein in a glass of milk. Other healthful choices include Brazil nuts, cashews, chestnuts, hazelnuts, pecans, and pine nuts, as well as pumpkin seeds, sesame seeds, and sunflower seeds.[20]

Spill the beans—on your plate. Beans are among the most versatile of protein sources.[21] Though they aren't complete proteins, they do supply essential amino acids. One of these amino acids, lysine, supports the synthesis of carnitine, which is used by cells to generate energy.

Beans are also rich in soluble fiber, which helps balance blood sugar. Because of their fiber content, beans help prevent the insulin resistance that can lead to fat gain.

Aim for three or four ½-cup servings per week of beans and other legumes. Among the most popular varieties are black, pinto, navy, lima, and great Northern beans, as well as chickpeas (garbanzo beans) and lentils. Just take care not to prepare them in saturated fat, such as butter, lard, or vegetable shortening. For some delicious recipe ideas, see Part 6.

CHAPTER 23

■ ■ ■

Right Carbs, Right Times

I magine that you're spending a cold winter's night in a mountain cabin with only a small wood-burning stove to provide heat. You have two kinds of fuel on hand—a can of kerosene, and a pile of dry oak logs. Which fuel would you use if you wanted to stay warm?

If you pour on the kerosene, you'll get an explosion of heat, but it won't last very long. Light the logs, and as every camper knows, you'll have a slow-burning fire to last until morning.

By now you might be wondering just what heat sources have to do with carbohydrates. The standard American diet has its own version of kerosene—fast-burning, flash-in-the-pan simple carbs like candy and soda, as well as refined breads and pastas. Complex carbohydrates— such as whole grains, legumes, fresh fruits, and vegetables—are the oak logs. By comparison, they're a far better energy source.

Your Meta-Stat responds very well to complex carbohydrates and very poorly to the simple variety. There's a reason for that. Our ancestors ate mostly plant foods that they had foraged from field and forest. Plant foods are complex carbs. So the Meta-Stat evolved with complex carbs as its primary fuel. The body metabolizes them in a way that creates a nice, steady fire as an energy source.

As we humans introduced simple carbohydrates into our diet, The Meta-Stat didn't know how to respond. Much of this fast-burning,

Become an Occasional Fruitophile

Are you hungry right now? If it's about time for a snack and you're feeling like something sweet, reach for an orange, peach, tangerine, or some berries. These and other fruits are rich in natural fiber. Research suggests that a small dose of the natural sweetness in fruit may quash cravings for refined sugar or fat.[1]

What's more, because a piece of fresh fruit takes up a lot of space in the stomach, you won't feel hungry as quickly after eating one. In fact, a Pennsylvania State University research team led by Barbara Rolls, PhD, determined that eating an apple before each meal can produce substantial fat loss, even without dieting.[2]

short-term fuel goes to waste. Or perhaps I should say waist, since overindulging in simple carbs can lead to fat retention and weight gain.

Still, it's important not to lump together all carbohydrates and label them as bad. Unfortunately, this is what many popular diets do. If you give up carbs completely, you might lose some water weight, but your body fat will stay put. The real secret to successful fat loss—not to mention energy production—is eating the right kind of carbohydrates in the right amounts. This will keep your Meta-Stat functioning at its peak.

CARBOHYDRATES: A QUICK PRIMER

Carbohydrates are the primary source of glucose, or blood sugar—the essential fuel of every cell. Glucose helps maintain the body's temperature and powers many of its processes, from respiration and digestion to immune function and tissue repair.

Carbohydrates take three basic forms, each named for the complexity of its molecular structure: monosaccharides, disaccharides, and polysaccharides. Of these, polysaccharides are the most complex. They consist of long chains of sugar units that have bonded together.

Since Neolithic times 12,000 years ago, most humans have survived on diets that feature an abundance of complex carbohydrates and a few simple carbohydrates. In fact, these diets are such good sources of nutrients that the World Health Organization Expert Committee on Cardiovascular Disease has noted them for contributing to "a good life expectancy at all ages."[3]

On the other hand, simple carbohydrates—primarily refined sugar and white flour and the foods that contain them—contribute to a host of health problems. For example, simple carbs are known to elevate blood fats and cholesterol.[4] One particular kind of simple carb, a sugar known as sucrose, appears to deplete the trace mineral chromium. A shortage of chromium can contribute to heart disease and diabetes,[5] as well as breast cancer.[6]

The trouble with simple carbohydrates is that they enter the bloodstream swiftly, spiking blood sugar to far above healthy levels. In response, the body releases extra insulin to remove all the sugar from the bloodstream. Blood sugar levels plummet back to normal, but not without depleting energy and stirring up appetite.

Even so-called natural sugars—maple syrup, maple sugar, date sugar, barley malt, honey, brown rice syrup, molasses, fruit juice, and fruit concentrates—aren't the healthy alternatives they may seem to be. Some are modest sources of minerals, but that doesn't outweigh their effect on blood sugar.

MAXING OUT ON SWEETS?

According to the US Surgeon General, the average intake of simple sugars rose by 74 percent from 1962 to 2000. Sodas and juice drinks account for as much as 80 percent of this increase.

In fairness, we really can't cut back on simple sugars if we don't know where they're coming from or how much we're consuming. The Nutrition Facts labels on foods list sugars as a factor of "Total Carbohydrate," but not all foods carry these labels. Even when they do, you have nothing against which to compare the sugar content, since there's no official Daily Value for sugar.

According to the USDA, people who follow a 2,000-calorie diet

The Hazards of a "Sugar High"

Sodas and many juice drinks get their sweetness from large quantities of high-fructose corn syrup, a simple sugar. Researchers are finding evidence that constant exposure to sugars such as fructose can cause cravings much like an addictive drug. One Princeton University scientist found that taking rats off a high-sugar diet threw them into a state of anxiety much like what's seen in withdrawal from morphine.[7]

Research suggests that high levels of dietary fructose (as well as dietary fat) confuse the brain chemistry, muting the signals that normally would produce a sense of fullness after a meal.[8] Usually, these satiety signals come from peptides, messenger chemicals that are regulated by hormones such as insulin, leptin, and ghrelin. But when we consume foods and drinks that are loaded with fructose, the overzealous sweetener throws off the regulation of these key hormones. As the brain loses its ability to respond to these hormones, body fat increases.

If you must drink soda, it makes sense to choose sugar-free varieties. Some studies suggest that switching from regular soda to diet can contribute to significant fat loss over a period of 10 weeks.[9] In general, though, it's much healthier to drink water—perhaps with a squeeze of lemon or lime for flavor—or unsweetened tea.

should limit themselves to about 40 grams of added sugars a day. That's the equivalent of 10 teaspoons of sugar. For comparison, a typical megasize soda contains as much as 25 teaspoons of corn syrup or refined sugar. That's more than double the added-sugar "cap" for a single day.

Of course, added sugars aren't the only sources of refined carbohydrates. Others include white-flour breads and pastas, as well as all processed foods. The refined carbs from these foods contribute to fatigue and fat gain.[10]

WHEN SIMPLE ISN'T BETTER

The human body can't handle more than a few grams of refined carbohydrate at a time without ramping up its fat-making and fat-storing processes. The surge in insulin that follows the rapid breakdown of refined carbs is a known contributor to fat gain, not to mention fatigue.

Along the timeline of human evolution, the introduction of refined carbohydrates is a relatively recent phenomenon. The body simply hasn't developed the mechanisms to handle the sugar overload. It reacts the only way it knows how—by clearing the bloodstream of the excess sugar as quickly as possible.

"People simply do not stop gaining weight by eating large quantities of pasta or white rice," says Louis Aronne, MD, director of the Comprehensive Weight Control Center at New York Weill Cornell Medical Center.[11] Like a growing number of other physicians and nutritionists, Dr. Aronne advocates a transition away from large quantities of refined carbs to moderate amounts of complex carbs such as vegetables, fruits, legumes, and whole grains. Because these foods break down slowly, they don't trigger such sharp spikes in blood sugar and insulin, so the body can continue to focus on burning fat rather than storing it.[12]

Another benefit of complex carbohydrates is that they're high in fiber, so they're more satisfying than refined carbohydrates. This means you'll feel full on less food, which further supports fat loss.

In a study at the University of Leeds in England, researchers presented participants with an assortment of low-fat complex carbohydrates and, on a separate occasion, a selection of higher-fat fare—meats, cheeses, creamy casseroles, and pastries. On average, the men and women ate half as much of the complex carbs. This is because complex carbs are more effective in stimulating the satiety signal, which tells the brain "I'm full."[13] As you make the transition from refined to complex carbohydrates, you should notice that you don't feel hungry as often.

This raises an important point: While you definitely should cut back on refined carbs, you definitely *shouldn't* give up carbohydrates altogether. Your body needs complex carbs to burn fat. Without them, fat molecules recombine to form what are known as ketone bodies. The ketones become a substitute brain fuel and, in the process, dramatically alter the body's all-important acid-base balance. This leads to ketosis, a serious medical condition that can precipitate potentially life-threatening illness.

Fiber: The Fat-Fighting Advantage

One of the reasons that complex carbohydrates are so important to the MSOn Eating Plan is that they're superior sources of dietary fiber. The phrase "dietary fiber" refers to all plant material that resists digestion. Technically, it isn't roughage, though you may hear it described as such. Rather, it ensures the smooth transit of food through the digestive tract.

Dietary fiber takes one of two primary forms: soluble and insoluble. The soluble fibers include pectin and mucilage. As the name suggests, they dissolve in water to form a gel-like substance that prevents cholesterol from being absorbed into the bloodstream.[14] The insoluble fibers—such as cellulose and hemicellulose—*absorb* water, swelling up and adding bulk to waste in the intestines. With help from insoluble fiber, waste passes much more easily.

Because they are bound to the digestible carbohydrates in whole foods, both kinds of dietary fiber slow the absorption of sugar into the bloodstream. This is why, in general, people with diabetes fare best on high-fiber diets.[15] But all of us can benefit from stable blood sugar levels, which promote fat burning rather than fat storage.

If you've been avoiding carbohydrates, you may not have been getting as much dietary fiber as you need. In my opinion, it's one reason that low-carb diets often fail. So how much fiber should you aim for? The National Cancer Institute recommends 20 to 35 grams per day, much

GET TO KNOW THE GLYCEMIC LOAD

If complex carbohydrates drive fat loss and a steady energy supply, while refined carbohydrates promote fat gain and fatigue, you obviously want more of the former and less of the latter. But how can you be sure which is which?

As a rule of thumb, complex carbohydrates tend to be whole foods like the ones that discussed throughout this chapter—vegetables, fruits, legumes, and whole grains. Anything that's manufactured or processed more likely falls into the refined carbohydrate category.

A more precise tool for evaluating the healthfulness of a carbohy-

more than the average intake of 10 grams. Other experts go even higher, to 30 to 60 grams per day.[16]

The MSOn Eating Plan emphasizes a varied diet of fresh, whole foods to ensure a plentiful supply of soluble and insoluble fiber. In general, fruit, vegetables, legumes, and whole grains are the best sources.[17] In the following list, the number of grams of fiber is per 100 grams of food.

Soluble Fiber Sources

- All-Bran (24.9)
- Shredded wheat (10.2)
- Barley (7.4)
- Asparagus (2.8)

- Brussels sprouts (2.7)
- Green beans (2.3)
- Carrots (1.9)
- Broccoli (1.7)

Insoluble Fiber Sources

- Dry oat bran (7.2)
- Dried white beans (1.7)
- Dried split peas (1.6)
- Cooked rolled oats (0.8)

- Strawberries (0.8)
- Apples (0.7)
- Bananas (0.6)

drate source is what's known as the glycemic index. Developed by David Jenkins, MD, PhD, DSc, and his colleagues at the University of Toronto, the glycemic index measures how much and how quickly a given food can raise blood sugar. It was an invaluable first step in quantifying what happens in the body when we eat certain foods.

Since its inception, the glycemic index has drawn some criticism because it uses 50-gram carbohydrate portions of foods rather than actual serving sizes. For a food like carrots, for example, you'd need to eat an entire pound to get 50 grams of carbohydrates. So researchers have revised and refined the glycemic index into a new rating system called the glycemic load. According to Walter Willett, MD, chairman of

Feel the (Calorie) Burn

Seasoning your meal or snack with a spicy seasoning may boost your metabolic rate, so you produce more energy and burn more fat. For one study that appeared in the journal *Human Nutrition/Clinical Nutrition*, participants ate identical 766-calorie meals—only some meals contained 3 grams of chili powder and 3 grams of mustard sauce, while the rest were free of spices. Researchers tracked the participants' metabolic rates for 3 hours postmeal. Their conclusion: The spicy meals raised metabolism by 25 percent, on average.[18]

In a separate study, Australian researchers found that people who ate spicy foods stayed energetic and alert significantly longer during the day than those who ate more bland fare.[19] So try adding a dash of chili powder or Tabasco or a dab of spicy mustard to your next meal or snack—any of which may rev up your postmeal metabolic rate.[20] You'll also be less likely to overeat because the flavor is so intense.

the department of nutrition at Harvard School of Public Health, "The glycemic load better reflects a food's effect on your body's biochemistry than either the amount of carbohydrate or the glycemic index alone."[21]

To determine the glycemic load of a particular food, the researchers used a more realistic portion. Again using carrots as an example, the glycemic load reflects a typical 2-ounce serving, which is much more realistic than a full pound. (For a sampling of glycemic load values for various foods, see page 228.)

There is evidence that eating foods with lower glycemic loads for breakfast can help prevent overeating for the rest of the day.[22] Still, while the glycemic load is helpful for comparing and choosing foods, especially carbohydrates, "don't plan your whole diet around it," advises Dr. Willett, who is widely regarded as one of the nation's foremost nutrition experts. He points out that "some carbohydrate-rich foods deliver far more than just blood sugar. Fruits and vegetables offer fiber, vitamins, minerals, and plenty of active phytochemicals. The same is true for intact or slightly processed grains."[23]

CARB POWER FOODS

If you've dramatically reduced your consumption of carbohydrates, now is the time to invite these nutritionally vital foods back into your meals and snacks. Just be sure to choose the right kinds of carbs in the right quantities.

As a starting point, I've put together a list of what I call Carb Power Foods. All are complex carbohydrates that supply an abundance of all-important vitamins, minerals, phytonutrients, and fiber. All have a modest effect on blood sugar and insulin, maintaining both at relatively stable levels. When consumed in moderation as part of the MSOn Eating Plan, the Carb Power Foods promote fat burning and energy production. Let's look at each one in turn.

Beans. Besides being rich in protein, beans are a top-notch source of complex carbohydrates, vitamins, minerals, and soluble fiber.

Berries. Packed with antioxidants, berries—including blueberries, blackberries, boysenberries, cherries, cranberries, currants, raspberries, and strawberries—help protect against disease and may slow the aging process. I try to eat a small serving of one of these fruits on most days. When fresh berries aren't in season, frozen are just as good.

In my family, a favorite snack is dried organic blueberries. A very small handful supplies a wealth of nutrients and a boost to energy.

Broccoli. Along with other cruciferous vegetables, broccoli is among the most nutrient-dense complex carbohydrates around. It supplies calcium to build strong bones, plus a host of vitamins and other minerals to support the body's fat-fighting and energy-enhancing processes.

Cantaloupe. It's a superb source of vitamins A and C, with some soluble fiber but relatively few calories and virtually no fat. If you're not fond of cantaloupe, peaches and plums are terrific alternative choices.

Garlic and onions. Beyond their potent flavor, garlic and onions contain substances that not only help burn fat but also lower blood cholesterol.[24] They add zing to any almost any entrée or side dish.

Oats and other whole grains. Whole grains are an excellent source of fiber, plus healthy fats and a host of vitamins and minerals. These

(continued on page 230)

Get to Know the Glycemic Load

The following chart allows you to compare at a glance the glycemic loads of various foods. In general, the lower a food's GL value, the better. A GL of less than 16 is ideal.

Still, you can't make your food choices on GL values alone. Calories count, too. Take peanuts as an example. With a GL of 1 per ½ cup serving, they may seem like a smart snack. But the 330 calories is a tad on the high side.

By the same token, foods with high GL values aren't automatically off-limits. Simply pair them with foods that have low GLs. It's the overall glycemic load of a meal that's key. So look for foods in the low to moderate GL range, watch your portion sizes, and—above all—choose for taste!

Food	Serving Size	Glycemic Load	Calories
Fruits			
Apple	1 average	6	75
Apricots	4 medium	6	70
Banana	1 average	12	90
Cherries	15 cherries	3	85
Grapefruit	1 average	5	75
Grapes	40 grapes	13	160
Kiwi	1 average	6	45
Mango	1 small	14	110
Orange	1 average	5	65
Papaya	1 cup cubes	9	55
Peach	1 average	7	70
Pear	1 medium	10	125
Pineapple	1 cup cubes	7	75
Plums	2 medium	5	70
Pumpkin	1 cup, mashed	3	85
Raisins	½ cup	42	250
Strawberries	1 cup	1	50
Watermelon	1 cup cubes	7	50
Fruit Juices			
Apple juice	1 cup	12	135
Grapefruit juice	1 cup	9	115
Orange juice	1 cup	15	110

Food	Serving Size	Glycemic Load	Calories
Pineapple juice	1 cup	15	130
Tomato juice	1 cup	4	40

Vegetables

Food	Serving Size	Glycemic Load	Calories
Corn	1 ear, 1 cup kernels	20	130
Potato, baked	1 small	34	220
Yam	1 cup, cooked	13	160

Legumes

Food	Serving Size	Glycemic Load	Calories
Black beans	1 cup, cooked	82	35
Garbanzo beans	1 cup, cooked	13	285
Kidney beans	1 cup, cooked	10	210
Lentils	1 cup, cooked	72	30
Peas	1 cup	31	35
Soybeans	1 cup, cooked	1	300

Grains

Food	Serving Size	Glycemic Load	Calories
Barley	1 cup, cooked	11	190
Brown rice	1 cup	16	215
White rice	1 cup, cooked	23	210
Whole grain bread	1 slice	14	80–120

Cereals

Food	Serving Size	Glycemic Load	Calories
Cream of wheat	1 cup, cooked	22	350
Raisin bran	1 cup	29	185
Shredded wheat	1 cup mini squares	15	110

Dairy Products

Food	Serving Size	Glycemic Load	Calories
Ice cream, low-fat	1 cup	13	220
Milk, whole	1 cup	3	150
Pudding, vanilla	1 cup	16	250
Yogurt, with fruit	1 cup	9	200+

Nuts

Food	Serving Size	Glycemic Load	Calories
Cashews	½ cup	4	395
Peanuts	½ cup	1	330

Snack Foods

Food	Serving Size	Glycemic Load	Calories
Corn chips	2 ounces	21	350
Pizza	1 large slice	20	300
Popcorn	2 cups	16	110
Pretzels	1 ounce	33	115

Sources: *American Journal of Clinical Nutrition,* July 2002; 76: 5–56.
Heber, D. *The L.A. Shape Diet* (Regan Books, 2004).

Go for Color

As scientists learn more about the disease-fighting compounds in fruits and vegetables, it's becoming clear that the more vibrant the color of a food, the more potent the protection against fat gain and disease. Skins of vivid red, orange, blue-purple, and dark green hues reveal a wealth of phytochemicals beneath. In fact, the nutrients in fruits and vegetables are so important to optimal health that a number of leading scientists now recommend 9 to 10 servings a day rather than the standard 5 servings.[25] Incorporating these foods into your meals and snacks whenever possible is vital to energy production and fat loss.

days, you can choose from many different whole grains, from the common whole wheat and rye to the more exotic buckwheat and quinoa.

Oats, in particular, appear to offer important health benefits. For example, they have a very beneficial effect on blood sugar and insulin,[26] which can keep metabolism in fat-burning mode. Oats also are among the few good sources of the trace mineral selenium, which is vital to hormone balance.

When shopping for whole grains, pay very careful attention to the ingredients list. You should see the word *whole* with any grain. Often what appears to be whole in fact is refined.

If you're partial to hot cereal in the morning, try steel-cut or old-fashioned oats or Kashi. (Instant oatmeal has a higher glycemic load.) Among cold cereals, look for brands with minimal sugar and other sweeteners. And don't overlook whole grain pasta, which is now widely available.

Oranges. Oranges, as well as other citrus fruits, are rich in fiber and vitamin C. I suggest eating one whole fruit, or even two, a day.

Pumpkin and other orange, red, and yellow vegetables. These veggies get their color from carotenoids, potent antioxidants that play important roles in disease prevention. One well-known carotenoid, beta-carotene, is converted to vitamin A in the body.

Soy. Soybeans and soybean products are rich in both complex carbohydrates and protein, not to mention fiber.

Spinach. Spinach has more documented health benefits than almost any other food. Beyond its supplies of antioxidants and omega-3s, it's an important source of coenzyme Q_{10}, which is vital to cellular energy production and fat burning.[27]

Tomatoes. Tomatoes are nutritional powerhouses. They may be best known for lycopene, a carotenoid that may help protect against heart disease and certain kinds of cancer. Interestingly, cooked tomatoes contain up to eight times as much lycopene as raw. (Watermelon also has lycopene, but it's a bit too high in fructose, a natural sugar.)

CHAPTER 24

■ ■ ■

Good Fats Aren't Fattening

Through all the years of debate about why we gain weight and how we should lose it, at least one fact is irrefutable: Excess dietary fat leads to excess body fat. According to Robert E. T. Stark, MD, author of *Controlling Fat for Life* and past president of the American Society of Bariatric Physicians, more than 90 percent of dietary fat calories end up in the body's fat deposits.[1]

That said, not all dietary fat is the enemy. Recent scientific studies show that a modest amount of the right kind of dietary fat is absolutely vital to fat burning and energy production, as well as to hormone balance and overall health.[2] It's too much of the wrong kind of dietary fat that causes trouble.

Different fats have different effects on your Meta-Stat. The fat from, say, a chuck roast takes one route through the body; the fat from salmon, another. I'll say more about the chemical structure and absorption of various fats later in the chapter. For now, suffice it to say that you don't need much beef fat to turn your Meta-Stat from on to off. On the other hand, the essential fatty acids in coldwater fish like salmon are excellent for your Meta-Stat.

Improving the proportion of good fats to bad in your diet is important not just for weight management but for general health. Still, it isn't the only factor that influences the number on the scale. Consider that in the United States, the average fat intake has dropped from 40 percent of calories to 34 percent—while the rate of weight gain and obesity is on the rise. And according to European population surveys, women who eat the least fat are the most likely to weigh more than they should.[3] Clearly, other factors beyond dietary fat are at work.

In this chapter, you'll learn how to distinguish the good fats from the bad ones and how to increase the former while reducing the latter. Even with the good fats, though, moderation is key.

THE BAD FATS

Bad fats seem to be lurking almost everywhere—in cheeses and red meats, in fried and processed foods. The most harmful are the trans fatty acids, also known as trans fats. They contribute to high cholesterol as well as obesity, both serious risk factors for heart disease.

Trans fats are by-products of hydrogenation, the manufacturing process by which liquid vegetable oil becomes solid. Though they're most common in margarine, spreads, and dressings, they occur in virtually every processed food. In fact, as many as 40 percent of all foods on supermarket shelves contain trans fats.

Beyond the trans fat dilemma, most foods that are high in bad fats are also high in sugar.[4] This potent combination—found in ice cream, baked goods, and chocolate candies, among other traditionally favorite foods—may be especially hazardous to your health, not to mention your waistline. Eating too many fatty, sugary foods can disrupt the metabolic processes that keep your Meta-Stat in balance.

Just as sugar is stimulating the production of insulin, large quantities of fat are entering the bloodstream. Insulin sensitizes fat cells for fat storage. Sugar also boosts the activity of lipoprotein lipase (LPL), a fat-storing enzyme. So just as insulin is opening up the fat cells, LPL drives the circulating fat right in.[5]

Essentially, in the presence of sugar, fat calories are more likely to end up in storage than burned for fuel. The net effect is a dramatic increase in fat gain, with much of it preferentially deposited around the waist and abdomen.[6] And as abdominal fat builds up, the Meta-Stat dials down.

If that doesn't convince you to curtail your consumption of bad fats, perhaps this will: Eating too much fat contributes to mental and physical fatigue.[7] "The viscosity [thickness] of blood measurably increases" after a high-fat meal or snack, explains Neil Barnard, MD, faculty member at George Washington University School of Medicine. "This may be a contributor to the mental and physical slowdown that many people feel after eating."[8]

"Fat seems to slow processes like thought and movement," agrees Judith J. Wurtman, PhD, a nutritional researcher at MIT. "It makes people very lethargic. During the long digestive process that follows a high-fat meal, more blood is diverted to the stomach and intestines and away from the brain."[9]

This is why you're much better off spending your daily fat calories on good fats rather than bad fats. Where bad fats disrupt energy production and fat burning, good fats actually support these processes.

THE GOOD FATS

You may know the good fats by their more formal name: essential fatty acids (EFAs). They're essential because their unique chemical structure allows for their use in the production of prostaglandins. These hormonelike substances regulate key biochemical processes and are vital to metabolism and nerve function.

In the body, EFAs help regulate fat levels, water balance, and a wide range of metabolic functions. Recent research also suggests that these good fats reduce triglycerides and improve insulin sensitivity, benefits that collectively reduce the risk of fat gain.[10]

Unlike sluggish saturated fats and harmful trans fats, EFAs have unique properties that enhance rather than hinder metabolism. True, EFAs are high in calories, and just like bad fats, they can contribute to weight gain if you overdo. Still, they are able to metabolize in ways that are beneficial rather than detrimental to your health, and your Meta-Stat.

The EFAs take two forms: alpha-linolenic acid, an omega-3 fatty acid, and linolenic acid, an omega-6 fatty acid. Both EFAs, and especially the omega-3s, play essential roles in energy balance and blood sugar metabolism. Researchers have observed a phenomenon known as fuel partitioning, in which the EFAs direct blood sugar toward the muscles for use as fuel. Simultaneously, they're directing other fatty acids away from triglyceride synthesis and fat storage.

Research has shown that omega-3 fatty acids are able to increase the size of mitochondria, the cellular structures that generate energy and burn fat. Each cell has two sets of mitochondria, and omega-3s build up both of them.[11] EFAs in general enhance the production of enzymes such as carnitine palmitoyltransferase, which assists in the transport of fatty acids into the mitochondria for use as fuel while inhibiting the production of enzymes that contribute to fat storage.[12]

Omega-3 fatty acids also have the ability to enhance thermogenesis, the all-important process by which the body burns fat to produce energy and heat. Thus, the higher percentage of omega-3s you consume, the more you elevate your fat-burning power.[13]

The typical dietary ratio of omega-6 to omega-3 fatty acids is between 10:1 and 100:1. That's way out of proportion. The World Health Organization recommends a ratio between 5:1 and 10:1. A growing number of scientists advocate a more even split between the two EFAs, with the optimal ratio somewhere in the neighborhood of 3:1.

The human body cannot manufacture its own EFAs, so you need to be sure to get enough from your diet. This requires careful planning. Your goal is to raise your omega-3 consumption while cutting back on omega-6s. Unfortunately, while omega-6s are quite abundant in foods, omega-3s are harder to come by. Unless you eat significant amounts of whole grains, nuts, and seeds, you're likely to come up short.

Certain vegetable oils, such as soy and walnut, do contain omega-3 fatty acids, but processing and storage reduce the omega-3 content. From a chemical perspective, EFAs are quite fragile. They will spoil rapidly if they aren't stored properly.

To enhance your EFA intake, especially of omega-3s, I recommend the following:

- Eat wild salmon or another type of fatty fish at least twice a week. Salmon—along with mackerel, trout, and sardines—are among the best dietary sources of omega-3 fatty acids.

Olive Oil (in Moderation) Burns Fat, Too

Like the essential fatty acids, monounsaturated fats support fat burning rather than fat storage. Australian researchers have found that the body uses more fat as fuel when we eat meals prepared with a monounsaturated fat, such as olive oil, rather than a saturated fat.[14]

During metabolism, the body breaks down various fuel sources in chemical reactions that release energy. Then other chemical reactions determine the appropriate use of this energy. Any excess energy molecules can be burned off simply by switching on what are known as uncoupling proteins, or UCPs. Researchers have determined that olive oil increases the activity of UCPs in fat and muscle tissue, thereby boosting metabolism.[15]

Include olive oil or another monounsaturated fat, such as canola oil or avocados, in your diet. Just pay attention to serving sizes, since too much of even a good fat can inhibit fat burning and energy production.[16]

- Sprinkle fresh sunflower or pumpkin seeds on salads.

- Enjoy a snack of walnuts, almonds, pecans, or hazelnuts. Just be careful not to overdo.

- Replace any refined grains in your diet with whole grains. For example, the wheat germ in whole wheat is a good source of EFAs.

- Choose free-range chicken or turkey whenever possible. It may contain higher amounts of EFAs.

- Look for eggs from free-range chickens. They have up to 30 percent more omega-3s than traditional eggs. Plus, the egg whites are a superb protein source.[17]

- Don't rely too heavily on low-carbohydrate foods. Too many are high in calories but devoid of EFAs.

SET YOUR FAT BUDGET—AND SPEND WISELY

So how much dietary fat can you consume to support your body's vital processes while preventing the accumulation of body fat?

Government agencies such as the National Cancer Institute and organizations such as the American Heart Association have been rather consistent in recommending a "fat cap" of 30 percent of total calories. Yet according to the latest research, this limit may be a little conservative. While it may slow the development of heart disease, it won't necessarily prevent it.[18] Nor will it deter fat gain.

In a study at Cornell University, researchers tracked the weights of 13 women whom they had randomly assigned to follow either a control diet (supplying 35 to 40 percent of calories as fat) or a low-fat diet (20 to 25 percent of calories as fat).[19] Eleven weeks into the study, the women took a 7-week break, then switched diets.

Most of the women showed increases in body fat while on the control diet, which contained a more moderate amount of fat. On the low-fat diet, they lost 5½ pounds of body fat, on average. Interestingly, the only variable was the fat content. The women didn't limit their calories or portion sizes. This suggests that the lower dietary fat intake is at least partly responsible for the body fat loss.

"Our research confirms that people can lose weight without dieting," says David Levitsky, PhD, professor of nutrition and psychology at Cornell. "The weight loss is relatively slow, but it's persistent. It should result in about a 10 percent loss of body fat per year."[20] Although men didn't participate in the study, there's no reason to think they would respond any differently to a lower fat intake, according to Dr. Levitsky.

Consistent with this research, the MSOn Eating Plan advocates a daily fat intake in the range of 20 to 25 percent of total calories. No more than one-third of those fat calories should come from saturated fat, with the remaining calories about evenly split between polyunsaturated and monounsaturated fats.[21]

What about the lower end of the fat calorie range? Just how low can you safely go, in terms of your fat intake?

In fact, the body needs only about 4 to 6 percent of its daily calories as fat in order to support various biochemical functions.[22] Still, while some studies seem to confirm the value of extremely low fat diets for therapeutic purposes—for patients with severe heart disease, for example—there's little evidence to support the long-term benefits of these diets. In fact, some research suggests that very low fat diets may stimulate the body to produce more fat from blood sugar[23] and to increase appetite.[24]

A reasonable dietary goal of between 20 and 25 percent of total daily calories as fat will support fat loss. Your metabolism will surpass your overall calorie intake, which means you'll be burning fat rather than storing it.

In order to determine your target fat intake, you can use the chart on page 215 as a starting point. Then follow these steps:

1. Multiply your daily calorie limit by 0.20 and 0.25 to determine the lower and upper ends of your personal dietary fat range.

   _____ total calories × 0.20 = _____ fat calories

   _____ total calories × 0.25 = _____ fat calories

2. Divide both figures by 9—the number of calories in 1 gram of fat—to calculate your daily fat budget.

   _____ fat calories ÷ 9 = _____ fat grams

   _____ fat calories ÷ 9 = _____ fat grams

WHERE TO TRIM THE FAT

Once you know your daily fat budget, you can set out to slim down your meals and snacks. Use these strategies as your jumping-off point.

Go "light" on dips, and be picky about chips. You can save a boatload of fat calories just by bypassing the sour-cream dips, deep-fried nachos, and other popular appetizer fare. Try serving ¼ cup fresh guacamole on 100 percent whole grain crackers, pita chips, or—on occasion—fat-free tortilla chips. Avocados are rich in fat, but it's the beneficial monounsaturated kind. Still, be careful not to overdo.

Know your soups. Research suggests that eating soup helps to reduce fat cravings and total calorie intake.[25] I suggest gazpacho—which has a tomato base—over other soups with beef, pork, or cream bases. Or try ordinary tomato soup made with fat-free or 1 percent milk.

Give your salads a makeover. If you're a fan of salad bars, feel free to pile your plate with a variety of vegetables—from popular fixings such as tomatoes, green peppers, and mushrooms to "exotic" greens such as arugula, radicchio, and watercress. Just be careful not to spoil your salad by coating it with a creamy full-fat dressing. Instead, lightly spritz your creation with olive or canola oil and vinegar.

New research shows that a small amount of healthy oil on salad actually helps the body absorb more of the vital nutrients from the vegetables. These days, you can choose from any number of flavorful vinegars. My family's favorite is balsamic. Try several to find one that pleases your palate.

Slim down subs and sandwiches. Skip the croissant, which could contain up to 50 grams of fat, for the more modest 2 to 3 grams in a slice of 100 percent, unrefined whole grain bread. Go open face—meaning one slice of bread instead of two—and choose lean meat such as sliced turkey breast over ham, bologna, or salami. For taste and texture, add lots of veggie toppings, such as romaine lettuce, spinach, tomato, onions, red or green peppers, and jalapeños. Forgo the mayo and finish with a dash of spicy mustard and a splash of vinegar.

Hold off on high-fat dairy foods. These include full-fat milk, cheese, cream cheese, and yogurt. The good news is, all of these have fat-free or low-fat alternatives. Just be sure to read labels, as some fat-free or low-fat dairy products may contain trans fats.

Try a nonburger burger. A grilled chicken breast, ground turkey burger, or garden burger can be a tasty alternative to a traditional all-beef hamburger. If you must have the real thing, get the stripped-down version—one patty without the fatty add-ons like bacon, cheese, and mayo. Dress it with mustard and/or ketchup, plus lots of veggies.

Hold the fries. No matter what oil they're prepared in, french fries are fattening. Actually, so is any food that's deep fried or batter fried. Think of the batter or breading as a high-carb, white-flour sponge that soaks up fat and grease—sending fat calories through the roof.

Be smart when treating your sweet tooth. Bypass the usual high-fat, high-sugar desserts in favor of fresh fruit or low-fat plain yogurt. You can try something a bit more decadent on occasion. Just limit yourself to a few bites, and chew each bite *very* slowly. Immediately afterward, brush your teeth, which can help end the craving for more sweets.

Be honest with yourself. If you know in your heart that—at least for now—you can't bear to give up your favorite fatty food, then don't force yourself. You'll only set yourself up for failure and guilt. Go ahead and indulge, but cut the portion in half. As long as it's an occasional treat, it won't do any harm.

CHAPTER 25

Calories Still Count

In the MSOn Eating Plan, the size and timing of your meals and snacks is critical. You might rationalize a large dinner by vowing to add an extra mile to your evening walk, or to skip your evening snack. That doesn't matter to your Meta-Stat. All it knows is that it's facing more calories than it's accustomed to processing. You won't like what it does with the excess.

When you eat often, you also need to eat light. It's the how that goes along with the when of the MSOn Eating Plan. In this chapter, we're going to explore what "light" means and why it matters so much. The key is to keep flavors high and quantities moderate.

We humans have an inborn tendency to overeat. We inherited it from our hunter-gatherer forebears. For them, it made sense. They were much more active than we are, and they didn't always know where their next meal was coming from. We, of course, simply head to the nearest supermarket or restaurant.

The combination of too much food and too little physical activity all but shuts down the Meta-Stat rather than stoking it. We end up paying a huge price, in terms of fatigue and excess body fat.

If your goal is to burn fat, you need to reduce your daily calorie intake—even if only slightly—while elevating your daily activity level. Cutting calories can take some getting used to. After all, we're living in the era of supersizing, in which restaurants routinely serve food in

body releases in response. The presence of so much insulin means that your body will burn carbohydrate for fuel rather than tapping into its fat stores. By comparison, small meals and snacks demand less insulin. In the absence of excess insulin, the body will burn fat as it should.

WATCH OUT FOR THE MEAL'S END

It takes about 20 minutes from the start of a meal or snack for your body to get the "I'm full" signal. Turn this to your advantage by slowing down your fork, taking more moderate-size bites, and thoroughly chewing each one. You'll eat less and still feel satisfied.

If you finish your meal or snack before reaching the 20-minute mark, excuse yourself from the table. Walk around for a few minutes, take a few sips of ice water or unsweetened tea, and maybe go brush your teeth. By then your satiety signal should have kicked in. Slow down and give it the time it needs.

When choosing your meals and snacks, keep in mind that whole foods such as fresh vegetables and fruits and whole, unrefined grains tend to be most filling because of the fiber they contain. As a bonus, they're low in calories and fat.

Also seek out foods that are pleasing to your palate. Research suggests that the sight, smell, and taste of your favorites may stimulate your body to burn more calories[2], a sign that you're turning your Meta-Stat to a higher setting.

Canadian researchers performed a series of studies—first with rats, then with people—to compare meals that were identical nutritionally but quite different flavor-wise. The researchers determined that the more flavorful food seemed to stimulate a thermic effect. In other words, it increased the rate at which the body burns calories.[3]

Think about your favorite meals and snacks. After you pinpoint the flavors you love, seek out recipes that accentuate them while reducing fat, sugar, and calories. If you focus first on savory flavors and second on the nutrient profile, you'll have a much easier time consistently eating in a way that supports your Meta-Stat.

portions that are two, three, or even four times what the averag
son needs for sustenance.

As discussed in Chapter 21, the human body runs better on
but frequent meals and snacks. Yet it also has the ability to acco
date food beyond reasonable capacity. Every time you overeat
trigger hormonal reactions that jump-start emergency fat makin
fat storage. Specifically, the standard American diet—consisti
three large meals a day—stimulates the production of insulii
body's most potent profat hormone.[1]

Because your body can't utilize all the extra calories, they a
more likely to end up as body fat. That's your metabolic heritag
by trading the standard three square meals a day for smaller but
frequent meals and snacks, you'll be able to work with your Met
rather than fighting it. Before you know it, you'll be looking ba
what you now consider a meal and wondering how you managed
through that much food at a single sitting!

THE RISKS OF ACCIDENTAL OVEREATING

To avoid overeating, you need an eating plan that doesn't r
willpower. If you try to control your calorie intake through will
alone, it may work fine . . . for a while. Eventually, your resistan
wane. You may feel the urge to eat a little extra, but "a little" tur
to be an entire day's worth of calories.

Even fat-free foods can ramp up the body's fat-making process
they're eaten to excess. I'm not kidding. These foods trigger hor
and enzymatic reactions that convert nonfat calories into fat an
pack the fat into your body's fat cells. So those chocolate-d
cream-filled, caramel-laced minicakes could end up on your hi
matter if the label says they're "100 percent fat-free."

The bottom line is this: Overeating is a boon to fat cells. Wh
a meal or snack tops your body's limit of 600 calories in a single :
the excess calories—even from fat-free foods—stimulate fat s
rather than fat burning. To put this limit in perspective: Some fas
"meal deals"—the typical double burger/mammoth fries/monste
combination—supply 1,500 calories!

Remember, too, that the larger a meal is, the more insulii

PART

Set Your Course for Success

FIVE

CHAPTER 26

The Meta-Stat Success Map

By now you should have a good sense of what the Meta-Stat is, how it works, and how you can activitate it throughout the day for optimal fat burning and energy production. Now you need to make choices. Which switches should you use to turn on your Meta-Stat, and when?

I could give specific recommendations for an average person. The catch is, there is no such thing as an average person. We are each, and all, biochemically unique. Renowned biochemist Roger Williams, PhD, conducted research 40 years ago showing that differences in anatomy and metabolism from person to person can dramatically influence individual energy, strength, and health.[1]

The Meta-Stat approach is the first to make this research one of its cornerstones. It is completely flexible and easily tailored to your own goals, needs, and preferences. The more you tune in to yourself, the better and longer lasting your results will be.

The Meta-Stat approach is a lifestyle *rhythm*. Once you establish that rhythm and make it part of your daily life, you won't need to worry about whether or not you're following the rules or breaking them. Consider something that you probably do automatically, like driving the car. Once you're accustomed to driving, do you contemplate your

(continued on page 248)

Your Meta-Stat Success Map

Name: _____

Date: _____

28-Day Goals

Clear, specific, actionable.   It's important to me because:

1.   1.

2.   2.

MSOn Minutes

Which switches did you activate today? Circle all that apply.

#1: Wake up on the right side of the bed

#2: Create activity momentum

#3: Catch light to boost energy

#4: Take in more oxygen

#5: Seek ideal fluid intake

#6: Rise up and stand tall

#7: Turn down the heat, turn up your energy

#8: Improve hormone balance, hour after hour

#9: Stay calm in an uptight world

#10: Stop the stress response

#11: Ramp up your evening Meta-Stat setting

#12: Get plenty of good-quality rest

Meta-Stat Workout

Circle one:

- Abs and legs (days 1 and 4) • Upper body (days 2 and 5)
- Aerobic (days 3 and 6) • Flexibility and balance (days 1, 2, 4, and 5)
- Muscle tone-ups (anytime)

Body part	Exercise	Duration/# of repetitions	Resistance level

Meta-Stat Eating Plan

	Time	Food
Meal #1		
Snack		
Meal #2		
Snack		
Snack		
Meal #3		
Snack		

Fluids (in cups)

Circle one:

I   2   3   4   5   6   7   8

Daily Energy Wave

Chart your energy level on the following grid, using I as low energy and 10 as high.

10																				
9																				
8																				
7																				
6																				
5																				
4																				
3																				
2																				
1																				
A.M.	4	5	6	7	8	9	10	11	12	1	2	3	4	5	6	7	8	9	10	11 P.M.

Progress Markers

I.

2.

3.

4.

actions every time you press the accelerator or put on the brake? You simply get in the habit of doing those things, along with a lot of other actions like braking at a stop sign, using your turn signal, and checking your mirrors. Your actions are automatic.

So why should a weight-loss or exercise program be any different? Once you get past the "learner" stage, your day-to-day lifestyle habits should be as worry-free as driving a car. And that's exactly what will happen when you get used to the Meta-Stat approach.

To integrate the different switches and reset your Meta-Stat, it helps to have a day-to-day plan that you can monitor and review. That's where the Meta-Stat Success Map comes in.

WHAT THE SUCCESS MAP CAN DO FOR YOU

The Meta-Stat Success Map is an adaptation of a tool that I've used in various forms with thousands of people to help them achieve remarkably high-level goals in their personal and professional lives. Using the map, you can customize the three core components of the Meta-Stat approach—the MSOn Switches, the MSOn Workout, and the MSOn Eating Plan—into a program that's just right for you.

With the Meta-Stat Success Map, you have the perfect tool to help you reach your goals. It helps you stay organized. It takes the guesswork out of achieving new results every single day. It documents your progress, reveals what you learn in your daily life, shows the gaps that you need to fix, and records each of your personal achievements.

This is where you can assemble actions that seem to best fit your lifestyle. You can draw from any of the hundreds of tips and tools throughout the book. You can devise others that are uniquely your own. Then get going!

To make the program work for you—to maximize the energy-enhancing, fat-burning, feel-good power of the MSOn Switches—you need to personalize your Meta-Stat program. Here's how to begin.

1. Make copies of the map on pages 246 and 247. Start with 28 copies—enough to cover the first 4 weeks of your program.

2. Date each copy, starting with tomorrow.

3. Save all copies of your Success Map. I keep mine in a three-ring binder, along with blank sheets of paper for taking notes. These comprise a record of your success. By keeping a record and reviewing it frequently, you can identify and track the MSOn Switches that are most effective in your personal program.

A GUIDE TO THE MAP

The Meta-Stat Success Map provides a quick and easy way to remind yourself of all the Meta-Stat components and how they fit together. It gives you a visual incentive because you can see at a glance whether you're balancing the components of the program to maximize results. As you begin to reach for new goals, you can adjust your program accordingly.

To show you how this works, let's look individually at each part of the Success Map. I'll guide you through it.

28-Day Goals

Under this heading, you'll list two specific changes you wish to accomplish in the next 4 weeks and give a few specific reasons why this success would mean a lot to you. This "anchors" the commitment and also makes it easier to give a rationale to others if they ask why you're changing your actions, attitudes, or behaviors. (For tips on setting actionable, achievable goals, see Chapter 27.)

To the right of your goals, I ask you to write down why each goal is important to you. A vital success factor is to have no regrets. You can't go backward. You can only build your life forward. But you can notice and modify the actions you're taking to fit your own upcoming needs and challenges.

MSOn Minutes

The MSOn Minutes are quick and easy. No preparation required! Your body needs these minutes to tone up your muscles, catch the light, de-stress and loosen up, and take a strategic pause or break. To get the maximum benefit from MSOn Minutes, just use the switches in Part 2. You can keep track of when you turned on those switches and how they helped.

For optimal fat burning and energy production, you should activate one of the MSOn Switches every 15 to 30 minutes throughout the day. That way, you're constantly stimulating your Meta-Stat so it keeps working 24 hours a day.

The MSOn Workout

In the Meta-Stat approach, you maximize your strength and metabolic power with a series of intensely focused, brief exercise sessions. I discussed the components of the MSOn Workout in Part 3. Here's a brief recap.

- 20 minutes of aerobic activity 3 days a week

- Muscle tone-ups any time throughout each day

- Core strength training (abs and legs) twice a week

- Upper-body strength training (chest, back, shoulders, and arms) twice a week

- Balance and flexibility 4 days a week

In the Meta-Stat Success Map, I've assigned the various components to specific days of the week. This is just a suggestion; feel free to do what works for you. The idea is to work your body differently on successive days for maximum fat-burning, energy-generating benefit. Each day, be sure to note the exercises you've done, the duration or number of repetitions and the resistance level.

You'll notice that the Meta-Stat Workout covers 6 days rather than 7. The seventh day is a day off for relaxing and invigorating yourself in ways other than formal exercise. Following this simple, proven approach, you'll cover all the essentials for whole-body health in minimal time.

Remember, this is not an Olympic athlete's workout regimen, designed to max out your muscle power or create awesome endurance. Your notes on duration, resistance level, and peak intensity are personal reminders, not the scorecard of a competitor-in-training. As happens with everyone who follows the Meta-Stat program, the MSOn Workout helps you steadily develop strength and muscle tone for optimal results. But you never have to compare these results to anyone else's!

The MSOn Eating Plan

Good nutrition fuels fat loss and energy production. Use this section of the Meta-Stat Success Map to make notes about your eating plan and its results.

For example, next to each of your three light to moderate meals (breakfast, lunch, and dinner), you'll enter the time and your food choices. You also may want to note whether a snack is high-fiber, high-protein, or high-carb.

To make the map work for you, it's important to be accurate. Even if you just have three crackers, it's important to write it down. Did you go out for a smoothie in the afternoon? Be sure to mention that as well.

Of course, sufficient fluid intake is crucial to building energy and burning fat. Simply circle the appropriate number of servings each day.

Notice that the map is set up so that you easily compare the MSOn Eating Plan with the Daily Energy Wave. Over time, you'll be able to see at a glance how your energy level is related to—and influenced by—your food choices and dietary habits.

Daily Energy Wave

In order to catch energy and metabolism whenever they start to fall, and then bring them up again, research shows that self-monitoring of energy waves is important.[2] In this part of the Meta-Stat Success Map, you will note the high points of your energy and calmness levels as well as the low points of fatigue- and tension-related pressures.

By tracking your energy wave, you have the opportunity to become an objective observer of your mental and physical well-being. Of course, it's hard to look back at the end of the day and remember whether your energy was high or low at any particular time, so I recommend keeping the map near at hand and jotting down reminders of your energy wave during the day. All it takes is a pencil mark on this chart to remind you that "I really had a surge of energy around 11 o'clock," or "At 2:30, I was ready to fall asleep in my chair." If you keep daily copies of the map like a journal, you'll be able to see patterns emerge over time.

Progress Markers

One of the crucial determinants of success is whether you can focus on signs of progress instead of perfection. Your approach needn't be all or nothing. Let it be *something* or nothing. At day's end, review your map and reflect on what progress you made. Note four things you did very well today that helped you move toward increased success in your 28-day goals.

THE POWER OF THE MAP

After a few days you'll find, as most people do, that completing the Meta-Stat Success Map becomes an easy and satisfying daily habit. Remember, this isn't an audit or a report card. It's a simple tool to help you become an objective observer of your own energy patterns, eating habits, exercise routines, and sleep patterns. The better you understand these patterns, the more effectively you'll be able to manage each day to reach your goals.

It's not likely that you'll make use of all the MSOn Switches in a single week, or even a month. You'll find that some switches seem far more powerful and effective than others, and naturally you'll have personal preferences. But I believe it's still important to be familiar with all of them, so you can make the best possible day-to-day selection for your own health, energy, and well-being.

True, some switches are so simple you will want to use them many times during the day for a quick pick-me-up. In almost an instant, they can rev up your metabolic powers. Other switches require more time and planning. Now, which ones are right for you?

Of course, you're the best person to answer that question. As you read this book and test each switch yourself, you'll find your own best sequence for weaving them into your day, anywhere, anytime. But if you're not quite sure where to begin, the following sample "starter programs" might help.

To Jump-Start Fat Loss

1. Begin with MSOn Switch #11 to stimulate your evening metabolism.

2. Follow with MSOn Switch #1, which provides a fat-burning boost from the first thing in the morning.
3. Increase the active moments throughout your day with MSOn Switch #2.

To Get Off a Fat-Loss Plateau

1. First turn to MSOn Switch #2 for brief but frequent pulses of activity that raise your Meta-Stat.
2. Add MSOn Switch #3, harnessing a few minutes of light to rev up your body's fat-burning power.
3. Be sure to try MSOn Switch #5; sipping ice water can increase fat-burning metabolism by 30 percent.

To Ease into a More Active Lifestyle

1. Start with MSOn Switch #2, which shows you how to be more active in your daily routine.
2. Try the muscle tone-ups in the MSOn Workout to ease your body into strength training.
3. If you have a sedentary job, don't overlook the benefits of proper posture, as described in MSOn Switch #6.

To Build Energy Now

1. Turn up cellular energy production with MSOn Switch #4, which improves oxygen intake.
2. Add MSOn Switch #9, which quickly builds reserves of calm energy, the lasting source of new vitality.
3. Of course, take steps to ensure a good night's sleep, as recommended in MSOn Switch #12.

As you learn the Meta-Stat approach, you will find many other ways to tailor this one-of-a-kind program to your one-of-a-kind metabolic needs and goals. And you'll get in the habit of using the Meta-Stat Success Map to keep track of your daily progress. That way, you can observe the habits and daily patterns that move you along toward your goals.

Before the first month is over, most people find that the Meta-Stat approach has become automatic and inseparable from their daily lifestyles. As your energy and fat-burning power steadily increase, the results that you get and the goals that you achieve are sure to be lasting.

CHAPTER 27

■　　■　　■

Choosing the Right Goals for You

The exceptional life depends not on working harder, but
on different and even opposite actions from habit
and the crowd.

—Ralph Waldo Emerson

Goals. They're a dime a dozen. We post them. Memorize them. Proclaim them. We implore ourselves to achieve them. But too often, with too few exceptions, we don't pursue those goals long enough or persistently enough to achieve them.

All around the world, lives and jobs end up as highways littered with goals that never came true.

You can change that. Starting today, right now.

THE CRITICAL IMPORTANCE OF GOALS

What can you actually achieve using the Meta-Stat approach? To answer that question, it's essential to appreciate the importance of setting personal goals.

According to researchers, people who grasp their own original goals in distinctive and specific ways are 50 percent more likely to take confident actions to achieve those goals. And they are 30 percent more likely to feel a sense of control under stressful conditions.[1]

In my years of research with star performers around the world, there is one simple formula for goals that work. For the 1 percent of people who actually succeed in achieving the goals they set for themselves, this formula explains their success. It has four components.

- Goals

- Obstacles

- Mechanisms

- Measurements

Goals

Goals are not dreams. Goals are specific, practical tasks that you choose to accomplish within a well-defined time period. It's vital to make sure that each and every goal is focused on what you want rather than what you don't want. For instance, I don't consider fighting fatigue a goal. I urge people to set goals that are based on *exactly what they want to have happen*—for example, achieving more strength or having more energy.

Your goals are unique to you. They should be things that you consider worthy of individual pursuit. In general, good goals share the following characteristics.

They are specific. Your goals should be particular enough for you to know whether or not you have made progress. Will you actually be able to tell when you have met a goal? The more details you can include in your goal setting, the better.

Goals should be just as original as you are. In the millions of years of life on Earth, there has never, ever been another being exactly like you, and there never will be. This is your time. This is your chance. And your goals need to match.

They are constructive and positive. If you allow yourself to focus on preventing a bad outcome instead of bringing about a good one, you become entrapped by the negative. That makes a bad outcome even more likely to occur.[2]

The fact is, we humans can't dwell on the reverse of an idea. When we try to "prevent," "avoid," or "block" something, our brains can't interpret that sort of message. Instead, the habit of negative suggestion brings to fruition the concerns and challenges we're imagining. Whenever you set a goal, make it constructive as well as clear.

They are believable. Your goals should be believable—to *you*. To others, they may seem unlikely or even impossible. That's fine. A goal in which you believe need not be realistic or even probable by another person's standard. Keep in mind that many of the greatest breakthroughs in history—both big ones that changed the world and small ones that changed individual lives—were shrugged off by others as folly.

They are challenging. Generally, your goals should keep you stretching to achieve more of what's possible in your life and work. But you need small challenges as well as big ones. Sometimes, small victories promote progress in the most powerful ways, even while we're striving to make big victories happen.

They are measurable. Your goals don't necessarily require a deadline. But whether they're short term or long term, they should contain some sort of benchmark by which you can measure progress at regular intervals. I advise that you do your progress checks no more than 1 week apart.

Vague goals are everywhere, and they can be a real problem. "I want to lose weight" is a good example of a vague goal. It can mean that you stop eating, or you become ill—neither of which is desirable.

Setting lofty, abstract goals with pronouncements about changing your life for the better may feel good at first. When you pull yourself up to your full height and announce your new direction, you may even experience a sense of excitement or euphoria. But it's unlikely to last. For about 9 of every 10 people, declarations and expectations of self-change produce a temporary improvement in self-image, but within a few weeks, disappointment invariably sets in. Then self-image takes a beating, ending up worse than it was before.[3]

Research published in *Peak Performance Journal* confirms that vague goals such as "get fit," "be healthy," or "do my best" almost never work.[4] So zero in on the details and notice the difference!

They emphasize development over performance. Most people define their goals in terms of performance improvement. And that's a mistake, researchers say. According to a study of mental imagery in *Peak*

Performance Journal, personal development goals lead to greater progress than do personal performance goals.

When you set a performance goal such as winning a trophy or defeating an opponent, you're likely to pursue it simply by putting a temporary twist on your existing routine. Then once you achieve it, you revert to your old habits. So even if you "win," it won't bring about permanent change. And permanent change is essential for lasting results.

Obstacles

What could stand between you and your goals? Too often, we're reluctant to acknowledge potential challenges and pitfalls, as though ignoring them might make them go away. Only they don't. Eventually we realize that we need to identify them so we can find ways to overcome them.

Sometimes you can climb over obstacles. More often, though, you need to blaze a path around them or chip away at them a little at a time. Your success at breaking through may hinge not on your talents and worthiness but on your ability to handle problems along the way.

Consider the most common obstacles you will run into when you're pursuing a goal. Old habits, for instance. The brain has an inherent tendency to crave routine and therefore reinforce old behaviors. Thus, you'll want to give some thought to the kinds of habits that may impede your progress.

Here are some other common obstacles to be aware of.

- Stress and tension

- Distractions

- Time constraints

- Fatigue or low energy

- Narrow mindset

- Rigid attitudes

- Hidden or unchallenged presumptions

- Lack of social support

Mechanisms

One good mechanism beats a hundred good plans. Mechanisms are simple, specific strategies for navigating obstacles and achieving desired results. Simplicity is critical. The reason: A small but very powerful structure of the brain, the amygdala, prefers the world to run on routine. It resists *any* change, even a minor one. Instead, it relentlessly urges you toward the familiar, the tried and true. It wants you to be what you have been and to remain just as you are.

Star performers devise mechanisms to consciously override the amygdala's "don't change a thing" message. They know they need to do it; otherwise, they would remain stuck in the present, forever repeating the past. They'd never achieve their goals.

When contemplating possible mechanisms, focus on subtle shifts in behavior. For example, if your goal is to engage in more physical activity every day, you might schedule a walk in your calendar, just as you would any other appointment. By using this mechanism, you build momentum in the right direction. Mechanisms become leverage points, propelling you toward your goal. Think of it this way: The goal is what you want to happen; the mechanism is what you use to make it happen.

Measurements

All advancement in life and work depends to one degree or another on measurements. Otherwise, you'd have no idea whether you're moving forward or marking time. Studies show that people who regularly monitor their progress toward their individual goals are 32 percent more likely to make strides than those who don't.[5]

With mechanisms, in particular, you need to be able to assess whether and how well they're working. This information determines whether you should continue in the same direction or try a different approach.

You should be able to see a tangible, positive result from each chosen mechanism within a week. Sometimes you can get a sense of your progress much more quickly—in a day, an hour, or even a minute.

KEEP UP THE MOMENTUM

Momentum matters. One of the key reasons for unrealized goals is that people who start off with good intentions often skip the daily actions that cultivate new habits and forward momentum.[6] For anyone who stops, restarting is a major hurdle. It requires energy and resolve, and it can be quite draining. In fact, if you stop and start often enough, you may get tired of trying.

That's just one reason why I recommend photocopying and using the Meta-Stat Success Map (see page 246) in 28-day installments. It helps create momentum. You take simple, specific actions every day; measure results every week; and build a bridge from where you are to where you want to be over a 4-week period.

Four weeks is a manageable and motivating timeframe. Go much longer, and your goals lose their clarity. Go less, and you won't develop the necessary momentum to pursue your goals in the first place.

HOW TO CREATE GOALS THAT WORK

Here is a quick sampling of four goals that I often hear from my clients. See if at least one of them matches one of your own.

1. Exercise more often during the day, every day.

2. Overcome cravings to make better food choices.

3. Tone all of your muscles.

4. Stay on top of stress all day long.

Let's look at each of these with the goal-setting formula in mind.

1. Exercise More Often during the Day, Every Day

This is one of the key priorities in the Meta-Stat approach: turning up your Meta-Stat with signals from active minutes throughout the day so you're burning more calories and body fat while producing more energy.

Obstacles: Daily routine, busy schedule, no free time, overload, stress, lack of energy

Mechanism: Create a simple reminder system to prompt you to get up and move every 15 to 30 minutes. For example, you might set your watch alarm to beep every half hour. Remember to use your Meta-Stat Success Map to track your active minutes—standing up while talking on the telephone, taking the stairs between floors, performing simple muscle-toning exercises. The increase in energy and alertness, and the corresponding increase in effectiveness, will more than make up for any "lost" time.

Measurement: At the end of the day, did it work? Did you exercise? Did you feel more energetic and more effective because of these embellishments to your daily routine?

2. Overcome Cravings to Make Better Food Choices

This is another of the Meta-Stat priorities: building meals and snacks to support energy production and fat burning, without overeating or overindulging in unhealthy foods.

Obstacles: Old habits, deep-seated love for certain "forbidden" foods, poor perception of healthy alternatives, eating on the run, skipping meals and snacks

Mechanism: Preplan midmorning, midafternoon, predinner, and evening snacks (and track them on the Meta-Stat Success Map); test at least two new Meta-Stat recipes each week; clear the refrigerator and pantry of all foods that don't support the MSOn Eating Plan; create a strategy for nipping cravings in the bud, such as chewing a piece of sugarless mint gum or sipping ice water or unsweetened tea.

Measurement: Did you eat four nutritious snacks a day? Did you test at least two new recipes? When a craving came on, were you able to stop it?

3. Tone All of Your Muscles

The more muscles you tone, the more energy you have and the more fat you burn—even while you sleep.

Obstacles: No time, can't afford gym membership, don't like exercise to begin with

Mechanism: Make exercise easier than you ever imagined. Invest in hand weights or resistance bands and leave them where you'll all but trip over them; choose a no-equipment dynamic visualized tension exercise (see Chapter 17) for every major muscle group; take at least four brief "toning breaks" every day.

Measurement: Did you fit in your four toning breaks per day? Which body parts are showing results?

4. Stay on Top of Stress All Day Long

Stress is a major saboteur of energy production and fat burning. It has become such a fact of modern life that it seems normal. You may even come to depend on the false energy from epinephrine, cortisol, and other fat-making stress hormones. They produce a buzz that can feel like the effects of caffeine. But it isn't healthy. Learning how to cope with stressful situations, and how to minimize their physical and psychological effects is vital.

Obstacles: Too many "hot buttons" that can trigger stress; too few opportunities to relax and recharge

Mechanism: Identify one or two of your worst hot buttons—for example, getting stuck in traffic, waiting in line, meeting deadlines. Whenever you find yourself facing one of these stressful situations, practice the instant calming sequence (see page 128).

Measurement: Did you spot your hot button? How quickly did you respond to it? How quickly were you able to calm yourself?

NOW IT'S YOUR TURN

Using the formula in this chapter, you can create your own goals. Be sure to make note of them in the Meta-Stat Success Map. Then they're yours to follow through. A simple check-in at the end of each day will help determine what's working, what isn't, and what you might do differently tomorrow. Keep the switches that are effective for you, and toss the rest. Really.

The human brain loves to hoard information, even bits that aren't useful. They can distract you from achieving your goals. That's when a little mental housecleaning is in order. Do your best to avoid information overload. Sometimes less is more.

As you pursue your goals, be prepared for those obstacles that you have identified—and perhaps a few that you haven't. When you encounter one, simply call upon your MSOn switches (plus any other tools and techniques in your personal inventory) to overcome it. You'll clear the way to continue on the path to success.

CHAPTER 28

▪ ▪ ▪

Guide Your Success Instincts

O ne of the fundamental principles driving the Meta-Stat approach is that none of us can succeed with our minds alone. That's a primary reason so many weight-loss programs fail.

When we try to *think* our way to new results—with commitments, checklists, and plans—it can go fine for a while, for an hour or most of a day or even a few days. But then, invariably, it falls apart. We aren't making the necessary changes in our habits and behaviors that automatically stoke the Meta-Stat to burn fat and boost energy. Instead, we rely on willpower to achieve these same results. And it gets tiring. Eventually, we give in to a craving, or we skip a workout . . . and we lose ground toward our goals.

The truth is, it's maddeningly hard for the human mind to control habits and behaviors on its own.[1] The Meta-Stat evolved to rely on many other mechanisms—especially the instincts and feelings of the gut and heart—to keep it functioning at an optimal level.

WISDOM FROM WITHIN

The human capacity to survive and thrive is driven less by the brain in the head than by newly discovered intelligence centers in the gut and in the heart. The highest reasoning and brightest ingenuity involve all three of these "brains" working together.

In the old view of how brain one—the brain in the head—influences human behavior, any direct life experience enters the nervous system through the five senses. In this traditional model, each experience travels right to the brain, which processes the information and determines an appropriate response. Everything happens in the head.

The new view, as you will see in a moment, is nothing like that. In fact, whenever too much brain activity is drawn off into thinking and remembering, not enough energy is left for feeling and experiencing what's new right now. As a result, performance that could be ingenious and practical becomes clumsy and irrelevant. Sometimes reliance on the thinking brain is not only insignificant to the acquisition and expression of knowledge and expertise, it actually interferes with this process.[2]

Research has proven that intelligence is distributed throughout the body. Whenever we have a direct experience, it does *not* go directly to the brain to be deciphered and contemplated. Instead, it travels to the neurological networks of the intestinal tract and heart.

The Brain in the Gut

Every contact point with life creates a gut feeling. You may notice it as "butterflies" in your stomach or a "knot" of intestinal tension or excitement. Or, depending on how intensely you have been trained to always stay in your head, you may not notice it at all.

But it is there. And it is asking a lot of questions, whether or not you realize it. Not just asking them—answering them, too, in ways that will affect your actions. "How important is this situation? Is there an opportunity here? Is there a threat? What, exactly, do I need right now to sustain my energy and strength?"

Known as the enteric nervous system, this "second brain" in the intestines is independent of but also connected to the brain in the head.[3] Scientists who study the elaborate system of nerve cells inside the intestinal tract report that it has more neurons than the entire spinal column—about 100 million of them.[4] The complex circuitry enables it to act with lightning speed—many thousands of times faster than the brain in the head—and to operate independently, learning, remembering, and influencing your perceptions and behaviors.

Whether or not you acknowledge your "gut reactions," they are shaping everything you do, just as they shape everything everyone around you does, all the time. So begin to tune in. Ask yourself, What am I feeling right now? What's most important to my energy and concentration? What's the best choice I can make at this moment? Let your gut instincts help determine how you can support your Meta-Stat's fat-burning, energy-producing power. Pay attention as they note which new habits are working best and when you should fire up your Meta-Stat throughout the day.

The Brain in the Heart

After each experience has been digested by the enteric nervous system, the heart steps in to ponder it. Most of us think of the heart as a pump—which it is—but it's so much more. Aristotle once observed, "The brain is in the heart." He may have been ridiculed for his statement then, but not anymore.

In the 1990s, scientists in the emerging field of neurocardiology discovered the true brain in the heart, which acts independently of the one in the head. And it's comparable in size, with a distinctive set of more than 40,000 nerve cells called baroreceptors as well as a complex network of neurotransmitters, proteins, and support cells.[5] The brain in the heart has powerful, highly sophisticated computational abilities.[6] And just like the brain in the gut, it uses its neural circuitry to learn, remember, and dictate actions.

In a fetus, the human heart develops before the nervous system and thinking brain. The electrical energy in every heartbeat, and the information contained therein, pulse to every cell of the body.[7] And every beat prompts billions of cells to fire in a perfectly synchronized rhythm. Recent studies on learning and emotional response show that the coherence of the rhythms in the heart brain can change the effectiveness of the thinking brain, often dramatically.[8]

With every heartbeat, there is instantaneous whole-body communication, a wave that travels through the arteries many times faster than actual blood flow.[9] This creates another language of interior communication, as pressure waves vary with each intricate pattern of heartbeat rhythm.[10] Each one of the trillions of cells feels this pressure wave and is dependent on it in a number of ways.

The heart also communicates with the rest of the body through the messenger chemicals of the hormonal system. One such chemical is atrial peptide, a primary driver of motivated behavior.[11] If we don't *feel* our goals and priorities, we can't *live* them.[12] It's the heart, not the head, that plays a dominant role in moving us to excel.

In terms of human ingenuity and initiative, your heart is not only open to new possibilities, it actively scans for them, ever seeking a new, intuitive understanding of what matters most to you. Then it instantaneously searches for new opportunities that support your aspirations,[13] rather like a far-reaching sensory system or a personally meaningful radar.

Just as your gut processes far more than your food, your heart circulates far more than your blood. Every single heartbeat speaks an intelligent language to your body that deeply influences how you perceive your world and how you react to it.[14]

With this new understanding of the heart comes the realization that the oft-heard call to "keep emotions out of it" ends up being a sure track to poor choices and misguided efforts. Of course you must think with your brain, as clearly and insightfully as you can. Yet without the active involvement of your heart, you may fall short of achieving your full potential—whether in fat burning, energy production, or something else.[15]

LISTEN TO YOUR BODY

As you tune in to your Meta-Stat every 15 to 30 minutes throughout the day, be sure to tap *all* of your sources of wisdom and insight. Let your three brains—the one in your head, the one in your gut, and the one in your heart—help you navigate the vital choice points that you encounter over the course of a day. These are critical moments at which you can gain or lose momentum. Ask yourself, What does my gut say about this? My heart? My head? Then listen carefully to each of those three streams of intelligence before deciding how to act.

With practice, this will not in any way slow your ability to make on-the-spot choices. Rather, it will deepen and improve such choices. In this way, you will gain vital momentum to sustain fat loss and energy production at optimal levels.

PART

Meta-Stat Recipes

SIX

The recipes in the pages that follow build on the principles of the MSOn Eating Plan. They supply lean protein, complex carbohydrates, and healthy fats in the right proportions for optimal Meta-Stat function. Most are easy to prepare—and of course, they taste great!

Feel free to mix-and-match the recipes to create your own menus. Just remember to follow the 3 + 4 formula: 3 meals averaging 600 calories each, plus 4 snacks averaging 300 calories each, per day. If certain meals or snacks surpass these calorie limits, don't worry. Simply balance them with lower-calorie choices through the rest of the day. The key is to eat at regular intervals, and to keep meals and snacks roughly the same size. This provides proper fuel for your Meta-Stat, so it runs at peak efficiency throughout the day.

You will notice that some recipes are higher in sodium than others. If you're watching your sodium intake, simply leave out any added salt or replace it with another favorite seasoning.

Enjoy!

—*Leslie Cooper*

Starters and Snacks

KALAMATA OLIVE SPREAD

Makes 36 servings (¾ cup)

Prep time: 10 minutes

Olives are rich in monounsaturated fat, the type that is beneficial to health in small quantities. Kalamatas are the most popular variety of olive in Greece. One of our favorite ways to eat this spread is with crostini, or toasted bread slices. Because of its intense flavor, it can add extra zest to pastas, sauces, soups, and even chicken or fish.

1	cup pitted kalamata olives
1	clove garlic, minced
¼	cup packed fresh basil leaves
1	tablespoon lemon juice
	Freshly ground black pepper
1	tablespoon olive oil

In a food processor, combine the olives, garlic, basil, and lemon juice. Pulse until the ingredients are coarsely chopped, scraping down the sides of the bowl as needed. Season with the pepper.

Add the olive oil. Pulse until the mixture is finely chopped but not pureed. Store in a covered container in the refrigerator.

Per 1 teaspoon serving: 16 calories, 0 g protein, 1 g carbohydrates, 2 g total fat, 0 mg cholesterol, 0 g dietary fiber, 73 mg sodium

ROASTED EGGPLANT SPREAD

Makes 6 servings (1½ cups)

Prep time: 10 minutes

Baking time: 30–45 minutes

This low-fat version of a Mediterranean favorite has a light texture, with hints of lemon and garlic. It's delicious when served at room temperature and spread on crusty bread or crackers. You also can serve it as a dip with cut-up vegetables such as carrots and broccoli.

2	tablespoons olive oil
1	teaspoon kosher salt
1	small to medium eggplant, halved lengthwise
2	cloves garlic, halved
1	teaspoon chopped fresh parsley
½	teaspoon grated lemon peel
	Salt
	Freshly ground black pepper

Preheat the oven to 500°F.

Line with foil or coat with cooking spray a baking pan just large enough to hold the eggplant. Add 1 tablespoon of the oil and sprinkle with the kosher salt.

Add the eggplant, cut side down, and the garlic. Bake for 30 to 45 minutes, or until the eggplant is very soft. Remove from the oven and cool on a rack.

Place the garlic in a food processor or blender. Scoop the pulp from the eggplant and add to the processor. Puree until smooth. Add the parsley, lemon peel, and the remaining 1 tablespoon oil. Season to taste with the salt and pepper.

Per serving: 60 calories, 2 g protein, 5 g carbohydrates, 5 g total fat, 0 mg cholesterol, 3 g dietary fiber, 322 mg sodium

ROASTED GARLIC HUMMUS

Makes 8 servings (2 cups)

Prep and cooking time: 35 minutes

Hummus is a Middle Eastern spread that uses chickpeas and tahini (sesame seed paste) as its base. Serve it as an appetizer or snack with hunks of fresh bread, crackers, or raw vegetables for dipping. To make a sandwich, spread the hummus on pita bread or wraps and top with your choice of lettuce, tomato, sliced onion, roasted peppers, cucumbers, sprouts, and shredded carrots.

5	cloves garlic, unpeeled
1	16-ounce can chickpeas, drained and ½ cup liquid reserved
4	tablespoons tahini
3	tablespoons fresh lemon juice
½	teaspoon dried parsley
¼	teaspoon ground cumin
	Pinch of cayenne pepper
	Salt
	Freshly ground black pepper

Preheat the oven to 400°F.

Place the garlic in a square of foil and lightly coat with cooking spray. Wrap the foil around the garlic and bake for 30 minutes. Allow to cool, then unwrap and discard peel.

In a food processor or blender, combine the garlic, reserved chickpeas liquid, tahini, lemon juice, parsley, cumin, and cayenne pepper. Puree until smooth.

Season to taste with the salt and black pepper.

Per serving: 98 calories, 4 g protein, 11 g carbohydrates, 5 g total fat, 0 mg cholesterol, 3 g dietary fiber, 174 mg sodium

SAVORY SPINACH BALLS

Makes 48

Prep time: 20 minutes

Baking time: 10 minutes

I received the original recipe for these spinach balls from a friend who loved to take them to parties because they didn't require much work, and they always were a hit. Unfortunately, they were loaded with fat, especially saturated fat. This healthier version is delicious served alone or with a marinara sauce for dipping. The spinach balls also make a great vegetarian substitute for meatballs.

2	10-ounce packages frozen chopped spinach, thawed
1	cup grated Parmesan cheese
1	cup liquid egg substitute
2	eggs, beaten
4	tablespoons unsalted butter, melted
2	tablespoons chopped fresh parsley
2	teaspoons Italian seasoning, crushed
1	teaspoon garlic powder
¾	teaspoon salt
3	cups fresh whole wheat bread crumbs (about 3 slices bread)
	Freshly ground black pepper

Preheat the oven to 350°F. Line a baking sheet with foil or parchment paper and lightly coat with cooking spray.

Place the spinach in a colander and squeeze to remove most of the liquid. Transfer to a medium bowl. Add the cheese, egg substitute, eggs, butter, parsley, Italian seasoning, garlic powder, and salt. Mix well. Stir in the bread crumbs and season to taste with the pepper.

Divide the mixture into 48 balls and place on the prepared baking sheet. Lightly coat the balls with cooking spray.

Bake for 10 minutes or until lightly browned. Serve warm or at room temperature.

Per ball: 32 calories, 2 g protein, 2 g carbohydrates, 2 g total fat, 13 mg cholesterol, 1 g dietary fiber, 95 mg sodium

TZATZKIKI
(GREEK CUCUMBER-YOGURT SPREAD)

Makes 8 servings (2 cups)

Prep time: 20 minutes

Tzatzkiki originated in Greece, where it's made with a thick, rich yogurt. To achieve this texture with low-fat or fat-free yogurt, I drain it to remove some of the liquid. The longer the yogurt drains, the thicker it will become. Serve this dip with chunks of whole grain bread or pita bread.

2	cups low-fat or fat-free plain yogurt
I	large hothouse cucumber, peeled
½–I	teaspoon kosher or regular salt
I	clove garlic, minced
	Freshly ground black pepper

Place the yogurt in a funnel or strainer lined with cheesecloth. Set over a bowl to catch the drippings. Refrigerate for several hours to overnight, discarding the drained liquid as needed.

Grate the cucumber. Place in a colander, sprinkle with the salt, and allow to drain for 20 minutes. Squeeze out the excess liquid.

In a medium bowl, mix the yogurt and garlic. Fold in the cucumber and season with the pepper. Cover and refrigerate until ready to serve.

Per serving: 45 calories, 4 g protein, 6 g carbohydrates, I g total fat, 4 mg cholesterol, I g dietary fiber, I63 mg sodium.

Smart Cooking: Hothouse cucumbers are the ones you see wrapped in plastic in the supermarket. They're great to use when you don't want the watery center and seeds of a regular cucumber.

SICILIAN CAPONATA

Makes 12 servings (3 cups)

Prep and cooking time: 45 minutes

An Italian relish, caponata traditionally is served warm or at room temperature as a side dish or a spread. It makes a wonderful rustic-style sauce for pasta and grilled chicken breasts. It will keep in the refrigerator for up to a week; the flavors actually blend and deepen as it sits.

3	tablespoons olive oil
I	large onion, cut into ½" cubes
2	ribs celery, cut into ½" cubes
I	red bell pepper, cored, seeded, and cut into ½" cubes
4	cloves garlic, minced
1½	pounds eggplant, peeled and cut into ½" cubes
I	14½-ounce can diced tomatoes, drained
3	tablespoons tomato paste
2	teaspoons dried oregano
¼	cup chopped pitted kalamata olives
3	tablespoons red wine vinegar
2	tablespoons drained capers
2	tablespoons chopped basil leaves
2	teaspoons sugar
2	tablespoons pine nuts (optional)
	Salt
	Freshly ground black pepper

In a large nonstick skillet, heat the oil. Add the onion and cook for 2 minutes. Stir in the celery and bell pepper. Cook over medium heat for 5 minutes.

Add the garlic, eggplant, tomatoes, tomato paste, and oregano. Reduce the heat to medium-low, cover, and cook for 20 minutes, stirring occasionally.

Remove from the heat and stir in the olives, vinegar, capers, basil, sugar, and pine nuts, if using. Season to taste with the salt and black pepper.

Let stand at room temperature for at least 3 hours before serving, or cover and store in the refrigerator.

Per serving: 76 calories, 2 g protein, 9 g carbohydrates, 4 g total fat, 0 mg cholesterol, 3 g dietary fiber, 200 mg sodium

TUSCAN WHITE BEAN SPREAD

Makes 12 servings (¾ cup)

Prep time: 10 minutes

This versatile spread makes a flavorful butter substitute when served with thickly sliced whole grain bread. Another option is to thin it with a little reserved bean liquid or low-sodium chicken or vegetable broth and use it as a dip for vegetables.

1	15-ounce can cannellini, navy, or great Northern beans, rinsed and drained
1	large clove garlic
1	tablespoon lemon juice
2	teaspoons white wine vinegar
2	sprigs fresh parsley
2	basil leaves
1	teaspoon Dijon mustard
¼	teaspoon dried oregano
	Red pepper flakes to taste
2	tablespoons olive oil
	Salt
	Freshly ground black pepper

In a food processor or blender, combine the beans, garlic, lemon juice, vinegar, parsley, basil, mustard, oregano, and pepper flakes. Puree until smooth.

With the processor or blender running, slowly pour in the oil. Season to taste with the salt and black pepper.

Store in a covered container in the refrigerator. Serve at room temperature.

Per serving: 45 calories, 1 g protein, 5 g carbohydrates, 2 g total fat, 0 mg cholesterol, 1 g dietary fiber, 73 mg sodium

WILD MUSHROOM RAGU

Makes 32 servings (2 cups)

Prep time: 15 minutes

Cooking time: approximately 1 hour 10 minutes

This is a very versatile recipe. You can serve the ragu over fish or chicken, toss it into pasta, add it to soups, or spread it on crostini (toasted bread slices) and top with fresh mozzarella cheese. It's perfect for just about any dish that could use a dash of concentrated mushroom flavor.

2	tablespoons olive oil
¼	cup chopped shallots
4	cloves garlic, minced
2	pounds mixed mushrooms, thinly sliced
1	cup reduced-sodium vegetable, mushroom, or chicken broth
¼	cup dry red wine
2	tablespoons balsamic vinegar
1	teaspoon dried thyme
½	teaspoon dried sage
2	tablespoons chopped fresh parsley
	Salt
1	teaspoon dry sherry
	Freshly ground black pepper

In a large saucepan, warm the oil over medium heat. Add the shallots and garlic and cook for 2 to 3 minutes. Stir in the mushrooms and cook for 5 minutes, or until they begin to soften.

Add the broth, wine, vinegar, thyme, sage, and 1 tablespoon of the parsley.

Reduce the heat to medium-low. Simmer, stirring occasionally, for about 1 hour, or until most of the liquid has been absorbed and the mushrooms are thick and rich.

Stir in the sherry and the remaining 1 tablespoon parsley. Season to taste with the salt and pepper. Simmer for 5 minutes. Serve immediately or refrigerate until ready to use.

Per 1 teaspoon serving: 20 calories, 1 g protein, 2 g carbohydrates, 1 g total fat, 0 mg cholesterol, 0 g dietary fiber, 4 mg sodium

QUICK AND EASY HOMEMADE GUACAMOLE

Makes 24 servings (1½ cups)

Prep time: 5 minutes

Yes, avocados are high in fat. But it's mostly monounsaturated fat, the healthy kind. With this recipe, you have a tasty way of incorporating avocado into your diet.

2	ripe avocados, peeled, pitted, and halved lengthwise
2	tablespoons reduced-fat sour cream
1	tablespoon salsa
1	tablespoon lime juice
¼	teaspoon garlic powder
	Salt
	Freshly ground black pepper

In a small bowl, combine the avocados, sour cream, salsa, lime juice, and garlic powder. Using a knife, chop the avocados until the mixture is creamy, with small chunks. Season with the salt and pepper. Stir before serving.

Per 1 teaspoon serving: 14 calories, 0 g protein, 1 g carbohydrates, 1 g total fat, 0 mg cholesterol, 1 g dietary fiber, 3 mg sodium

- -

Smart Cooking: Shopping for avocados can be a bit tricky. They can look nice on the outside but be brown and mushy on the inside. Here's a foolproof method for getting perfectly ripe avocados every time.

Look for fruits that are hard and green or just beginning to turn black. Place them in a paper bag on your kitchen counter and check them each day for several days. When the skin is black and the avocados feel slightly soft when pressed, they are ready to use. You can store them in the refrigerator for several more days, if you wish.

If you can't wait for the avocados to ripen, choose ones that have black skin and yield slightly to your touch. Avoid those that are mushy or shriveled or have soft spots.

If you don't intend to serve your guacamole right away, tightly seal the bowl with a cover or with plastic wrap so no air can get into it. This will prevent the avocado from turning brown.

FRESH CORN SALSA

Serves 4

Prep time: 10 minutes

When fresh corn isn't in season, frozen works just as well. Turn up the heat by using a larger jalapeño or Tabasco sauce.

1	large ear corn
3	plum tomatoes, diced
2	scallions, chopped
1	small jalapeño pepper, finely chopped
3	tablespoons lime juice
1–2	tablespoons chopped fresh cilantro
	Salt
	Freshly ground black pepper

Grill, steam, or boil the corn until just cooked through. Be careful not to overcook. Set aside to cool.

Cut the kernels from the cob and place in a medium bowl. Add the tomatoes, onions, jalapeño, lime juice, and cilantro. Season to taste with the salt and pepper.

Per serving: 46 calories, 2 g protein, 11 g carbohydrates, 1 g total fat, 0 mg cholesterol, 2 g dietary fiber, 6 mg sodium

Bakery-Fresh Breads and More

HIGH-PRO ENERGY BREAD

Makes 2 loaves (24 slices)

Prep time: 30 minutes

Baking time: 40–45 minutes

Homemade bread is such a treat. This recipe yields two loaves—one to serve right away, the other to freeze for later. The higher-protein ingredients make for a soft, chewy bread that you can toast for breakfast or a snack, topped with a dollop of reduced-fat cream cheese, peanut butter, or fruit spread.

1¼	cups warm (110°–115°F) fat-free milk or soy milk
1	package (2¼ teaspoons) active dry yeast
¼	cup honey
1½	cups bread flour or unbleached flour
¾	cup soy flour
¾	cup coarsely chopped walnuts
½	cup cottage cheese
2	eggs
3	tablespoons wheat gluten
¾	teaspoon salt
2¾	cups whole wheat flour

In a large bowl, combine the milk, yeast, and honey. Set aside for 5 minutes, or until foamy.

Add the bread flour or unbleached flour. Using an electric mixer, beat well for 3 minutes. Stir in the soy flour, walnuts, cottage cheese, eggs, gluten, salt, and 2 cups of the whole wheat flour.

Turn out onto a floured surface and knead in enough of the remaining ¾ cup whole wheat flour to form a soft dough. Knead for 10 minutes, or until smooth and elastic. Form the dough into a ball.

Coat a large bowl with cooking spray or a little olive oil. Transfer the dough to the bowl and turn to coat all sides. Cover and let rise in a warm place for about I hour, or until doubled in size.

Coat 2 loaf pans (9" x 5") with cooking spray. Punch down the dough and divide into 2 pieces. Shape into 2 loaves and place in the prepared pans. Cover and let rise in a warm place for 35 to 45 minutes, or until doubled in size.

Preheat the oven to 350°F. Transfer the loaves to the oven and bake for 40 to 45 minutes, or until brown on top. Remove the loaves from the pans and tap on the bottom. They should sound hollow; if not, return to the oven for a few minutes. Cool on a wire rack.

Per slice: 136 calories, 6 g protein, 21 g carbohydrates, 4 g total fat, 19 mg cholesterol, 3 g dietary fiber, 102 mg sodium

MULTIGRAIN CLOVERLEAF ROLLS

Makes 20

Prep time: 30 minutes

Baking time: 10 minutes

These hearty rolls go great with soup or salad.

1¼	cups warm (110°–115°F) fat-free milk or soy milk
I	package (2¼ teaspoons) active dry yeast
I	tablespoon honey or sugar
2	eggs, beaten
I	cup multigrain flour such as soy, spelt, oat, and/or barley
I	tablespoon wheat gluten
¾	teaspoon salt
2	tablespoons unsalted butter, melted
2	cups whole wheat flour

In a large bowl, combine the milk, yeast, and honey or sugar. Set aside for 5 minutes, or until foamy.

Add the eggs, multigrain flour, gluten, salt, and I tablespoon of the butter. Using an electric mixer, beat well for 3 minutes. Stir in 1½ cups of the whole wheat flour.

Turn out onto a floured surface and knead in enough of the remaining ½ cup whole wheat flour to form a soft dough. Knead for 10 minutes, or until smooth and elastic. Form into a ball.

Coat a large bowl with cooking spray or a little olive oil. Transfer the dough to the bowl and turn to coat all sides. Cover and let rise in a warm place for about 1 hour, or until doubled in size.

Coat 2 muffin pans (12-cup) with cooking spray.

Punch down the dough and divide into 20 pieces. Shape each piece into 3 balls and place all 3 balls in 1 muffin cup. Continue with the remaining pieces until you have 20 muffin cups with 3 balls each. Cover and let rise in a warm place for 30 to 45 minutes, or until doubled in size.

Preheat the oven to 425°F. Brush the tops of the rolls with the remaining 1 tablespoon butter. Bake for 10 minutes, or until lightly brown on top. Remove from the pans and cool on a wire rack.

Per roll: 94 calories, 4 g protein, 15 g carbohydrates, 2 g total fat, 24 mg cholesterol, 2 g dietary fiber, 102 mg sodium

PUMPKIN CRANBERRY LOAF

Makes 1 loaf (10 slices)

Prep time: 15 minutes

Baking time: 1 hour

For variety, you can prepare this recipe as muffins instead of a loaf. Simply reduce the baking time by about 15 to 25 minutes, depending on the size of the muffins. If you prefer, you can leave out the cranberries, too.

2	cups whole wheat pastry flour or unbleached flour
2	teaspoons baking powder
½	teaspoon salt
¼	teaspoon baking soda
¼	teaspoon ground cinnamon
¼	teaspoon ground ginger
¼	teaspoon ground cloves
2	large eggs

1	cup sugar
1	cup canned solid-pack pumpkin
¼	cup canola oil
¼	cup orange juice
1	teaspoon vanilla extract
¾–1	cup fresh or frozen cranberries, halved
¼–½	cup chopped walnuts

Preheat the oven to 350°F. Lightly coat a large (8½" x 4½" x ¾") loaf pan with cooking spray.

In a large bowl, combine the flour, baking powder, salt, baking soda, cinnamon, ginger, and cloves.

In a medium bowl, whisk the eggs until lightly beaten. Add the sugar, pumpkin, oil, orange juice, and vanilla, beating after each addition.

Fold the egg mixture into the flour mixture, stirring just enough to incorporate the ingredients. Fold in the cranberries and walnuts.

Pour the batter into the prepared pan. Bake for 1 hour, or until a toothpick inserted into the center comes out clean or with fine crumbs on it. Remove from the pan and cool on a wire rack.

Per slice: 263 calories, 5 g protein, 42 g carbohydrates, 9 g total fat, 42 mg cholesterol, 3 g dietary fiber, 277 mg sodium

BRAN MUFFINS WITH APPLES AND PECANS

Makes 12

Prep time: 20 minutes

Baking time: 15 minutes

These muffins are packed with nutrients. They are much lower in fat but a lot more flavorful than traditional bran muffins.

3	tablespoons unsalted butter, softened, or canola oil
½	cup packed brown sugar
⅓	cup fat-free plain yogurt

3	tablespoons honey
I	egg
I	teaspoon grated orange peel
1¼	cups wheat bran
I	cup whole wheat pastry flour or unbleached flour
1½	teaspoons baking soda
½	teaspoon salt
¼	teaspoon grated nutmeg
¼	teaspoon ground cinnamon
I	small apple, peeled, cored, and diced
¼	cup finely chopped pecans

Preheat the oven to 375°F. Line a 12-cup muffin pan with paper liners or coat with cooking spray.

Place the butter or oil in a large bowl. If using butter, beat with an electric mixer until smooth. Add the brown sugar and beat until creamy. Add the yogurt, honey, egg, and orange peel, beating after each addition.

In a medium bowl, combine the wheat bran, flour, baking soda, salt, nutmeg, and cinnamon.

Fold the flour mixture into the yogurt mixture, stirring just enough to incorporate the ingredients. Fold in the apple and pecans.

Spoon the batter into the prepared muffin pan. Bake for 15 minutes, or until a toothpick inserted into the center of a muffiin comes out clean or with moist crumbs. Remove from the pan and cool on a wire rack.

Per muffin: 148 calories, 3 g protein, 24 g carbohydrates, 5 g total fat, 25 mg cholesterol, 4 g dietary fiber, 268 mg sodium

OLD-FASHIONED GINGERBREAD MUFFINS

Makes 12

Prep time: 10 minutes

Baking time: 15 minutes

These muffins only taste like the ones Grandma used to make. This updated version is low in fat and filled with whole grain goodness—a moist, flavor-packed treat for gingerbread lovers.

1½	cups whole wheat pastry flour
1½	teaspoons ground ginger
¾	teaspoon ground cinnamon
½	teaspoon salt
½	teaspoon baking powder
¼	teaspoon ground nutmeg
¼	teaspoon ground cloves
¼	teaspoon baking soda
1	egg, beaten
¼	cup molasses
¼	cup maple syrup or honey
4	tablespoons unsweetened applesauce
2	tablespoons canola oil

Preheat the oven to 350°F. Line a 12-cup muffin pan with paper liners or coat with cooking spray.

In a medium bowl, combine the flour, ginger, cinnamon, salt, baking powder, nutmeg, cloves, and baking soda. Stir well.

In a small bowl, combine the egg, molasses, maple syrup or honey, applesauce, and oil.

Pour the liquid mixture into the dry mixture, stirring just enough to incorporate the ingredients. Be careful not to overmix.

Spoon the batter into the prepared muffin tin. Bake for 15 minutes, or until a toothpick inserted into the center of a muffin comes out with moist crumbs. Remove from the tin and cool on a wire rack.

Per muffin: 109 calories, 2 g protein, 19 g carbohydrates, 3 g total fat, 18 mg cholesterol, 1 g dietary fiber, 150 mg sodium

MULTIGRAIN SOFT PRETZELS

Makes 12

Prep time: 25 minutes

Baking time: 10 minutes

Preparing these pretzels is fast and easy. Although the recipe calls for yeast, the dough doesn't need to rise. Experiment with any variety of whole grain flour. If you have a countertop mixer with a dough hook, try using it to knead the dough.

1	package (2¼ teaspoons) rapid-rise active dry yeast
¼	cup whole grain flour such as soy, spelt, barley, or oat
1	tablespoon wheat gluten
½	teaspoon salt
1¾–2¼	cups whole wheat flour
¾	cup warm (120°–130°F) fat-free milk or soy milk
2	tablespoons honey
2	eggs, beaten
1	tablespoon sesame seeds
1	teaspoon coarse kosher salt (optional)

Preheat the oven to 425°F. Line a baking sheet with parchment paper or coat with cooking spray.

In a large bowl, combine the yeast, whole grain flour, gluten, salt, and 1¾ cups of the whole wheat flour. Add the milk, honey, and all but 1 tablespoon of the eggs. Set aside the remaining egg. Stir to mix well.

Turn out onto a floured surface and knead for 10 minutes, adding more whole wheat flour as needed to form a smooth, elastic dough. The dough should be slightly sticky. If it seems too wet, knead in a little more flour. Cover the dough and let rest for 10 minutes.

Divide the dough into 12 pieces and roll each piece into a 15" log. Shape each log into a pretzel and place on the prepared baking sheet. Brush each pretzel with the remaining 1 tablespoon egg and sprinkle with the sesame seeds and kosher salt, if using.

Bake for 10 minutes, or until just lightly browned. Remove from the baking sheet and cool on a wire rack.

Per pretzel: 103 calories, 5 g protein, 18 g carbohydrates, 2 g total fat, 36 mg cholesterol, 3 g dietary fiber, 118 mg sodium

Cheddar-Filled Multigrain Soft Pretzels: To make these pretzels, you can use the recipe on page 285, with one additional ingredient: 6 ounces reduced-fat sharp Cheddar cheese, cut into 12 cubes. After dividing the dough into 12 pieces, roll each piece into a ball rather than a log. Press a cheese cube into each ball, reshaping to seal well. Place the balls on the prepared baking sheet and cut an X on the top of each. This will prevent the cheese from bursting out the bottom as the pretzels bake. Continue as directed in the original recipe.

Per pretzel: 148 calories, 8 g protein, 19 g carbohydrates, 5 g total fat, 46 mg cholesterol, 3 g dietary fiber, 238 mg sodium

Sumptuous Salads

BEET AND APPLE SALAD WITH CHEESE AND WALNUTS

Serves 4

Prep and cooking time: 30 minutes

You can enjoy this unique salad any time of year, but it's best in autumn, when apples and beets are freshest. Be sure to assemble the salad just before serving. Otherwise, the apples will turn brown and the beets will color everything pink. If you must grate the apples ahead of time, try tossing them with a little lemon juice, to help prevent discoloration.

I	pound beets, tops trimmed
2	tart apples, peeled, cored, and grated
2	tablespoons walnut oil
2	tablespoons champagne or white wine vinegar
	Salt
4	large leaves bib lettuce
4	tablespoons low-fat soft goat cheese or feta cheese
4	tablespoons toasted walnut pieces
	Freshly ground black pepper

In a medium saucepan, cook the beets on high for 25 minutes, or until soft when pierced with a sharp knife. Drain and set aside to cool.

Peel and grate the beets. Transfer to a medium bowl and add the apples, oil, and vinegar. Toss to mix. Season to taste with the salt.

Place I leaf of the lettuce on each of 4 salad plates. Spoon an equal amount of the beet mixture onto the lettuce leaves. Top each salad with a tablespoon each of the cheese and walnuts. Season to taste with the pepper. Serve immediately.

Per serving: 208 calories, 4 g protein, 21 g carbohydrates, 13 g total fat, 2 mg cholesterol, 5 g dietary fiber, 139 mg sodium

CHOPPED CHICKEN SALAD

Serves 8

Prep time: 20 minutes

This salad is a meal in itself. To shorten the prep time, buy precooked or rotisserie chicken, precut carrots, and preshredded cabbage. Serve with light Italian dressing or another low-fat dressing of your choice.

10	cups romaine lettuce hearts, torn into small pieces
4	cups shredded cooked chicken breast
3	cups shredded carrots
2	cups shredded red cabbage
20	pitted black or green olives, sliced
2	large tomatoes or 4 Roma tomatoes, diced
8	ounces feta cheese, crumbled
½	cup toasted sunflower seeds
6	scallions, sliced
2	cups Terra Stix or broken tortilla chips

In a large salad bowl, combine the lettuce, chicken, carrots, cabbage, olives, tomatoes, cheese, sunflower seeds, and scallions. Toss gently. Top with the Terra Stix or broken tortilla chips. Serve immediately.

Per serving: 380 calories, 27 g protein, 22 g carbohydrates, 21 g total fat, 78 mg cholesterol, 5 g dietary fiber, 602 mg sodium

- -

Smart Cooking: Terra Stix are crunchy vegetable chips, similar to potato chips but cut into thin strips. They're available in many supermarkets and gourmet markets. If you can't find them, broken tortilla chips work just as well.

GREEK CHOPPED SALAD

Serves 6

Prep time: 20 minutes

You can make this salad in a snap. The bright colors of the ingredients enhance the presentation.

4	cups romaine lettuce, chopped into small pieces
2	cups cubed cucumbers
I	15-ounce can chickpeas, rinsed and drained
4	ounces feta cheese, crumbled
¼	cup finely chopped red onion
18	pitted kalamata olives, sliced
¼	cup roasted red peppers, chopped
¼	cup chopped fresh parsley
2	tablespoons drained capers
3	tablespoons fresh lemon juice
2	tablespoons olive oil
½	teaspoon dried oregano, crushed
	Salt
	Freshly ground black pepper

In a large bowl, combine the lettuce, cucumbers, chickpeas, cheese, onion, olives, red peppers, parsley, and capers. Sprinkle with the lemon juice, oil, and oregano. Season to taste with the salt and black pepper. Serve immediately.

Per serving: 210 calories, 8 g protein, 17 g carbohydrates, 12 g total fat, 17 mg cholesterol, 4 g dietary fiber, 759 mg sodium

GREEN BEAN, TOMATO, AND FRESH MOZZARELLA SALAD WITH PASTA

Serves 8

Prep and cooking time: 25 minutes

You can serve this salad as a light entrée or a side dish with a piece of fish or poultry. It has lots of flavor and texture. Leftovers keep extremely well in the refrigerator for several days.

1½	pounds fresh green beans, washed and trimmed
10	ounces thin spiral or penne pasta
2	tablespoons olive oil
2	tablespoons lemon juice
1	tablespoon red wine vinegar
	Red pepper flakes to taste
1	pint grape tomatoes, halved
4	ounces fresh mozzarella cheese, cut into small cubes
¼	cup finely chopped red onion
3	tablespoons freshly grated Parmesan or Asiago cheese
3	tablespoons toasted pine nuts
2	tablespoons chopped fresh basil
	Salt
	Freshly ground black pepper

Fill a sink or large pan with ice water.

Bring a large saucepan of water to a boil. Add the green beans and cook for approximately 4 minutes, or until bright green.

With a slotted spoon or small colander, remove the beans and immediately put them into the ice water to stop the cooking. When chilled, dry and set aside.

Bring the water in the pan back to a boil and add the pasta. Cook for approximately 8 to 10 minutes, or until al dente. Drain, reserving ¼ cup of the cooking water.

In a small bowl, whisk together the oil, lemon juice, vinegar, pepper flakes, and reserved cooking water.

In a large bowl, combine the beans, pasta, tomatoes, mozzarella, onion, cheese, pine nuts, and basil. Add the oil and vinegar mixture and toss gently. Season to taste with the salt and black pepper. Refrigerate until ready to serve.

Per serving: 272 calories, 11 g protein, 36 g carbohydrates, 10 g total fat, 12 mg cholesterol, 4 g dietary fiber, 138 mg sodium

ITALIAN CHOPPED SALAD

Serves 8

Prep time: 15 minutes

A chopped salad like this one is a bounty of color and texture. Experiment with the ingredients, using whatever vegetables and cheeses you have on hand. You can make this salad up to an hour ahead of time; just keep it in the refrigerator and don't add the dressing until ready to serve. Use the low-fat dressing of your choice; my personal favorite is a tablespoon or two of olive oil and balsamic vinegar.

1	head romaine lettuce, coarsely chopped (about 3 cups)
2	heads Belgian endive, cored and chopped
1	small head radicchio, chopped (about 2 cups)
8	ounces fresh mozzarella cheese, cubed
½	red onion, finely chopped
½	cup roasted red peppers, chopped
12	green or black pitted olives, quartered lengthwise
2	tablespoons toasted pine nuts
1	tablespoon chopped fresh parsley
1	tablespoon chopped fresh basil
	Salt
	Freshly ground black pepper

In a large salad bowl, combine the lettuce, endive, radicchio, mozzarella, onion, red peppers, olives, pine nuts, parsley, and basil. Season to taste with the salt and black pepper. Toss with dressing and serve immediately.

Per serving: 166 calories, 9 g protein, 10 g carbohydrates, 10 g total fat, 20 mg cholesterol, 4 g dietary fiber, 463 mg sodium

ITALIAN COUNTRY RICE SALAD

Serves 6

Prep and cooking time: 50 minutes

Although wild rice is an American food, it adds nice color and texture to this flavorful Italian-style salad. It makes an ideal picnic dish because none of the ingredients will spoil even if left at room temperature for several hours.

2½	cups water
¾	cup brown rice
½	cup wild rice
3	tablespoons olive oil
1	clove garlic, minced
1	tablespoon balsamic vinegar
1	tablespoon red wine vinegar
1	teaspoon grated lemon peel
½	teaspoon dried oregano
¼	teaspoon red pepper flakes
6	sun-dried tomatoes, soaked in hot water to soften, drained, and chopped
½	cup finely chopped red onion
1	red bell pepper, cored, seeded, and chopped
9	black olives, pitted and sliced
9	green olives, pitted and sliced
¼	cup toasted slivered almonds or pine nuts
2	tablespoons drained capers
2	tablespoons freshly grated Parmesan cheese
2	tablespoons minced fresh parsley
1	tablespoon chopped fresh basil
	Salt
	Freshly ground black pepper

In a medium saucepan, bring the water to a boil. Add the brown rice and wild rice. Reduce the heat to medium-low, cover, and cook for 45 minutes, or until the water has been absorbed. Remove from the heat, cover, and set aside for about 5 minutes. Do not stir.

In a small bowl, combine the oil, garlic, balsamic vinegar, red wine vinegar, lemon peel, oregano, and pepper flakes.

In a large bowl, combine the tomatoes, onion, bell pepper, black olives, green olives, almonds or pine nuts, capers, cheese, parsley, and basil.

Gently fluff the rice with a fork. Add the rice and dressing to the vegetables and toss. Season to taste with the salt and pepper. Serve chilled or at room temperature.

Per serving: 258 calories, 6 g protein, 33 g carbohydrates, 13 g total fat, 1 mg cholesterol, 4 g dietary fiber, 379 mg sodium

ITALIAN INSALATA MISTA

Serves 6

Prep time: 15 minutes

This is a basic Italian green salad, but it always is a hit. Using greens with varying textures and flavors is key.

8	cups baby salad greens such as mache, romaine, spinach, or mesclun
1	large carrot, grated
½	large seedless cucumber, cubed
3	tablespoons toasted sunflower seeds or pine nuts
3	tablespoons freshly grated Parmesan cheese
3	tablespoons extra-virgin olive oil
1½	tablespoons red wine vinegar
1½	tablespoons balsamic vinegar
½	teaspoon grated lemon peel
	Salt
	Freshly ground black pepper

In a large bowl, combine the greens, carrot, cucumber, sunflower seeds or pine nuts, and cheese.

In a small bowl, whisk together the oil, red wine vinegar, balsamic vinegar, and lemon peel. Season to taste with the salt and pepper.

Pour the dressing onto the salad and toss gently. Serve immediately.

Per serving: 122 calories, 3 g protein, 6 g carbohydrates, 10 g total fat, 2 mg cholesterol, 3 g dietary fiber, 6 mg sodium

JICAMA SLAW

Serves 6

Prep time: 15 minutes

This salad is the perfect accompaniment to a Mexican meal. It's cool, crunchy, and juicy, with just a hint of chili powder and lime.

1	medium jicama, peeled and cut into julienne slices (about 4 cups)
1	cup shredded carrot
1	cup shredded red cabbage
¼	cup diced red bell pepper
¼	cup finely chopped red onion
1	tablespoon chopped fresh cilantro
2	tablespoons olive oil
2	tablespoons lime juice
2	tablespoons white wine vinegar
1	teaspoon grated lime peel
½	teaspoon sugar
¼	teaspoon chili powder
	Salt
	Freshly ground black pepper

In a large bowl, combine the jicama, carrot, cabbage, bell pepper, onion, and cilantro.

In a small bowl, whisk together the oil, lime juice, vinegar, lime peel, sugar, and chili powder.

Pour the dressing over the vegetables and season to taste with the salt and black pepper. Refrigerate until ready to serve.

Per serving: 90 calories, 1 g protein, 12 g carbohydrates, 5 g total fat, 0 mg cholesterol, 5 g dietary fiber, 21 mg sodium

----

Smart Cooking: Jicama (HICK-uh-muh) is a large, round root vegetable with sand-colored skin and crisp, juicy, slightly bland, white flesh. It's popular throughout Mexico, Asia, and the American Southwest, where it often is eaten raw or stir-fried. Jicama will keep unwrapped in your refrigerator's vegetable bin for up to 3 weeks. Once you cut it, cover the unused portion with plastic wrap and refrigerate for up to a week.

Asian Jicama Slaw: Finding something to serve with Asian dishes can be a challenge, so I came up with this Asian version of the Jicama Slaw on the opposite page. Use the same recipe, with the following ingredient substitutions.

• 1 tablespoon each regular and toasted sesame oil for the olive oil

• Equal amounts lemon juice and peel for the lime juice and peel

• Equal amount rice wine vinegar for the white wine vinegar

• ¼ teaspoon grated fresh ginger for the chili powder

Serves 6

Prep and cooking time: 40 minutes

Although this recipe calls for quite a few ingredients, it's divided into three steps for fast and easy preparation. Once you taste the results, I'm sure you'll agree it's well worth the effort! Because the seafood marinates in the vinaigrette, it will stay fresh for 2 days without turning fishy. This means you can get several meals from one salad.

Vinaigrette

⅓	cup lemon juice
3	tablespoons olive oil
2	tablespoons white wine vinegar
I	clove garlic, minced
	Grated peel of I lemon
I	teaspoon sugar
¾	teaspoon salt
	Freshly ground black pepper

Salad

I	rib celery, finely diced
½	orange or yellow bell pepper, seeded and finely diced
½	cup roasted red peppers, finely chopped
8	pitted kalamata olives, slivered
3	scallions, halved lengthwise and sliced
2	tablespoons chopped fresh parsley
I	tablespoon chopped fresh basil
I	tablespoon chopped fresh dill

Seafood

I½	cups water
½	cup white wine or lemon juice

10	sprigs parsley
6	whole black peppercorns
2	long strips lemon peel
½	teaspoon salt
½	pound medium shrimp, rinsed
½	pound sea scallops, muscle removed, cut into quarters or eighths
½	pound calamari, body sliced into rings, tentacles cut into bite-size pieces
8	ounces precooked crabmeat

To make the vinaigrette: In a large bowl, combine the lemon juice, oil, vinegar, garlic, lemon peel, sugar, and salt. Season to taste with the pepper.

To make the salad: Add the celery, bell pepper, red peppers, olives, scallions, parsley, basil, and dill to the vinaigrette and toss to mix.

To make the seafood: Fill a large bowl with ice water. Set aside.

In a medium saucepan, combine the water, wine or lemon juice, parsley, peppercorns, lemon peel, and salt. Bring to a boil. Reduce the heat to medium, keeping the liquid at a steady simmer.

Add the shrimp and cook for 1 minute. Add the scallops and cook for 1 minute. Add the calamari and cook for 30 seconds to 1 minute.

Remove the pan from the heat and drain the liquid. Place the seafood in the ice water to stop the cooking.

Remove the seafood from the water. Peel the shrimp and add to the salad along with the scallops, calamari, and crabmeat. Refrigerate until ready to serve.

Per serving: 262 calories, 28 g protein, 11 g carbohydrates, 10 g total fat, 180 mg cholesterol, 1 g dietary fiber, 877 mg sodium

----

Smart Cooking: This recipe calls for a total of 2 pounds of seafood. If you prefer, you can use just one variety, such as clams or mussels. Experiment with your favorites.

Many people, especially children, don't like to see the squid's tentacles in their salad. Ask your fishmonger for just the body, which you can slice into rings.

MEDITERRANEAN LENTIL SALAD

Serves 6

Prep and cooking time: 50 minutes

This salad is equally delicious whether served chilled atop a bed of greens, at room temperature with crackers or crusty bread, or warm as a side dish with chicken or fish. Any leftovers should stay fresh in the refrigerator for several days.

2	cups water
I	cup small French green lentils or regular green lentils
2	tablespoons olive oil
2	tablespoons lemon juice
I½	tablespoons red wine vinegar
I	small clove garlic, minced
I	teaspoon grated lemon peel
½	teaspoon Dijon mustard
½	cup chopped red or yellow bell pepper
½	cup shredded carrot
½	cup diced cucumber
I0	kalamata olives, slivered
2	tablespoons finely chopped red onion
I	tablespoon chopped fresh dill
I	tablespoon chopped fresh basil
	Salt
	Freshly ground black pepper
	Crushed red pepper flakes

In a medium saucepan, bring the water to a boil. Add the lentils and return to a boil. Reduce the heat to medium-low, cover, and cook for 40 to 45 minutes, or until the lentils are soft.

In a medium bowl, whisk together the oil, lemon juice, vinegar, garlic, lemon peel, and mustard. Add the bell pepper, carrot, cucumber, olives, onion, dill, and basil.

When the lentils are cooked, drain in a colander if necessary. Stir into the salad. Season to taste with the salt, black pepper, and pepper flakes and toss well. Let marinate until ready to serve, or refrigerate.

Per serving: 169 calories, 8 g protein, 21 g carbohydrates, 6 g total fat, 0 mg cholesterol, 5 g dietary fiber, 131 mg sodium

ROASTED CHICKEN SALAD WITH MANGO AND PISTACHIOS

Serves 6

Prep and cooking time: 35 minutes

You can vary this recipe by substituting peaches, apricots, grapes, or other fruits for the mango. I've even used fresh pears and apples in autumn, with wonderful results. Roasting and shredding the chicken gives the salad added flavor and texture. Serve on a bed of greens or as a sandwich in pita bread, a roll, or a wrap.

4	bone-in chicken breast halves
	Salt
	Freshly ground black pepper
½	cup reduced-fat mayonnaise
½	cup reduced-fat sour cream
2	tablespoons lemon juice
1	teaspoon dried tarragon
1	teaspoon Dijon mustard
½	teaspoon grated lemon peel
2	ribs celery, diced
½	red bell pepper, seeded and diced
1	mango, peeled and cut into cubes
½	cup shelled unsalted pistachios, coarsely chopped
¼	cup fresh parsley, chopped

Preheat the oven to 400°F. Line a baking dish with foil.

Place the chicken in the baking dish. Coat with cooking spray and season with the salt and black pepper. Roast for approximately 30 minutes, or until cooked through. Set aside to cool.

In a large bowl, combine the mayonnaise, sour cream, lemon juice, tarragon, mustard, and lemon peel.

Remove the skin and bones from the chicken and shred by hand into bite-size pieces. Fold into the dressing, along with the celery, bell pepper, mango, pistachios, and parsley. Season with the salt and black pepper. Refrigerate until ready to serve.

Per serving: 200 calories, 12 g protein, 15 g carbohydrates, 11 g total fat, 31 mg cholesterol, 2 g dietary fiber, 249 mg sodium

SHRIMP AND PASTA SALAD WITH SNOW PEAS

Serves 4

Prep and cooking time: 45 minutes

Light but satisfying, this pasta salad is a favorite at parties. Leftovers will keep in the refrigerator for 1 to 2 days.

½	pound snow peas, cut on the diagonal
8	ounces penne pasta
2	tablespoons olive oil
2	tablespoons lemon juice or to taste
1½	teaspoons Dijon mustard
1	small clove garlic, minced
1	teaspoon grated lemon peel
½	teaspoon dried tarragon, crumbled
	Salt
	Freshly ground black pepper
1	pound medium shrimp, cooked and peeled
4	ounces feta cheese, crumbled

1	red or orange bell pepper or a combination, cored, seeded, and thinly sliced
¼	cup chopped red onion
1	tablespoon finely chopped fresh parsley
1	tablespoon finely chopped fresh basil

Bring a large saucepan of water to a boil. Fill the sink or a large pan with ice water.

Add the snow peas to the boiling water and blanch for 1 to 2 minutes, or until bright green. Scoop out the peas with a strainer or colander and plunge into the ice water to stop the cooking. Once the peas have cooled, dry on a paper towel.

Return water to a boil. Add the pasta and cook according to the package directions or until al dente. Be careful not to overcook. Drain, reserving 2 tablespoons of the cooking water. Transfer the pasta to a large bowl.

In a small bowl, combine the oil, lemon juice, mustard, garlic, lemon peel, and tarragon. Add the reserved cooking water. Season to taste with the salt and black pepper.

Pour the dressing over the pasta and toss well. Add the shrimp, cheese, bell pepper, onion, parsley, and basil. Toss well. Season to taste with the salt, black pepper, and additional lemon juice, if desired. Cover and refrigerate until ready to serve.

Per serving: 503 calories, 37 g protein, 53 g carbohydrates, 16 g total fat, 198 mg cholesterol, 4 g dietary fiber, 538 mg sodium

SOUTHWESTERN THREE-BEAN SALAD

Serves 6

Prep time: 20 minutes

Using canned beans in a marinated salad is a quick and easy way to add fiber and lean protein to your diet. Our favorite combination of beans is black, pinto, and kidney. You can use any type of beans you like. Create just the right amount of spiciness by adding more or less red pepper flakes.

3	15-ounce cans beans, rinsed and drained
1	cup frozen corn, thawed and drained
¼	cup finely chopped red onion
¼	cup chopped red bell pepper

1	tablespoon chopped fresh parsley
1	tablespoon chopped fresh cilantro
¼	cup low-fat chicken or vegetable broth
2	tablespoons olive oil
2	tablespoons tomato paste
	Juice of 1 lime
	Grated peel of 1 lime
1	tablespoon red wine vinegar
1	clove garlic, minced
1	teaspoon honey or sugar
1	teaspoon chili powder
½	teaspoon ground cumin
	Salt
	Freshly ground black pepper
	Red pepper flakes

In a large bowl, combine the beans, corn, onion, red pepper, parsley, and cilantro.

In a small bowl, combine the broth, oil, tomato paste, lime juice, lime peel, vinegar, garlic, honey or sugar, chili powder, and cumin.

Pour the dressing over the beans and toss. Season to taste with the salt, black pepper, and pepper flakes. Toss well and let marinate until ready to serve.

Per serving: 238 calories, 11 g protein, 36 g carbohydrates, 6 g total fat, 0 mg cholesterol, 12 g dietary fiber, 481 mg sodium

WILD RICE AND SWEET POTATO SALAD WITH PEAR VINAIGRETTE

Serves 8

Prep and cooking time: 50 minutes

If you're looking for a tasty addition to a holiday meal, try this salad. It can be made a day or so ahead, since the flavors blend as it marinates. Serve it on a bed of greens.

2½	cups water
1¼	cups wild rice, rinsed
2	pounds sweet potatoes, peeled and cut into small cubes
3	scallions, sliced
½	red bell pepper, seeded and finely diced
⅓	cup toasted pecans
¼	cup chopped fresh parsley
2	ripe pears, peeled and cored
3	tablespoons walnut oil
2	tablespoons white wine vinegar
2	tablespoons lemon juice
½–1	teaspoon dried sage
	Salt
	Freshly ground black pepper

In a large saucepan, bring the water to a boil. Add the rice. Reduce the heat to medium-low, cover, and simmer for 45 minutes, or until the rice is soft but not mushy.

While the rice is cooking, place the sweet potatoes in another large saucepan and fill with water. Bring to a boil, reduce the heat to medium-low, and cook for 5 minutes, or until the potatoes are just soft. Be careful not to overcook, or the potatoes will break apart in the salad. Drain and rinse under cold water to stop the cooking. Set aside.

In a large bowl, stir together the scallions, bell pepper, pecans, and parsley.

In a small processor or blender, puree 1 of the pears. Add the oil, vinegar, lemon juice, and sage. Puree until smooth. Season to taste with the salt and black pepper. Set aside.

When the rice is cooked, drain and transfer to the bowl. Toss with the vinaigrette. Chop the remaining pear and gently fold into the salad along with the sweet potatoes. Taste and season with the salt and black pepper, if desired. Refrigerate until ready to serve.

Per serving: 264 calories, 7 g protein, 46 g carbohydrates, 7 g total fat, 0 mg cholesterol, 6 g dietary fiber, 50 mg sodium

Soups by the Spoonful

BLACK BEAN SOUP WITH LIME

Serves 6

Prep time: 15 minutes

Cooking time: 1½ hours

This rich and hearty soup has lots of flavor. Serve it with cornbread and a salad or as a side dish or first course with a Mexican entrée. Using a food processor to chop the vegetables reduces the preparation time.

1	tablespoon olive oil
1	red onion, chopped
1	red bell pepper, cored, seeded, and chopped
1	carrot, chopped
1–2	jalapeño peppers, chopped
4	cloves garlic, chopped
1	bay leaf
1	tablespoon ground cumin
1	tablespoon ground coriander
1	teaspoon dried oregano
3	cups dried black beans, picked over, rinsed, and soaked overnight
8	cups low-sodium vegetable or chicken broth
1	teaspoon liquid smoke flavoring (optional)
2	tablespoons chopped fresh parsley
2	tablespoons chopped fresh cilantro
2	tablespoons dry sherry
1	tablespoon lime juice

1   teaspoon grated lime peel

Salt

Freshly ground black pepper

In a large soup pot, warm the oil over medium heat. Add the onion, bell pepper, carrot, jalapeños, and garlic. Cook for 10 minutes, stirring occasionally.

Add the bay leaf, cumin, coriander, and oregano.

Drain and rinse the beans. Add to the pot along with the broth and liquid smoke, if using. Bring to a boil, then reduce the heat to medium-low. Cook, partially covered, for 1 to 1½ hours, or until the beans are tender. Remove the bay leaf.

Stir in the parsley, cilantro, sherry, lime juice, and lime peel. Season to taste with the salt and black pepper.

Per serving: 392 calories, 22 g protein, 69 g carbohydrates, 4 g total fat, 0 mg cholesterol, 21 g dietary fiber, 645 mg sodium

BROCCOLI RABE AND WHITE BEAN SOUP

Serves 8

Prep and cooking time: 1½ hours

Broccoli rabe, also known as rapini or rape, is a plant in the mustard family. It looks a lot like broccoli, but has thinner stems, smaller florets, and more leaves. Look for bunches with thin stems but no yellow leaves. Use the whole plants, discarding only the lower 2 inches of the stems.

3   cups dried white beans (cannellini, navy, and/or great Northern), picked over, rinsed, and soaked overnight

2   tablespoons olive oil

1   onion, chopped

2   ribs celery, finely chopped

1   carrot, finely chopped

12   cloves garlic

1   bay leaf

1   teaspoon dried basil

1   teaspoon dried oregano

8	cups low-sodium chicken or vegetable broth
1½	pounds broccoli rabe, chopped into ¼" pieces
2	teaspoons sugar
¼	teaspoon red pepper flakes
1	Parmesan rind (see Smart Cooking)
1	teaspoon grated lemon peel
	Salt
	Freshly ground black pepper
	Freshly grated Parmesan, Romano, Pecorino, or Asiago cheese

Drain and rinse the beans.

In a large soup pot, heat 1 tablespoon of the oil. Chop 8 cloves of the garlic. Add the onion, garlic, celery, and carrot. Cook over medium-low heat for 10 minutes.

Add the beans, bay leaf, basil, oregano, and broth. Bring to a boil, then reduce the heat to low. Simmer, partially covered, for 45 minutes to 1 hour, or until the beans are al dente.

In a medium nonstick skillet, heat the remaining 1 tablespoon oil. Chop the remaining 4 cloves garlic. Add the garlic, broccoli rabe, sugar, and red pepper flakes. Cook for 3 minutes, stirring constantly, until the broccoli rabe is bright green. Remove from the heat and set aside.

When the beans are cooked, stir in the broccoli rabe, Parmesan rind, and lemon peel. Simmer for 30 minutes, or until ready to serve. Remove the bay leaf and Parmesan rind and season to taste with the salt and black pepper. Sprinkle with the cheese.

Per serving: 372 calories, 26 g protein, 39 g carbohydrates, 6 g total fat, 0 mg cholesterol, 13 g dietary fiber, 128 mg sodium

----

Smart Cooking: To save time, substitute two 15-ounce cans of white beans for the dried beans. Once you drain and rinse the beans, you can skip the soaking as well as the first 45 minutes to 1 hour of cooking. Add the canned beans at the same time as the broccoli rabe, Parmesan rind, and lemon peel, and continue with the recipe.

The rind of Parmesan cheese can add depth and dimension to soups and stews. After grating the cheese, instead of throwing out the rind, put it in a plastic bag and store it in the freezer until you're ready to use it.

CANNELLINI BEAN AND BACON SOUP

Serves 8

Prep time: 15 minutes

Cooking time: 1 hour

Cannellini is another name for white kidney beans. If you don't have time to soak the beans overnight, use the quick-soak method. Place the beans in a large pot of water and bring to a boil for 1 minute. Remove from the heat, cover, and let soak for at least an hour before draining and using.

1	tablespoon olive oil
1	onion, chopped
2	carrots, chopped
3	ribs celery, chopped
1	red bell pepper, cored, seeded, and chopped
6	cloves garlic, chopped
½	pound turkey bacon, chopped
1	bay leaf
1	teaspoon dried marjoram
1	teaspoon ground coriander
½	teaspoon dried thyme
3	cups dried cannellini beans or other white beans, picked over, rinsed, and soaked overnight
8	cups low-sodium chicken broth
1	tablespoon sherry vinegar
2	teaspoons grated lemon peel
	Salt
	Freshly ground black pepper

In a large soup pot, warm the oil over medium heat. Add the onion, carrots, celery, bell pepper, and garlic. Cook for 10 minutes, stirring occasionally. Stir in the bacon, bay leaf, marjoram, coriander, and thyme.

Drain the beans and add to the pot along with the broth. Bring to a boil, then reduce the heat to medium-low. Cook, partially covered, for I hour, or until the beans are tender. Remove the bay leaf.

Stir in the vinegar and lemon peel. Season to taste with the salt and black pepper.

Per serving: 461 calories, 31 g protein, 61 g carbohydrates, 12 g total fat, 28 mg cholesterol, 22 g dietary fiber, 759 mg sodium

TUSCAN LENTIL SOUP

Serves 8

Prep and cooking time: I hour

Small French green lentils give this soup a nice texture, but regular lentils work just as well. For variety, try substituting chopped escarole for the spinach. Be sure to cook the pasta until al dente.

I	pound small French green lentils, rinsed
7	cups vegetable broth
I	bay leaf
2	tablespoons extra-virgin olive oil
2	cloves garlic, chopped
I	large onion, chopped
I	large carrot, chopped
2	ribs celery, chopped
I	cup small pasta
8	ounces spinach, chopped
I	14½-ounce can diced tomatoes
I	tablespoon chopped fresh parsley
	Salt
	Freshly ground black pepper
	Freshly grated Parmesan cheese (optional)

In a large soup pot, combine the lentils, broth, and bay leaf. Bring to a boil, then reduce the heat to a simmer. Cook, partially covered, for approximately 45 minutes, or until the lentils are just tender.

In a small skillet, heat the oil. Add the garlic, onion, carrot, and celery. Cook over low heat, stirring often, until the vegetables are very soft but not browned. Set aside.

Bring a medium saucepan of water to a boil. Add the pasta and cook for about 5 minutes, or until just al dente. Drain and set aside.

Add the sautéed vegetables, spinach, tomatoes (with juice), and parsley to the lentils. Simmer for 15 minutes, stirring often.

Stir in the pasta and season with the salt and pepper. Remove the bay leaf. Sprinkle with the cheese, if desired.

Per serving: 432 calories, 24 g protein, 73 g carbohydrates, 6 g total fat, 0 mg cholesterol, 16 g dietary fiber, 827 mg sodium

SEAFOOD AND WHITE BEAN CHILI

Serves 6

Prep and cooking time: 45 minutes

For extra-spicy chili, use two jalapeños rather than one. Serve with Tabasco sauce and cayenne pepper on the side.

2	tablespoons olive oil
1	large onion, chopped
4	cloves garlic, minced
1	jalapeño pepper, finely chopped, or one 4½-ounce can chopped green chiles
2	tablespoons chili powder
1	teaspoon ground cumin
1	teaspoon dried oregano
1	14½-ounce can diced tomatoes, drained
1½	cups dry white wine
1	8-ounce bottle clam juice
½	cup fat-free chicken or vegetable broth
¾	cup half-and-half
3	tablespoons cornstarch or arrowroot

2	19-ounce cans cannellini beans, rinsed and drained
½	pound scallops, quartered
½	pound medium shrimp, shelled, butterflied, and halved
½	pound chopped shelled clams
½	pound fish (such as tilapia, swordfish, cod, or halibut), cut into bite-size pieces
2	tablespoons chopped fresh parsley
I	tablespoon lime juice
	Salt
	Freshly ground black pepper

In a soup pot, warm the oil. Add the onion and sauté for 2 minutes. Stir in the garlic and jalapeño or green chiles. Cook over medium heat for 3 minutes.

Stir in the chili powder, cumin, and oregano. Add the tomatoes, wine, clam juice, and broth. Bring to a boil, then reduce the heat to low. Simmer, covered, for 30 minutes.

In a small cup, stir together the half-and-half and cornstarch or arrowroot. Add a few tablespoons of the tomato mixture, then slowly pour into the pot, stirring constantly.

Add the beans, scallops, shrimp, clams, fish, parsley, and lime juice. Cook for 2 to 3 minutes, or until the fish is cooked through. Season to taste with the salt and black pepper. Serve immediately.

Per serving: 419 calories, 33 g protein, 37 g carbohydrates, 11 g total fat, 103 mg cholesterol, 8 g dietary fiber, 697 mg sodium

BUTTERNUT SQUASH AND CRAB CHOWDER

Serves 6

Prep and cooking time: 55 minutes

Serve this unique soup with a salad and a slice of crusty whole grain bread or cornbread for a complete meal. If you have access to fresh Dungeness crabs, they're perfect in this recipe. Otherwise, use the freshest-tasting canned crabmeat you can find.

2	tablespoons unsalted butter
I	onion, chopped

I	rib celery, chopped
I	carrot, chopped
I	butternut squash (3½ pounds) peeled, seeded, and cubed
4	cups low-sodium chicken or vegetable broth
¼	teaspoon dried thyme
¼	teaspoon ground coriander
¼	teaspoon ground nutmeg
I	12-ounce can fat-free evaporated milk
½	cup half-and-half
I	pound precooked crabmeat (or 2 Dungeness crabs, cleaned and meat removed)
2	tablespoons dry sherry
I	tablespoon chopped fresh parsley
I	teaspoon grated lemon peel
	Salt
	Freshly ground black pepper

In a large soup pot, melt the butter over medium heat. Add the onion, celery, and carrot. Cook for 5 to 10 minutes, or until softened.

Stir in the squash. Add the broth, thyme, coriander, and nutmeg and bring to a boil over high heat. Reduce the heat to medium-low, cover, and simmer for 20 minutes, or until the squash is soft.

Stir in the milk. Cook for 5 minutes, or until the squash begins to break up and the broth thickens slightly.

Reduce the heat to the lowest setting. In a cup, add a couple of spoonfuls of soup to the half-and-half, then slowly pour into the soup, stirring constantly.

Add the crabmeat, sherry, parsley, and lemon peel. Season to taste with the salt and pepper.

Per serving: 323 calories, 27 g protein, 40 g carbohydrates, 8 g total fat, 73 mg cholesterol, 6 g dietary fiber, 423 mg sodium

SEAFOOD CHOWDER

Serves 8

Prep and cooking time: 50 minutes

I've been making this recipe for years. It has rich flavor and creamy texture without the fat content that's typical of chowders.

1	pound medium shrimp
½	teaspoon dried rosemary
½	teaspoon dried thyme
1	large strip lemon peel
6	cups water
1½	tablespoons unsalted butter
4	shallots, chopped
1	cup chopped celery
3	cloves garlic, minced
4	large red potatoes, peeled and diced
1	8-ounce bottle clam juice
1	pound sea scallops, quartered
8	ounces chopped clams
3	tablespoons lemon juice
2	tablespoons chopped fresh parsley
2	tablespoons dry sherry
4	tablespoons arrowroot or cornstarch
1	cup half-and-half
	Salt
	Freshly ground black pepper

Remove the shells from the shrimp. Place in a large saucepan along with the rosemary, thyme, and lemon peel. Add the water and bring to a boil.

Reduce the heat to medium and simmer for 30 minutes. Chop the shrimp into bite-size pieces and set aside.

In a large soup pot, melt the butter over medium heat. Add the shallots, celery, and garlic, and cook for 3 minutes. Add the potatoes and stir.

Pour the shrimp broth through a strainer into the pot. Add the clam juice. Bring to a boil, then reduce the heat to medium. Cook for 10 minutes, or until the potatoes are tender.

Reduce the heat to the lowest setting. Add the shrimp, scallops, clams, lemon juice, parsley, and sherry.

In a cup, stir the arrowroot or cornstarch into the half-and-half, then add several spoonfuls of the hot broth. Pour into the pot, stirring constantly as it thickens. Season to taste with the salt and pepper.

Per serving: 273 calories, 27 g protein, 27 g carbohydrates, 7 g total fat, 128 mg cholesterol, 2 g dietary fiber, 419 mg sodium

CHICKEN CHIPOTLE CHILI

Serves 8

Prep time: 15 minutes

Cooking time: 55 minutes

The chipotle peppers in adobo sauce give this chili a wonderfully smoky flavor. If you prefer your chili a little milder, use only one-quarter of a can of chipotles. Spoon the remaining peppers and sauce into a plastic bag and freeze for later use.

2	tablespoons olive oil
2½	pounds boneless, skinless chicken breast, cubed
	Salt
	Freshly ground black pepper
2	onions, chopped
1	red or green bell pepper, cored, seeded, and chopped
6	cloves garlic, minced
2	15-ounce cans kidney and/or pinto beans, rinsed and drained
1	28-ounce can diced tomatoes

I	28-ounce can crushed tomatoes
¼–½	7-ounce can chipotle peppers in adobo sauce, chopped
3	tablespoons chili powder
I	tablespoon ground cumin
I	tablespoon dried oregano
I	tablespoon unsweetened cocoa powder
2	cups frozen corn kernels, thawed
2	tablespoons chopped fresh cilantro
2	tablespoons lime juice

In a large soup pot, warm I tablespoon of the oil over medium heat. Add the chicken and season with the salt and black pepper. Cook, stirring, for 5 minutes, or until lightly browned. Transfer to a medium bowl.

Add the remaining I tablespoon oil to the pot. Stir in the onion, bell pepper, and garlic. Cook for 5 minutes. Stir in the beans, diced tomatoes (with juice), crushed tomatoes, chipotle peppers and sauce, chili powder, cumin, oregano, and cocoa. Reduce the heat to medium-low and simmer, covered, for at least 30 minutes.

Stir in the chicken, corn, cilantro, and lime juice. Cook, uncovered, for I5 minutes. Season with the salt and black pepper.

Per serving: 390 calories, 43 g protein, 42 g carbohydrates, 7 g total fat, 82 mg cholesterol, II g dietary fiber, 806 mg sodium

CREAMY CHICKEN AND BARLEY SOUP

Serves 6

Prep and cooking time: I¼ hours

This recipe is reminiscent of mushroom and barley soup, but with a few twists. It's homestyle cooking at its best.

I	tablespoon + 2 teaspoons olive oil
I	pound boneless, skinless chicken breast, cubed
I	onion, chopped
I	carrot, finely chopped

1	rib celery, chopped
8	ounces mixed varieties of mushrooms, chopped
3	cloves garlic, minced
1	teaspoon dried thyme
1	teaspoon dried tarragon
2	tablespoons dry red wine
1	cup pearled barley
1	bay leaf
7	cups fat-free chicken broth
1	cup half-and-half
1	tablespoon dry sherry
	Freshly ground black pepper

In a large soup pot, heat the 2 teaspoons oil. Stir in the chicken and cook for 3 to 5 minutes, or until partially cooked and browned on the outside. Remove and set aside.

In the same pot, heat the remaining 1 tablespoon oil. Stir in the onion, carrot, and celery. Cook over medium-low heat for 4 to 5 minutes, or until the vegetables are softened and just beginning to brown.

Add the mushrooms, garlic, thyme, and tarragon. Reduce the heat to low, cover, and cook for 15 minutes, stirring occasionally. Uncover and increase the heat to high. Add the wine and stir until the liquid is absorbed, about 1 to 2 minutes.

Add the barley and bay leaf. Stir to coat the grains. Pour in the broth and bring to a boil. Reduce the heat to low, cover, and simmer for 50 minutes, or until the soup has thickened and the barley is soft. Add the chicken.

In a cup, stir spoonfuls of the soup into the half-and-half, one at a time, until warm. Slowly pour into the pot, stirring constantly to prevent curdling.

Remove the bay leaf. Stir in the sherry and season to taste with the pepper.

Per serving: 327 calories, 25 g protein, 34 g carbohydrates, 10 g total fat, 59 mg cholesterol, 7 g dietary fiber, 658 mg sodium

DUCK AND LENTIL STEW

Serves 4

Prep and cooking time: 1 hour

Duck can be a healthy and delicious alternative to chicken or red meat if it's prepared properly. This recipe uses just the breast meat, which creates a rich-tasting stew.

1	tablespoon olive oil
1½	pounds duck breast, skin removed, cut into ½″ cubes
	Salt
	Freshly ground black pepper
1	onion, chopped
2	carrots, chopped
4	ounces mushrooms, chopped
1	rib celery, chopped
½	red bell pepper, seeded and chopped
1	clove garlic, minced
3	cups chicken broth
1	cup small green French lentils
¾	cup white wine
1	bay leaf
1	teaspoon dried tarragon
1	teaspoon dried chives
½	teaspoon dried thyme
1	tablespoon grated orange peel
1	tablespoon chopped fresh parsley
1	tablespoon sherry vinegar

In a large soup pot, warm 1½ teaspoons of the oil over medium heat. Add the duck and season with the salt and black pepper. Cook for 5 minutes, or until lightly browned.

Transfer the duck to a plate. Cover and refrigerate until ready to use.

Add the remaining 1½ teaspoons oil to the pot along with the onion, carrots, mushrooms, celery, bell pepper, and garlic. Cook for 10 minutes, stirring occasionally.

Add the broth, lentils, wine, bay leaf, tarragon, chives, and thyme. Bring to a boil over high heat. Reduce the heat to medium-low, cover, and cook for 45 minutes, or until the lentils are tender and the broth has thickened.

Stir in the orange peel, parsley, vinegar, and the duck with any juices. Season with the salt and black pepper. Remove the bay leaf. Cook for 5 minutes, or until the duck is cooked through. Serve immediately.

Per serving: 482 calories, 48 g protein, 39 g carbohydrates, 11 g total fat, 135 mg cholesterol, 10 g dietary fiber, 884 mg sodium

GRANDMA'S CHICKEN NOODLE SOUP

Serves 12

Prep and cooking time: 2 hours

Chicken noodle soup is a staple during cold and flu season. Even if you aren't sick, just the aroma is certain to have a therapeutic effect. Any type and size of noodle will work. Removing the skin from the chicken before cooking reduces the fat but not the flavor.

2	small onions with skin, halved
4	cloves garlic, unpeeled
4	ribs celery, with leaves
4	carrots
10	sprigs parsley
3½	pounds chicken pieces, skin removed
2	bay leaves
20	whole peppercorns
1	teaspoon dried thyme
20	cups water
	Salt

Freshly ground black pepper

10–12   ounces noodles

In a very large soup pot, combine the onions, garlic, celery, carrots, parsley, chicken, bay leaves, peppercorns, thyme, and water. Season with the salt.

Bring the soup to a boil, then reduce the heat to medium-low. Simmer, partially covered, for 1½ hours.

Gently remove the chicken and carrots and set aside to cool.

Place a strainer or colander over another large pot. Pour the soup into the strainer so that the broth drains into the pot and the strainer catches the vegetables. Discard the vegetables.

Return the broth to the stove and bring to a boil. Add the noodles. Cook according to the package directions, or until just al dente. Be careful not to overcook.

Remove the chicken from the bone and shred into bite-size pieces. Slice the carrots. Add the chicken and carrots to the soup. Season to taste with the salt and pepper.

Per serving: 261 calories, 33 g protein, 22 g carbohydrates, 4 g total fat, 107 mg cholesterol, 2 g dietary fiber, 134 mg sodium

CURRIED YELLOW PEA AND SWEET POTATO SOUP

Serves 6

Prep and cooking time: 1 hour

This recipe will produce a mildly spicy soup. For extra heat, add the second jalapeño pepper or the hot curry powder. Be careful not to overdo it, though. You can always add seasonings once the soup is fully cooked.

1   tablespoon peanut oil or canola oil

1   large red onion, finely chopped

5   cloves garlic, minced

1–2   jalapeño peppers, finely chopped

½   red bell pepper, seeded and finely chopped

1"   chunk ginger, finely chopped

6   cups low-sodium vegetable or chicken broth

I	large sweet potato (about I pound), peeled and cubed
2	cups yellow split peas
3	teaspoons mild or hot curry powder
I	teaspoon chili powder
I	teaspoon ground cinnamon
I	bay leaf
I	14-ounce can reduced-fat coconut milk
2	tablespoons lemon juice
	Salt
	Freshly ground black pepper

In a large soup pot, warm the oil over medium heat. Stir in the onion, garlic, jalapeños, bell pepper, and ginger. Cook, stirring occasionally, for 10 minutes.

Add the broth, sweet potato, split peas, curry powder, chili powder, cinnamon, and bay leaf. Bring the soup to a boil, then reduce the heat to medium-low. Cover and simmer for 45 minutes, or until the peas are softened.

Stir in the coconut milk and continue cooking for 5 minutes, until the soup is smooth and creamy. Add the lemon juice and season to taste with the salt and black pepper. Remove the bay leaf.

Per serving: 435 calories, 24 g protein, 69 g carbohydrates, 9 g total fat, 0 mg cholesterol, 3 g dietary fiber, 114 mg sodium

CREAM OF ROASTED TOMATO–BASIL SOUP

Serves 6

Prep and cooking time: I hour

This recipe calls for plum or Roma tomatoes, which are available year-round in most supermarkets. The extra step of roasting the tomatoes deepens their flavor. It's easy and well worth the time.

4	pounds plum tomatoes, stem ends removed, halved lengthwise
	Salt

I	teaspoon butter or olive oil
I	red bell pepper, cored, seeded, and chopped
3	shallots, chopped
4	cloves garlic, minced
1½	cups low-sodium vegetable or tomato juice
I	cup fresh basil leaves, chopped
I	teaspoon sugar
I	cup half-and-half
	Freshly ground black pepper

Preheat the oven to 500°F.

Line 2 baking pans (13" x 9") with foil. Add the tomatoes, cut side up, in a single layer. Lightly coat with cooking spray and season to taste with the salt. Bake for 25 minutes. Remove from the oven and set aside to cool.

In a large soup pot, melt the butter or warm the oil over medium heat. Stir in the bell pepper, shallots, and garlic. Cook for 5 minutes.

When the tomatoes are cool enough to handle, remove the skins and discard. Place the tomatoes in the pot along with the vegetable juice, half of the basil, and sugar. Bring to a boil, then reduce the heat to medium-low. Cook, covered, for 20 to 25 minutes, or until the vegetables are soft.

Puree the soup with a stick blender or in a food processor until smooth. Reduce the heat to the lowest setting and stir in the remaining basil.

In a cup, add a few spoonfuls of the soup to the half-and-half. Slowly pour into the pot, stirring constantly. Season to taste with the salt and black pepper.

Per serving: 156 calories, 5 g protein, 24 g carbohydrates, 6 g total fat, 16 mg cholesterol, 4 g dietary fiber, 84 mg sodium

ITALIAN TOMATO-BREAD SOUP

Serves 6

Prep and cooking time: 45 minutes

This thick and hearty soup is wonderful on a cold winter's day. In the Italian tradition, the recipe uses day-old bread as a thickener. A whole grain Italian-style loaf is ideal.

2	tablespoons olive oil
I	onion, chopped
4	cloves garlic, minced
2	28-ounce cans whole peeled tomatoes
4	cups low-sodium vegetable or chicken broth
¾	pound (about 6 cups) whole grain Italian bread, crusts removed, cubed
½	cup fresh basil, chopped
I	tablespoon sugar
	Salt
	Freshly ground black pepper
	Crushed red pepper flakes
I	cup half-and-half

In a large soup pot, warm the oil over medium heat. Add the onion and cook until softened, about 5 minutes. Add the garlic and cook for 2 minutes.

Stir in the tomatoes, breaking them up with a spoon. Add the broth, bread, half of the basil, and sugar. Season to taste with the salt, black pepper, and pepper flakes.

Bring to a boil, then reduce the heat to medium-low. Cover and simmer, stirring occasionally, for 30 minutes. Using a food processor or blender, puree until smooth.

Reduce the heat to the lowest setting. In a cup, add several spoonfuls of the soup to the half-and-half. Slowly pour into the pot, stirring constantly.

Add the remaining basil. Add more salt, black pepper, and/or pepper flakes, if desired.

Per serving: 341 calories, 12 g protein, 48 g carbohydrates, 12 g total fat, 15 mg cholesterol, 6 g dietary fiber, 852 mg sodium

THICK AND ZESTY GAZPACHO

Serves 6

Prep time: 15–20 minutes

This recipe first appeared in our book *Low-Fat Living*. It has become such a favorite over the years that I've included a slightly modified version here. Although gazpacho originated in Spain, it appears in many cuisines and has just as many variations. Serve with a dollop of reduced-fat sour cream and chopped fresh chives, if you wish.

4	cups low-sodium tomato or vegetable juice
1	15-ounce can chickpeas, rinsed and drained
1	large onion, finely chopped
1	orange or yellow bell pepper, cored, seeded, and chopped
1	cucumber, chopped
2	tomatoes, chopped
¼	cup chopped roasted red peppers
2	cloves garlic, minced
2	tablespoons chopped fresh parsley
1	tablespoon chopped fresh basil
1	tablespoon chopped fresh dill
2	tablespoons red wine vinegar
1	tablespoon olive oil
1	tablespoon honey or sugar
½	teaspoon dried tarragon
¼	teaspoon ground cumin
	Salt
	Freshly ground black pepper
	Hot-pepper sauce

In a large bowl, combine the tomato or vegetable juice, chickpeas, onion, bell pepper, cucumber, tomatoes, red peppers, garlic, parsley, basil, and dill. Stir in the vinegar, oil, honey or sugar, tarragon, and cumin.

Season to taste with the salt, black pepper, and hot-pepper sauce. Refrigerate for at least 1 to 2 hours before serving.

Per serving: 176 calories, 6 g protein, 30 g carbohydrates, 3 g total fat, 0 mg cholesterol, 6 g dietary fiber, 392 mg sodium

TOFU EGG DROP SOUP WITH VEGETABLES

Serves 6

Prep and cooking time: 40 minutes

The base of this recipe is similar to Chinese egg drop soup. With the added vegetables and tofu, it becomes a meal in itself. You also can serve it as a first course for an Asian-inspired meal.

1	tablespoon toasted sesame oil
1	small onion, chopped
2	ribs celery, chopped
1	red bell pepper, cored, seeded, and chopped
5	cloves garlic, minced
1	carrot, grated
1	teaspoon grated fresh ginger
7	cups low-sodium chicken broth
1	pound extra-firm tofu, cubed
1	(16-ounce) package frozen corn, thawed
¼	cup Chinese rice wine (mirin)
3	tablespoons low-sodium soy sauce
2	tablespoons cornstarch or arrowroot
2	tablespoons water
4	scallions, chopped

I	tablespoon chopped fresh cilantro
½–1	teaspoon chili puree with garlic or to taste
4	eggs, beaten
	Salt
	Freshly ground black pepper

In a large soup pot, warm the oil. Add the onion and cook over medium heat for 3 minutes.

Stir in the celery and bell pepper and cook for 3 minutes. Stir in the garlic, carrot, and ginger and cook for 3 minutes more.

Add the broth, tofu, corn, wine, and soy sauce. Bring to a boil, then reduce the heat to medium-low and cook for 5 minutes.

In a small cup, combine the cornstarch or arrowroot and water. Stir until smooth. Add a small amount of the soup, then slowly whisk into the soup until it thickens slightly, about I minute.

Stir in the scallions and cilantro. Season with the chili puree.

While constantly stirring the soup with a fork, slowly add the eggs, pouring in a steady stream. Let set for I minute, then stir well.

Season to taste with the salt and pepper and add more chili puree, if desired. Serve immediately.

Per serving: 315 calories, 21 g protein, 34 g carbohydrates, 12 g total fat, 141 mg cholesterol, 4 g dietary fiber, 450 mg sodium

Poultry Entrées

CARIBBEAN JERK CHICKEN PITA WRAPS

Serves 4

Prep and cooking time: 20 minutes

Jerk seasoning originated in the Caribbean. It's a combination of various spices, hot peppers, and scallions. Many companies make a less spicy version for those who want the flavor with a little less heat.

I	pound boneless, skinless chicken breast, cut into thin slices
2–3	tablespoons Jamaican jerk sauce
I	teaspoon olive oil
4	large whole wheat pita breads
I	mango, peeled and sliced
I	cup mixed greens or lettuce
½	red bell pepper, seeded and thinly sliced
4	tablespoons chopped pistachio nuts
4	tablespoons shredded coconut

In a small bowl, combine the chicken and jerk sauce. Cover and refrigerate for several hours to overnight.

In a large nonstick skillet, warm the oil over medium-high heat. Add the chicken and cook for 3 minutes, stirring constantly, until cooked through. (The chicken can also be grilled or broiled, if desired.)

To assemble, place one-quarter of the chicken on one end of each pita. Top with equal amounts of mango, greens, pepper, pistachios, and coconut. Starting on the end with the filling, fold the pita over the filling and roll to form a wrap.

Roll the wrap in plastic and fold under the ends to keep closed until ready to serve. Slice in half diagonally and serve.

Per serving: 429 calories, 35 g protein, 53 g carbohydrates, I0 g total fat, 66 mg cholesterol, 7 g dietary fiber, 675 mg sodium

CHICKEN AND BROCCOLI WITH TORTELLINI

Serves 4

Prep and cooking time: 30 minutes

Here's a recipe that's quick, easy, and loaded with flavor. Serve with a simple salad, and you can have a meal on the table in less than 30 minutes.

8	ounces reduced-fat cheese or vegetable tortellini
2	bunches (about 3 pounds) broccoli, cut into florets and stems discarded
1	tablespoon olive oil
2	tablespoons chopped shallots
6	cloves garlic, chopped
4	ounces mushrooms, sliced
1	pound boneless, skinless chicken breast, cut into thin strips
	Salt
	Freshly ground black pepper
2	tablespoons pine nuts, toasted
2–4	tablespoons grated Parmesan cheese or crumbled Roquefort cheese

Bring a large saucepan of water to a boil. Stir in the tortellini, reduce the heat to medium-high, and cook according to package directions or until al dente. Drain and set aside.

Place the broccoli in a large saucepan with water. Bring to a boil and cook for 2 minutes, or until bright green. Drain and refill the pan with ice water. When the broccoli is chilled, drain and set aside.

In a large nonstick skillet, warm the oil over medium heat. Add the shallots and garlic and cook for 2 minutes. Add the mushrooms and cook for another 4 minutes, or until softened.

Push the vegetables to the sides of the pan and add the chicken in the center. Season with the salt and pepper. Cook, stirring often, for 5 minutes, or until all the chicken pieces are cooked through.

Stir in the pine nuts and tortellini toss to mix well. Sprinkle with the cheese and serve immediately.

Per serving: 431 calories, 44 g protein, 37 g carbohydrates, 14 g total fat, 141 mg cholesterol, 10 g dietary fiber, 342 mg sodium

INDONESIAN COCONUT-CRUSTED CHICKEN TENDERS

Serves 4

Prep time: 10 minutes

Baking time: 15 minutes

These chicken tenders will please an adult palate, yet kids will love them, too. To complete the Indonesian theme, serve with Peanut Dipping Sauce (page 328).

1½	cups packed coconut flakes, lightly chopped
1	pound boneless, skinless chicken breast, sliced into tenders or nuggets
	Salt
	Freshly ground black pepper
1	egg white, lightly beaten

Preheat the oven to 325°F. Line a baking sheet with foil.

Sprinkle the coconut onto the baking sheet and spread in a thin layer. Bake for 5 to 7 minutes, or until just beginning to turn golden brown. Transfer to a shallow bowl.

Increase the oven temperature to 450°F. Coat a 9" x 13" baking pan with cooking spray.

Place the chicken between 2 sheets of plastic wrap and gently pound to ¼" to ½" thickness. Season with the salt and pepper.

Dip each piece of chicken in the egg white to moisten well. Press into the coconut and turn to coat both sides.

Place the chicken in the prepared baking pan and lightly coat with cooking spray. Bake for 15 minutes, or until cooked through.

Per serving: 361 calories, 30 g protein, 20 g carbohydrates, 18 g total fat, 66 mg cholesterol, 3 g dietary fiber, 237 mg sodium

PEANUT DIPPING SAUCE

Makes 4 servings (½ cup)

Prep time: 10 minutes

You can make this sauce as mild or as spicy as you like by varying the amount of chili puree you use.

3	tablespoons fat-free chicken broth
2	tablespoons natural peanut butter
1	tablespoon toasted sesame oil
1	tablespoon reduced-sodium soy sauce
2	teaspoons lime juice
1–2	teaspoons chili puree with garlic
1	teaspoon honey or sugar
	Salt
	Freshly ground black pepper

In a small processor or blender, combine the broth, peanut butter, oil, soy sauce, lime juice, chili puree, and honey or sugar. Puree until smooth and creamy. Season to taste with the salt and pepper.

Per serving: 89 calories, 2 g protein, 4 g carbohydrates, 8 g total fat, 0 mg cholesterol, 1 g dietary fiber, 209 mg sodium

PISTACHIO-CRUSTED CHICKEN WITH GOAT CHEESE AND APRICOT-SHERRY SAUCE

Serves 4

Prep time: 25 minutes

Baking time: 20–25 minutes

This dish is elegant enough for a dinner party but simple enough for a family dinner. If you're not fond of goat cheese, you can use another variety, such as Boursin or reduced-fat cream cheese. The sauce is a nice complement to the other flavors.

Sauce

3	ounces dried apricots, cut into small pieces
1	cup water
¼	cup dry sherry
	Grated peel of ½ lemon
	Salt
	Freshly ground black pepper

Chicken

4	boneless, skinless chicken breasts (about 1½ pounds)
	Salt
	Freshly ground black pepper
4	tablespoons soft garlic-and-herb goat cheese
1	egg white, lightly beaten
½	cup finely chopped pistachio nuts

To make the sauce: In a small saucepan, combine the apricots, water, sherry, and lemon peel. Bring to a boil, reduce the heat to medium, and simmer for 20 minutes.

Transfer to a blender or food processor and puree until smooth. Season to taste with the salt and pepper. Keep warm on the lowest heat.

To make the chicken: Preheat the oven to 400°F. Line a 9" x 13" baking pan with foil and lightly coat with cooking spray.

Season each chicken breast with the salt and pepper. Make a pocket in each breast by cutting through its side lengthwise. Be careful not to cut all the way through.

Stuff each breast with a tablespoon of the cheese. Dip in the egg white and press into the chopped nuts, turning to coat both sides.

Place the chicken in the prepared pan, coat lightly with cooking spray, and cover loosely with foil. Bake for 20 minutes, or until cooked through. Be careful not to overcook, or the chicken will become dry.

To serve, drizzle a few spoonfuls of sauce onto each plate and top with the chicken.

Per serving: 376 calories, 46 g protein, 18 g carbohydrates, 12 g total fat, 104 mg cholesterol, 4 g dietary fiber, 230 mg sodium

- -

Smart Cooking: A good pair of kitchen shears comes in handy for cutting up dried apricots and other dried fruits that are too sticky to cut with a knife. They also are perfect for cutting fresh chives into small pieces.

ROASTED CHICKEN BREASTS WITH LENTIL RAGOUT

Serves 4

Prep and cooking time: I hour

A ragout (or ragu) consists of pieces of poultry, fish, meat, or vegetables cut into uniform sizes and slowly braised. Here the ragout is served on top of chicken, similar to a thick sauce. Try pairing the dish with a scoop of mashed sweet potatoes or winter squash, such as acorn or butternut.

I	tablespoon olive oil
I	slice turkey bacon, chopped
I	onion, finely chopped
I	carrot, finely chopped
I	rib celery, finely chopped
I	small leek, white and light green parts finely chopped
2	cloves garlic, minced
2	tablespoons tomato paste
3	cups low-sodium chicken broth
¾	cup lentils
I	sachet d'epices (see Smart Cooking)
4	bone-in chicken breast halves, with skin
	Salt
	Freshly ground black pepper
2	tablespoons sherry vinegar
2	teaspoons balsamic vinegar
	Red pepper flakes

In a large saucepan, warm the oil. Add the bacon and cook on low for 3 to 5 minutes, or until browned. Stir in the onion, carrot, celery, leek, and garlic. Cover and cook, stirring occasionally, until tender, about I0 minutes.

Add the tomato paste and cook, stirring, for 2 minutes. Add the broth, lentils, and sachet d'epices. Bring to a boil, then reduce the heat to medium-low and simmer for 45 minutes, or until the lentils are tender. Remove and discard the sachet.

While the sauce is cooking, preheat the oven to 400°F. Line a baking dish with foil and add the chicken. Coat with olive oil cooking spray and season with the salt and black pepper.

Roast for approximately 30 minutes, or until cooked through. Remove the skin, cover the chicken, and set aside until ready to serve.

Season the ragout with the sherry vinegar, balsamic vinegar, and the pepper flakes, salt, and black pepper to taste. To serve, put each chicken breast on a plate and top with the ragout.

Per serving: 299 calories, 28 g protein, 35 g carbohydrates, 6 g total fat, 37 mg cholesterol, 7 g dietary fiber, 181 mg sodium

----

Smart Cooking: A sachet d'epices is a blend of herbs and spices wrapped in a piece of cheesecloth. It is used to infuse a dish with a special flavor, then removed and thrown away. It usually contains dried thyme, bay leaves, peppercorns, and fresh parsley stems. It may also include rosemary, citrus peel, caraway seeds, and cumin seeds.

For the lentil ragout, combine I teaspoon thyme, I bay leaf, 10 peppercorns, a small handful of parsley stems, I teaspoon rosemary, and a thick strip of lemon peel. Place the ingredients in a piece of cheesecloth and tie with kitchen string.

SAUTÉED CHICKEN BREASTS WITH PORCINI MUSHROOMS

Serves 4

Prep and cooking time: 25 minutes

Simple but elegant, light but satisfying—this dish has it all. What more could you want from a chicken breast?

½	ounce (½ cup) dried porcini mushrooms
I	cup hot water
4	boneless, skinless chicken breasts (about I pound)

	Salt
	Freshly ground black pepper
l	tablespoon olive oil
½	cup whole wheat pastry flour
¼	cup chopped shallots
½	cup dry red wine
3	tablespoons half-and-half
l	tablespoon unsalted butter

Fill a small bowl with cool water. Add the mushrooms and swirl to remove any grit. Drain and discard the water.

Place the mushrooms back in the bowl and add the hot water. Set aside to soak for at least 20 minutes.

Place a paper towel in a strainer and drain the mushrooms, reserving the soaking liquid. Chop the mushrooms and set aside.

Preheat the oven to the lowest setting.

Place the chicken breasts between 2 sheets of plastic wrap and pound to ¼" to ½" thickness. Season with the salt and pepper.

Heat the oil in a large nonstick skillet over medium-high heat.

Place the flour on a large plate and dredge the chicken, shaking off the excess. Immediately place the chicken in the skillet and cook for approximately 2 minutes per side, or until just cooked through.

Remove from the heat and transfer the chicken to an ovenproof plate. Cover and place in the oven to keep warm.

Place the skillet back on the heat, add the shallots, and cook for l minute. Stir in the mushrooms and cook for l minute. Stir in the reserved mushroom liquid (about ½ cup) and cook until most of the liquid has been absorbed. Add the wine and cook until most of the liquid has been absorbed.

Remove from the heat and stir in the half-and-half and butter. Season to taste with the salt and pepper. Remove the chicken from the oven and spoon the mushrooms over the top. Serve immediately.

Per serving: 315 calories, 36 g protein, 23 g carbohydrates, 10 g total fat, 80 mg cholesterol, 4 g dietary fiber, 89 mg sodium

CARIBBEAN GRILLED TURKEY BREAST

Serves 8

Prep time: 10 minutes

Grilling or roasting time: Approximately 1½ hours

These days, you can find fresh or frozen boneless turkey breasts in many supermarkets. For this recipe, look for an all-natural breast. Try serving with Smashed Orange-Ginger Sweet Potatoes (page 359).

1	boneless turkey breast (3–4 pounds)
5	tablespoons olive oil
	Juice of 1 lime
	Grated peel of 1 lime
1	tablespoon kosher salt
1	teaspoon allspice
1	teaspoon chili powder
1	teaspoon garlic powder
1	teaspoon onion powder
½–1	teaspoon freshly ground black pepper
½	teaspoon ground nutmeg
¼	teaspoon ground cinnamon

Rinse the turkey in cool water and pat dry. Place in a gallon-size zipper-lock bag.

In a small bowl, combine the oil, lime juice, lime peel, salt, allspice, chili powder, garlic powder, onion powder, pepper, nutmeg, and cinnamon. Stir to combine well.

Pour the spice mixture into the bag and toss to coat the turkey. Remove as much air as possible from the bag, seal, and place on a plate. Refrigerate and let marinate for 5 hours to overnight.

Remove the turkey and discard the remaining marinade.

Grill, roast, or rotisserie the turkey for up to 1½ hours, or until the internal temperature reaches 165°F. Let stand for 10 minutes before carving.

Per serving: 272 calories, 41 g protein, 2 g carbohydrates, 11 g total fat, 119 mg cholesterol, 1 g dietary fiber, 564 mg sodium

FARFALLE WITH SAUSAGE AND WHITE BEANS

Serves 6

Prep and cooking time: 30 minutes

Chicken and turkey sausage comes in all flavors and varieties. Look for ones that are low in fat and have lots of taste. If you choose precooked sausage, add it after preparing the vegetables. You can also substitute boneless, skinless chicken breasts cut into strips, if you wish.

8	ounces farfalle (bowtie) pasta
I	tablespoon olive oil
¼	cup chopped red onion
8	ounces mushrooms, sliced
6	cloves garlic, minced
I	pound chicken or turkey sausage, removed from casings
I	14½-ounce can diced tomatoes, drained
4	ounces (about 3 cups) spinach, torn into pieces
I	15-ounce can white beans, drained and rinsed
½	cup dry white wine
½	cup half-and-half
2	tablespoons grated Asiago or Parmesan cheese
	Salt
	Freshly ground black pepper

In a large saucepan of water, cook the pasta for 10 minutes, or until al dente. Drain, reserving ½ cup of the cooking water.

In a large nonstick skillet, warm the oil over medium heat. Add the onion and cook for 2 minutes. Stir in the mushrooms and garlic and cook for 3 minutes. Add the sausage and tomatoes. Cook, chopping the sausage, for 5 minutes.

Stir in the spinach, beans, and wine. Cook for 5 minutes, or until the sausage is cooked through and the spinach has wilted. Add the pasta and toss.

In a cup, stir the reserved cooking water into the half-and-half. Pour into the skillet and mix well. Add the cheese and toss. Cook for 2 minutes, or until the sauce begins to thicken and the ingredients are mixed well.

Season to taste with the salt and pepper. Serve immediately.

Per serving: 425 calories, 27 g protein, 49 g carbohydrates, 12 g total fat, 66 mg cholesterol, 5 g dietary fiber, 513 mg sodium

BROCCOLI AND ITALIAN SAUSAGE FRITTATA

Serves 6

Prep time: 25 minutes

Baking time: 20–25 minutes

A frittata is an Italian version of an omelet. While this recipe calls for broccoli and chicken or turkey sausage, feel free to substitute any ingredients you have on hand—such as spinach, mushrooms, roasted peppers, olives, and onions. It's a great way to use up leftovers.

1	tablespoon extra-virgin olive oil
1	bunch broccoli, cut into small florets
4	cloves garlic, minced or thinly sliced
	Salt
4	tablespoons freshly grated Parmesan cheese
1	link (2–3 ounces) precooked Italian chicken or turkey sausage
6	eggs or 1 cup liquid egg substitute + 2 eggs
1	tablespoon fat-free milk or water
	Freshly ground black pepper

Preheat the oven to 325°F. Generously coat a 9" pie plate or 8" x 8" pan with olive oil or cooking spray.

In a large nonstick skillet, heat the oil. Add the broccoli and garlic. Cook, stirring, for 1 minute. Season with the salt. Cook, stirring occasionally, for another 2 to 5 minutes, or until the broccoli is bright green and still slightly crisp.

Transfer the broccoli to a large bowl and sprinkle with 2 tablespoons of the cheese. Set aside to cool.

Remove the sausage from its casing and crumble or chop into small pieces. Add to the broccoli.

In a blender or with a mixer, beat the eggs, milk or water, and the remaining 2 tablespoons cheese. Season with the salt and pepper. Mix until foamy.

Combine the egg mixture with the broccoli and stir well.

Pour into the prepared pan. Bake for 20 to 25 minutes, or until lightly browned at the edges and slightly set in the center.

Remove from the oven and let stand for 10 minutes. Cut into squares or wedges and serve hot or at room temperature.

Per serving: 168 calories, 12 g protein, 8 g carbohydrates, 10 g total fat, 220 mg cholesterol, 3 g dietary fiber, 211 mg sodium

Seafood Favorites

ASIAN CASHEW SHRIMP WITH BROWN RICE

Serves 6

Prep and cooking time: 50 minutes

The wonderful thing about making Asian food at home is that you can use whatever vegetables your family enjoys most. This recipe uses my family's favorite combination. Try substituting pieces of chicken breast, scallops, or tofu for the shrimp. If you don't own a wok, a large skillet will do.

4	cups water
2	cups brown rice
	Salt
⅓	cup low-sodium soy sauce
⅓	cup sweet rice wine
1	tablespoon toasted sesame oil
2	teaspoons grated fresh ginger
2	cloves garlic, minced
1½	pounds shrimp, peeled and deveined
1	tablespoon cornstarch
2	tablespoons peanut oil
1	small red onion, thickly sliced
1	8-ounce can sliced water chestnuts, drained
8	shiitake or white mushrooms, stems removed and sliced
½	pound snow peas, stem and strings removed
½	cup unsalted cashews, toasted

In a medium saucepan, bring the water to a boil. Stir in the rice and season to taste with the salt. Reduce the heat to medium-low, cover, and cook for 40 to 45 minutes, or until the water has been absorbed. Remove from the heat and let stand, covered, for 5 minutes.

In a large bowl, stir together the soy sauce, wine, sesame oil, ginger, and garlic. Add the shrimp and toss to coat. Cover and refrigerate until ready to use.

Remove the shrimp from the marinade and set aside. Stir the cornstarch into the marinade until blended well.

In a wok or large nonstick skillet, heat the oil on high heat. Add the onion, water chestnuts, and mushrooms. Cook, stirring constantly, for 2 minutes. Add the shrimp, snow peas, and cashews, and cook, stirring, for 2 minutes.

Pour in the marinade. Stir for I minute, or until the sauce is thickened and the shrimp is cooked through. Serve immediately, spooned over the rice.

Per serving: 523 calories, 31 g protein, 62 g carbohydrates, 16 g total fat, 172 mg cholesterol, 5 g dietary fiber, 647 mg sodium

- -

Smart Cooking: Grating ginger used to be a tedious task. Not anymore, thanks to the fine graters called microplanes now on the market. Just peel the ginger and slide it across the knifelike ridges. You'll end up with a pile of finely minced, juicy ginger. You can purchase microplanes in cooking stores and mail-order catalogs.

SEARED SCALLOPS WITH LEMON AND CAPERS

Serves 4

Prep and cooking time: 25 minutes

With this dish as your entrée, you can have a meal on the table in a flash. Prepare a salad and side vegetable first. Then gather all of the ingredients for this recipe and put a pot of water on the stove to boil before you begin preparation. Within 15 minutes, you'll be sitting down to dinner!

I   pound sea scallops

Salt

Freshly ground black pepper

12	ounces thin noodles or pasta
3	tablespoons unsalted butter
1	shallot, minced
1	cup dry white wine
1	teaspoon grated lemon peel
2	tablespoons chopped fresh parsley
2	tablespoons lemon juice
1	tablespoon drained capers

Rinse the scallops and pat dry. Season on both sides with the salt and pepper.

Bring a large saucepan of water to a boil. Add the pasta and cook according to package directions, or until al dente. Drain and set aside.

In a large nonstick skillet, warm 1 tablespoon of the butter over medium-high heat. Add the scallops and cook for 1 to 2 minutes. Turn the scallops with tongs and cook for 1 to 2 minutes longer. Remove the skillet from the heat and transfer the scallops to a bowl. Cover with foil and set aside.

Return the skillet to the stove, reduce the heat to medium, and add the shallot. Cook for 1 to 2 minutes. Add the wine and lemon peel. Simmer for 6 to 7 minutes, or until the liquid is reduced to about ⅓ cup.

Remove from the heat. Stir in the parsley, lemon juice, capers, and the remaining 2 tablespoons butter. Season with the salt and pepper.

Toss the pasta with the sauce and top with the scallops. Serve immediately.

Per serving: 548 calories, 31 g protein, 66 g carbohydrates, 13 g total fat, 141 mg cholesterol, 3 g dietary fiber, 269 mg sodium

PAN-SEARED JUMBO PRAWNS IN DIJON MUSTARD SAUCE

Serves 4

Prep time: 10 minutes

Cooking time: 10 minutes

Feel free to substitute medium to large shrimp or scallops for the prawns. Serve on a bed of wild rice with sautéed greens, steamed asparagus, or broccoli.

2	tablespoons butter
2	tablespoons chopped shallots
½	cup low-sodium chicken broth
3	tablespoons half-and-half
2	tablespoons Dijon mustard
½	teaspoon dried crushed tarragon
	Salt
	Freshly ground black pepper
12	jumbo prawns, peeled and tails left on
1	tablespoon olive oil
4	cloves garlic, minced

In a saucepan, melt the butter over medium-low heat. Add the shallots and cook for 2 minutes, or until softened.

Whisk in the broth, half-and-half, mustard, and tarragon. Cook for 5 minutes, or until slightly thickened. Season with the salt and pepper. Keep warm on low heat.

Rinse the prawns under cool water and pat dry. With a sharp knife, cut lengthwise down the back, about halfway through the meat of each prawn. Remove the vein, leaving the tail intact. Season with the salt and pepper.

In a large nonstick skillet, warm the oil over medium heat. Add the garlic and cook, stirring constantly, for 30 seconds. Don't let the garlic brown.

Add the prawns. Cook for 1 to 2 minutes on each side, depending on their size. Pour the sauce over the prawns and continue cooking until the prawns are cooked through. Be careful not to overcook. Serve immediately.

Per serving: 157 calories, 9 g protein, 6 g carbohydrates, 12 g total fat, 67 mg cholesterol, 0 g dietary fiber, 291 mg sodium

ROASTED SALMON IN PARCHMENT WITH LEMON AND DILL

Serves 6

Prep time: 5 minutes

Baking time: 30 minutes

This is my family's favorite way to eat salmon. It cooks to perfection—no fishy taste or dry texture. It just melts in your mouth. And it's equally good whether served warm straight from the oven or chilled on a bed of greens. Wrapped tightly, the fish should keep well in the refrigerator for up to 3 days.

1½	pounds salmon fillets, skin removed
	Juice of ½ lemon
	Peel of ½ lemon, sliced
	Salt
	Freshly ground black pepper
4	sprigs fresh dill

Preheat the oven to 400°F.

Lay a piece of parchment paper, at least double the size of the salmon, on a baking sheet. Place the fish in the center, drizzle with the lemon juice, and season with the salt and pepper. Place the dill and lemon peel on top of the fish.

Bring the long sides of the parchment together on top of the salmon and fold over several times. Fold the short sides in the same way and tuck under the fish. You should have a neat, tightly closed package.

Bake for 25 to 35 minutes, depending on the thickness of the fish. Be careful not to overcook. Let stand for 5 minutes before serving. The fish will continue to cook slightly.

Open the parchment carefully. Discard the lemon peel, dill, and parchment. Serve the fish warm or cover and refrigerate until well chilled.

Per serving: 161 calories, 17 g protein, 0 g carbohydrates, 9 g total fat, 51 mg cholesterol, 0 g dietary fiber, 52 mg sodium

SMOKED SALMON-WRAPPED SCALLOPS WITH BLOOD ORANGE-SAFFRON COULIS

Serves 4

Prep and cooking time: 45 minutes

For this recipe, you'll need 8 long, thin bamboo sticks to skewer the scallops. Soak them in water for 30 minutes to prevent the ends from burning. For an attractive presentation, serve the scallops over wild rice or brown rice pilaf.

¼	teaspoon crushed saffron threads
4	blood oranges, juiced with pulp
2	tablespoons sugar
	Salt
	Freshly ground black pepper
16	sea scallops
1	tablespoon olive oil
4	ounces smoked salmon, cut into 16 thin strips

In a small cup, soak the saffron in a few tablespoons of hot water. Set aside.

In a small saucepan, combine the orange juice with pulp and the sugar. Bring to a boil. Reduce the heat to medium and simmer for 25 minutes, or until the juice is thickened slightly.

Add the saffron and water. Season to taste with the salt and pepper. Reduce the heat to the lowest setting and keep warm.

Preheat a grill or broiler and coat with cooking spray.

Rinse and dry the scallops. Place in a bowl, toss with the oil, and season with the salt and pepper.

Wrap a thin strip of salmon around a scallop. Skewer the scallop with 2 bamboo sticks. This will allow you to turn the scallops halfway through cooking. Repeat with the remaining salmon, scallops, and skewers so that each pair of sticks has 4 scallops.

Cook for 2 minutes. Turn the skewers and cook for another 2 minutes, or until the scallops are cooked through.

Drizzle with the sauce and serve immediately.

Per serving: 210 calories, 16 g protein, 24 g carbohydrates, 5 g total fat, 26 mg cholesterol, 3 g dietary fiber, 664 mg sodium

---

Smart Cooking: A coulis is a French interpretation of a thickened sauce. The coulis in this recipe uses blood oranges, a sweet, seedless red-fleshed orange that originated in Sicily. Here they're available primarily from November through March. You can substitute other sweet, seedless oranges if necessary.

FRESH SALMON CAKES

Makes 12

Prep time: 20 minutes

Cooking time: 5–10 minutes

A fillet of fresh salmon, finely chopped by hand, creates a moist and flavorful cake. I like to serve these on a bed of greens with Fresh Corn Salsa (page 278). Although the recipe has a long ingredient list, the cakes are mixed in one bowl and can be assembled in minutes.

2	eggs, lightly beaten
½	cup reduced-fat mayonnaise
¼	cup diced red onion
¼	cup diced red bell pepper
2	scallions, chopped
3	cloves garlic, minced
1	tablespoon chopped fresh parsley
1	tablespoon chopped fresh basil
1	tablespoon chopped fresh dill or 1 teaspoon dried
1	tablespoon fresh lemon juice
2	teaspoons Old Bay seasoning
1	teaspoon Tabasco sauce
⅓	teaspoon salt
	Freshly ground black pepper

1½	pounds salmon fillets, skin and bones removed, chopped by hand
2	cups fresh whole wheat bread crumbs
1–2	tablespoons olive oil

Preheat the oven to 250°F. Line a baking sheet with foil and place in the oven to warm.

In a large bowl, combine the eggs, mayonnaise, onion, bell pepper, scallions, garlic, parsley, basil, dill, lemon juice, Old Bay seasoning, and Tabasco sauce. Season with the salt and black pepper. Mix well.

Gently fold in the salmon and ½ cup of the bread crumbs. Be careful not to overmix. The mixture should be very wet, with lumps of salmon.

Warm 1 tablespoon of the oil in a nonstick griddle or skillet.

Place the remaining 1½ cup bread crumbs in a bowl. Divide the salmon into 12 portions and form each portion into a loose cake. Drop it into the bread crumbs and lightly coat both sides. Shake off the excess crumbs.

Gently place each cake in the preheated pan. Cook for 2 to 3 minutes on each side, or until lightly browned and cooked though. Remove from the pan and place on the baking sheet in the oven to keep warm.

Repeat with the remaining cakes, adding the remaining 1 tablespoon oil if necessary.

Per cake: 138 calories, 10 g protein, 5 g carbohydrates, 8 g total fat, 64 mg cholesterol, 1 g dietary fiber, 223 mg sodium

FRESH TUNA CAKES WITH SWEET MUSTARD-LIME SAUCE

Makes 8

Prep time: 15 minutes

Cooking time: 2–6 minutes

To make these cakes, buy the best fresh tuna you can find. Serve on plates drizzled with Sweet Mustard-Lime Sauce (page 345). Leftovers are great warm, chilled, or at room temperature.

2	scallions, finely chopped
2	tablespoons chopped fresh parsley

1	tablespoon black sesame seeds
1	clove garlic, minced
1	teaspoon grated fresh ginger
1	pound tuna, cut into cubes
1	tablespoon rice wine (mirin)
1	tablespoon reduced-sodium soy sauce
3	tablespoons dry whole grain breadcrumbs or panko
1	tablespoon peanut or sesame oil

In a medium bowl, combine the scallions, parsley, sesame seeds, garlic, and ginger. Stir to mix well.

Place the tuna on a cutting board and mince by hand.

Very gently fold the tuna, rice wine, and soy sauce into the onion mixture. Don't overmix, or the cakes will be dense.

Lightly pat the tuna mixture into 8 cakes, each 1" thick. Gently press both sides of each cake into the breadcrumbs.

In a medium nonstick skillet, warm the oil over medium-high heat. Add the cakes and cook for 1 to 3 minutes per side, or according to taste. Serve immediately.

Per cake: 115 calories, 14 g protein, 2 g carbohydrates, 5 g total fat, 22 mg cholesterol, 0 g dietary fiber, 98 mg sodium

SWEET MUSTARD-LIME SAUCE

Makes 8 servings (⅓ cup)

Prep time: 5 minutes

This tangy sauce makes a wonderful accompaniment to almost any type of fish dish.

1	tablespoon stone-ground mustard
1	tablespoon reduced-sodium soy sauce
1	tablespoon honey
1	tablespoon rice wine (mirin)

1	teaspoon lime juice
1/2	teaspoon chili puree with garlic
1/4	teaspoon grated lime peel

In a small cup, combine the mustard, soy sauce, honey, wine, lime juice, chili puree, and lime peel. Stir well.

Per serving: 14 calories, 0 g protein, 3 g carbohydrates, 0 g total fat, 0 mg cholesterol, 0 g dietary fiber, 164 mg sodium

MEDITERRANEAN TUNA STEAKS WITH ORZO

Serves 4

Prep and cooking time: 45 minutes

Mediterranean flavors abound in this dish. If grilling is either out of season or not an option, you can pan-sear or broil the tuna to your liking.

Marinated Tuna

2	tablespoons fat-free chicken or vegetable broth
1	tablespoon olive oil
1	tablespoon balsamic vinegar
1	teaspoon dried basil
1/2	teaspoon dried oregano
1/2	teaspoon grated lemon peel
1	pound tuna, cut into 4 pieces
	Salt to taste
	Freshly ground black pepper to taste

Orzo and Sauce

2	tablespoons olive oil
1	small onion, chopped
4	cloves garlic, minced
1	14½-ounce can diced tomatoes, drained

½	cup fat-free chicken or vegetable broth
¼	cup dry red wine
1	teaspoon dried oregano
1	teaspoon grated lemon peel
1	teaspoon sugar
10	ounces orzo pasta
3	tablespoons drained capers
1	tablespoon chopped fresh basil
1	tablespoon chopped fresh parsley
	Salt
	Red pepper flakes
4	tablespoons crumbled feta cheese or Parmesan cheese

To make the tuna: In a dish just large enough to hold the tuna in a single layer, combine the broth, oil, vinegar, basil, oregano, and lemon peel. Place the tuna in the dish and season with the salt and black pepper. Turn several times to coat with the marinade. Cover and refrigerate until ready to use.

To make the orzo and sauce: In a medium saucepan, heat the oil. Add the onion and garlic and cook over medium-low heat for 3 to 5 minutes, or until softened. Stir in the tomatoes, broth, wine, oregano, lemon peel, and sugar. Simmer for 15 minutes.

While the sauce is cooking, bring a large saucepan of water to a boil. Stir in the orzo and cook, stirring often, for 7 to 9 minutes, or until al dente.

Drain the orzo, reserving ¼ cup of the cooking water. Place the orzo in a large bowl and toss with the reserved cooking water.

Stir the capers, basil, and parsley into the sauce. Season to taste with the salt and pepper flakes.

To serve, remove the tuna from the dish and discard the remaining marinade. Grill for 2 to 4 minutes per side, according to taste.

Divide the orzo among 4 shallow bowls. Top with the sauce, tuna, and crumbled cheese.

Per serving: 583 calories, 39 g protein, 64 g carbohydrates, 18 g total fat, 51 mg cholesterol, 4 g dietary fiber, 631 mg sodium

MARINATED SWORDFISH WITH LEMON RISOTTO AND GARLIC GREEN BEANS

Serves 6

Prep and cooking time: 1 hour

Prepare a salad to go with this trio of recipes for a complete, elegant meal. Feel free to mix and match the recipes with other dishes as well.

Marinated Swordfish

1	clove garlic, minced
2	tablespoons olive oil
2	tablespoons fat-free chicken or vegetable broth
1	tablespoon balsamic vinegar
1	tablespoon lemon juice
1	teaspoon dried oregano
1	teaspoon chopped fresh basil
1	teaspoon Dijon mustard
1	pound swordfish, cut into 6 pieces
	Salt
	Freshly ground black pepper

Lemon Risotto

1	tablespoon unsalted butter
1	tablespoon olive oil
2	shallots, chopped
1½	cups arborio rice
½	cup white wine
4	cups fat-free chicken or vegetable broth, heated
1	tablespoon grated lemon peel
1	tablespoon chopped fresh basil

2–4	tablespoons freshly grated Parmesan cheese
	Salt
	Freshly ground black pepper

Garlic Green Beans

I	pound green beans
2	teaspoons olive oil
I	clove garlic, minced
2	teaspoons reduced-sodium soy sauce
	Freshly ground black pepper

To make the fish: In a dish just large enough to hold the fish in a single layer, combine the garlic, oil, broth, vinegar, lemon juice, oregano, basil, and mustard. Add the fish and season with the salt and pepper. Turn to coat with the marinade. Cover and refrigerate until ready to cook.

To make the risotto: In a heavy saucepan, warm the butter and oil over medium heat. Add the shallots and cook for 2 minutes. Pour in the rice and cook, stirring constantly, for I minute.

Add the wine and cook for I to 2 minutes. Gradually add the broth ½ cup at a time, stirring frequently after each addition until mostly absorbed.

Remove from the heat and stir in the lemon peel, basil, and cheese. Season to taste with the salt and pepper.

To make the green beans: While the risotto is cooking, steam the green beans for 4 to 5 minutes, or until bright green.

In a small skillet, warm the oil over medium-low heat. Add the beans, garlic, and soy sauce. Cook for 3 to 5 minutes, stirring often. Season to taste with the pepper.

To serve, heat the grill 25 minutes before serving. Remove the fish from the refrigerator I0 minutes before serving and grill for 3 to 5 minutes per side, depending on thickness. Discard the remaining marinade.

Spoon equal amounts of the risotto into the center of 4 individual soup bowls. Top with the grilled fish and place the green beans around the edges. Serve immediately.

Per serving: 436 calories, 24 g protein, 52 g carbohydrates, 14 g total fat, 36 mg cholesterol, 4 g dietary fiber, 605 mg sodium

HALIBUT ON A BED OF SPINACH WITH WHITE BEANS AND TOMATOES

Serves 4

Prep and cooking time: 35 minutes

Each of these recipes can stand on its own. Together, though, they create an attractive and flavor-packed entrée.

White Beans and Tomatoes

I	tablespoon olive oil
2	shallots, minced
2	large tomatoes, peeled, seeded, and drained
I	15-ounce can white beans, rinsed and drained
¼	cup dry white wine
2	tablespoons chopped fresh parsley
2	tablespoons chopped fresh basil
½	teaspoon sugar
I	teaspoon balsamic vinegar
	Salt
	Freshly ground black pepper

Spinach and Garlic Sauté

I	tablespoon olive oil
6	cloves garlic, finely chopped
I	pound baby spinach leaves
I	teaspoon sugar
	Salt
	Freshly ground black pepper

Halibut

I½	pounds halibut fillet, skin removed and cut into 4 pieces
I	tablespoon lemon juice

	tablespoon olive oil

Salt to taste

Freshly ground black pepper to taste

To make the white beans and tomatoes: In a small saucepan, warm the oil over medium heat. Add the shallots and cook for 1 minute.

Stir in the tomatoes, beans, wine, parsley, basil, and sugar. Cook for 10 minutes.

Add the vinegar and season to taste with the salt and pepper. Remove from the heat or keep warm on the lowest setting until ready to serve.

To make the spinach and garlic sauté: In a large nonstick skillet, warm the oil over medium heat. Add the garlic and cook for 1 minute, or until just beginning to brown.

Stir in the spinach a little at a time. As the spinach wilts, more will fit into the pan. Cook, tossing often, until all the leaves are bright green and wilted.

Add the sugar and season to taste with the salt and pepper. Toss well.

To make the fish: Rinse the fish under cool water and pat dry. Rub the fish with the lemon and oil. Season with the salt and pepper.

Grill or broil for approximately 5 minutes per side, depending on the thickness.

To serve, divide the spinach among 4 bowls. Place the fish on the spinach and top with the sauce. Serve immediately.

Per serving: 436 calories, 38 g protein, 41 g carbohydrates, 14 g total fat, 42 mg cholesterol, 10 g dietary fiber, 260 mg sodium

SOLE IN SHERRY BUTTER SAUCE

Serves 4

Prep time: 10 minutes

Baking time: 6–12 minutes

This particular dish is ideal for family-style dining or a small dinner party. The recipe calls for sole, but you can use any white fish, such as snapper, tilapia, flounder, or skate.

2	tablespoons extra-virgin olive oil
I	pound grey or Dover sole fillets
	Salt
	Freshly ground black pepper

3	tablespoons dry sherry
I	tablespoon unsalted butter
I	tablespoon finely chopped fresh parsley
10	ounces fresh linguini or other pasta
¼	cup freshly grated Parmesan cheese

Preheat the oven to 400°F. With the oil, coat a baking dish just large enough to hold the fish in a single layer.

Bring a large saucepan of water to a boil.

Rinse the fish and dry well with paper towels. Place in the baking dish and season with the salt and pepper. Drizzle with the sherry, dot with the butter, and sprinkle with the parsley.

Tilt the baking dish to coat the fish with the sauce. Bake for about 6 minutes per ½" thickness of fish.

Cook the pasta until al dente. Drain, reserving ¼ cup of the cooking water.

In a large serving bowl, toss the pasta with the reserved cooking water and the cheese.

Divide the pasta among 4 bowls. Place the fillets on the pasta and spoon the sauce over the top. Serve immediately.

Per serving: 425 calories, 31 g protein, 39 g carbohydrates, 14 g total fat, 118 mg cholesterol, 3 g dietary fiber, 189 mg sodium

On the Side

BASIC BLACK BEANS

Serves 6

Cooking time: 1 hour

The word *basic* is a nod to the versatility of this dish. It's delicious on its own, but you can also wrap the beans in tortillas, thin them with broth and serve them as a dip, or add them to soups or chili. Save any leftovers; they'll keep for up to 5 days in the refrigerator.

1½	cups dried black beans, picked over, rinsed, and soaked overnight
4	cups water
1	onion, chopped
2	cloves garlic, chopped
1	bay leaf
2	teaspoons chili powder
1	teaspoon salt or to taste
1	teaspoon grated lemon peel
1	teaspoon oregano
	Few drops of liquid smoke flavoring
1	tablespoon balsamic vinegar
1	tablespoon chopped fresh cilantro

Drain and rinse the beans.

Pour the water into a large saucepan. Add the beans, onion, garlic, and bay leaf and bring to a boil over high heat.

Reduce the heat to medium-low. Simmer, partially covered, for 45 to 60 minutes, or until the beans are tender.

Stir in the chili powder, salt, lemon peel, oregano, liquid smoke, vinegar, and cilantro. Cook, uncovered, for 5 minutes, or until the bean liquid reaches the desired thickness. Taste and adjust the seasonings as desired. Remove the bay leaf.

Per serving: 167 calories, 11 g protein, 32 g carbohydrates, 1 g total fat, 0 mg cholesterol, 10 g dietary fiber, 410 mg sodium

Spicy Black Beans: For extra kick, add a jalapeño pepper along with the onion and garlic. Season with Tabasco sauce and cayenne pepper.

BROCCOLI AND WHITE BEAN PUREE

Serves 4

Prep and cooking time: 20 minutes

Try this dish as an alternative to traditional steamed broccoli. The texture of the puree is similar to that of mashed potatoes.

1	bunch broccoli florets
1	tablespoon olive oil
2	cloves garlic, minced
1	19-ounce can cannellini or white beans
½	cup half-and-half
¼	cup reduced-fat sour cream
1	tablespoon unsalted butter
	Salt
	Freshly ground black pepper

In a saucepan with a steamer basket, bring a small amount of water to a boil. Add the broccoli, cover, and steam until bright green and just tender. Uncover and set aside.

In a medium nonstick skillet, warm the oil over medium heat. Add the garlic and cook for 1 to 2 minutes. The garlic should not turn brown. Add the beans, toss, and cook for an additional 2 minutes.

In a medium bowl, combine the beans, broccoli, half-and-half, sour cream, and butter. Season to taste with the salt and pepper.

In a blender, puree until smooth and creamy. Serve immediately.

Per serving: 234 calories, 8 g protein, 24 g carbohydrates, 12 g total fat, 24 mg cholesterol, 7 g dietary fiber, 317 mg sodium

CHICKEN AND VEGETABLE FRIED RICE

Serves 6

Prep and cooking time: 25 minutes

Traditional Chinese fried rice can be high in fat and calories. This healthier version eliminates much of the oil, substitutes brown rice for white, and incorporates a variety of crunchy vegetables. Use leftover rice or prepare the rice ahead of time and chill well. The cold prevents the grains from sticking together.

2	tablespoons reduced-sodium soy sauce
1	tablespoon rice wine (mirin)
1	teaspoon sugar
1	tablespoon peanut oil
1	red onion, chopped
1	red bell pepper, cored, seeded, and finely chopped
4	ounces shiitake mushrooms, thinly sliced
1	8-ounce can sliced water chestnuts, drained
1	cup shredded carrots
½	pound snow peas, halved diagonally
2	scallions, white and green parts sliced horizontally
1	tablespoon toasted sesame oil
1	pound boneless, skinless chicken breasts, sliced into ¼" slivers
3	cups brown rice, cooked and chilled
	Salt
	Freshly ground black pepper
3	eggs, beaten

In a small cup, combine the soy sauce, wine, and sugar. Set aside.

In a wok or large skillet, warm the oil over medium-high heat. Add the onion and cook for 3 minutes. Add the bell pepper, mushrooms, and water chestnuts and toss.

Cook, stirring constantly, for 3 minutes. Add the carrots, snow peas, and scallions. Cook for 2 minutes.

Push the vegetables to the sides of the pan. Increase the heat to high and pour the sesame oil into the middle of the pan. Add the chicken and season with the salt and black pepper. Cook, stirring constantly, for 3 minutes, or until the chicken is cooked through.

Add the rice and the soy sauce mixture. Stir well.

Move the rice to the sides of the pan and pour the eggs into the middle. Cook, stirring, for 1 minute, or until the eggs begin to set.

Stir the eggs into the other ingredients. Season with the salt and pepper and cook until mixed well. Serve immediately.

Per serving: 341 calories, 26 g protein, 38 g carbohydrates, 9 g total fat, 150 mg cholesterol, 5 g dietary fiber, 410 mg sodium

----

Smart Cooking: To make the 3 cups brown rice, boil 2 cups water and add the rice. Reduce the heat to medium-low, cover, and cook for 45 minutes. Remove from the heat and let stand for 10 minutes. Place in a covered bowl and refrigerate for several hours or until ready to use.

Shrimp and Vegetable Fried Rice: Replace the chicken with an equal amount of shrimp.

PEANUT SOBA NOODLES

Serves 4

Prep and cooking time: 15 minutes

This side dish complements most Asian-flavored entrées. For variety, try adding your choice of grated or matchstick carrots; steamed snow peas or sugar snap peas; steamed fresh soybeans (edamame); chopped peanuts; or cooked chicken, shrimp, or tofu cubes.

8	ounces soba noodles
2	tablespoons natural peanut butter
2	tablespoons rice vinegar

2	tablespoons rice wine (mirin)
2	tablespoons low-sodium chicken or vegetable broth
2	tablespoons reduced-sodium soy sauce
1	teaspoon chili puree with garlic
1	clove garlic, minced
½	teaspoon grated fresh ginger
1	tablespoon toasted sesame oil
2	scallions, chopped
1	tablespoon chopped fresh cilantro

Bring a large saucepan of water to a boil and add the noodles. Cook, stirring occasionally, for 8 minutes, or until al dente. Drain and rinse under cool water.

In a blender or small bowl, combine the peanut butter, vinegar, wine, broth, soy sauce, chili puree, garlic, and ginger. Blend or stir until smooth and creamy.

Add the oil to the noodles and toss well. Pour the dressing over the noodles and add with the scallions and cilantro. Toss well. Serve at room temperature or chilled.

Per serving: 301 calories, 11 g protein, 49 g carbohydrates, 8 g total fat, 0 mg cholesterol, 1 g dietary fiber, 773 mg sodium

- -

Smart Cooking: Soba noodles are made with nutritious whole grain buckwheat flour. They can be found in the Asian section of many supermarkets and natural food stores.

ROASTED ROOT VEGETABLE CASSEROLE

Serves 8

Prep time: 20 minutes

Baking time: 55–60 minutes

This is the perfect accompaniment to a roasted or rotisserie chicken. You can vary the dish by substituting your choice of root vegetables. The vegetables become sweet and flavorful from the roasting, and the toasted bread crumbs give them a little crunch.

I	red onion, cut into thick chunks
I	sweet potato, peeled and cubed
I	large parsnip, peeled and sliced
I	small rutabaga, peeled and cubed
5	cloves garlic, sliced
I	beet, peeled and cubed
4	sprigs fresh rosemary or thyme
3	tablespoons olive oil
	Kosher salt
	Freshly ground black pepper
I½	cups fresh whole wheat bread crumbs

Preheat the oven to 450°F. Coat a 3-quart or I3" x 9" shallow baking dish with cooking spray.

Add the onion, sweet potato, parsnip, rutabaga, garlic, beet, and rosemary or thyme. Toss with the oil and season well with the salt and pepper.

Bake on the bottom rack for 30 minutes. Remove from the oven and toss well. Bake for another I5 minutes, or until the vegetables are soft.

Remove from the oven and discard the rosemary or thyme sprigs. Spread the bread crumbs on top and coat with cooking spray. Bake for another I0 to I5 minutes, or until the crumbs are toasted.

Per serving: II2 calories, 2 g protein, I5 g carbohydrates, 5 g total fat, 0 mg cholesterol, 3 g dietary fiber, 53 mg sodium

----

Smart Cooking: To make fresh whole wheat bread crumbs, place a slice or two of whole wheat bread in a food processor with a knife blade. Process until fine crumbs form.

SMASHED ORANGE-GINGER SWEET POTATOES

Serves 8

Prep and cooking time: 25 minutes

Although the terms *sweet potato* and *yam* have become interchangeable in this country, they actually refer to different plants. If your supermarket carries garnet yams, try them. They have dark orange flesh that is especially sweet.

2½	pounds yams or sweet potatoes, peeled and cubed
¼	cup half-and-half
2	tablespoons unsalted butter
1	teaspoon grated orange peel
½	teaspoon grated fresh ginger
	Salt
	Freshly ground black pepper

Bring a large saucepan of water to a boil and add the yams or sweet potatoes. Boil for 10 minutes, or until soft. Drain and return to the pan.

Add the half-and-half, butter, orange peel, and ginger. Using a potato masher or large fork, mash until all the ingredients are mixed well and the potatoes are smooth. Season to taste with the salt and pepper. Serve immediately.

Per serving: 202 calories, 2 g protein, 40 g carbohydrates, 4 g total fat, 10 mg cholesterol, 6 g dietary fiber, 16 mg sodium

ROASTED RED PEPPER COULIS

Makes 6 servings (3 cups)

Prep time: 10 minutes

Cooking time: 30 minutes

This sauce is a staple in my kitchen. It's quick and easy to make with ingredients I keep on hand in the pantry. It's equally good with light summer dishes and hearty cool-weather recipes. Try using it as a substitute for tomato sauce in your favorite recipes.

1	tablespoon olive oil
1	onion, chopped
6	cloves garlic, minced
2	cups roasted red peppers, chopped
1	15-ounce can diced tomatoes
1	tablespoon balsamic vinegar
	Salt
	Freshly ground black pepper
	Crushed red pepper

In a medium saucepan, warm the oil over medium heat. Add the onion and cook for 5 minutes. Stir in the garlic and cook for 2 minutes. Add the red peppers, tomatoes (with juice), and vinegar.

Reduce the heat to medium-low, cover, and cook for 30 minutes. Season to taste with the salt, black pepper, and crushed red pepper.

Puree the sauce in a processor or blender until smooth. Keep warm on the lowest setting or refrigerate, covered, until ready to use.

Per serving: 142 calories, 4 g protein, 20 g carbohydrates, 2 g total fat, 0 mg cholesterol, 1 g dietary fiber, 951 mg sodium

Sweet Endings

BLUEBERRY WALNUT BISCOTTI

Makes 46

Prep time: 15 minutes

Baking time: 60 minutes

Dried blueberries, walnuts, and a hint of cinnamon flavor these crunchy twice-baked cookies. For an extra bit of sweetness, top with Cinnamon Icing (page 362).

1	cup dried blueberries
¾	cup hot water
2	cups whole wheat pastry flour or unbleached flour
1	cup sugar
1	teaspoon baking powder
½	teaspoon baking soda
½	teaspoon ground cinnamon
½	teaspoon salt
2	eggs
1	tablespoon vanilla extract
1	cup chopped walnuts

Preheat the oven to 325°F. Line a baking sheet with parchment paper.

Place the blueberries in a small bowl. Add the water and set aside.

In a large bowl, combine the flour, sugar, baking powder, baking soda, cinnamon, and salt. Stir to mix well.

In a small bowl, lightly beat the eggs and vanilla. Stir the eggs into the flour mixture until just combined.

Drain the blueberries. Fold the walnuts and blueberries into the batter until just combined.

Spread the dough onto the baking sheet in 3 thin rows, each about 12" long. Bake for 30 minutes. Remove from the oven and cool on a wire rack for 10 minutes. Reduce the oven temperature to 300°F.

Place the loaves on a cutting board. Using a sharp serrated knife, cut into ½" slices on the diagonal. Return the slices to the baking sheet, cut side down, and bake for 15 minutes.

Remove from the oven and turn the biscotti. Bake for an additional 15 minutes, or until dry and golden brown. Cool completely on a wire rack.

Per cookie: 65 calories, 1 g protein, 11 g carbohydrates, 2 g total fat, 9 mg cholesterol, 1 g dietary fiber, 51 mg sodium

CINNAMON ICING

Makes 46 servings

Prep time: 10 minutes

This icing is the perfect flavor complement to the Blueberry Walnut Biscotti. Allow it to cool completely before storing the biscotti; it will harden nicely.

1½	cups confectioners' sugar
1–2	tablespoons water
1½	teaspoons lemon juice
½	teaspoon vanilla extract
¼	teaspoon ground cinnamon

In a small saucepan, combine the sugar, water, lemon juice, vanilla, and cinnamon. Heat gently until lukewarm, stirring often. Thin with additional water or thicken with additional sugar if necessary.

Once the icing is slightly thick, use a knife to drizzle it over the biscotti in a zigzag pattern. Cool and store in an airtight container.

Per serving: 15 calories, 0 g protein, 4 g carbohydrates, 0 g total fat, 0 mg cholesterol, 0 g dietary fiber, 0 mg sodium

CHOCOLATE-RASPBERRY TAPIOCA PARFAITS

Serves 4

Prep time: 10 minutes

Cooking time: 15 minutes

Serve this chocolatey dessert on a warm summer day or after a hearty meal, when you want something cool and refreshing.

2¾	cups fat-free milk
1	egg, beaten
⅓	cup sugar
3	tablespoons quick-cooking tapioca
2	tablespoons cocoa powder
1	ounce chocolate, broken into pieces (see Smart Cooking)
2	teaspoons vanilla extract
1	pint fresh raspberries

In a medium saucepan, whisk together the milk, egg, sugar, tapioca, cocoa, and chocolate. Remove from the heat and set aside for 5 minutes.

Return the pan to the stove and cook over medium heat until the pudding comes to a full boil. Stir every few minutes so the bottom doesn't burn. Remove from the heat and stir in the vanilla.

Place a piece of plastic wrap on the surface of the pudding and set side to cool for 20 minutes. Remove the plastic and stir.

Place 3 or 4 raspberries at the bottom of each of 4 stem glasses. Divide half of the pudding among the glasses. Add 5 or 6 more raspberries on top of the pudding, placing the berries close to the edge of each glass. Divide the remaining pudding among the glasses. Top with the remaining berries, bottom side up. Cover and refrigerate for 1 hour to overnight.

Per serving: 239 calories, 10 g protein, 45 g carbohydrates, 5 g total fat, 56 mg cholesterol, 5 g dietary fiber, 89 mg sodium

----

Smart Cooking: For a dark chocolate pudding, use Dutch process cocoa powder and semisweet or bittersweet chocolate. For milk chocolate pudding, use regular cocoa powder and milk chocolate.

STRAWBERRY-VANILLA TAPIOCA PARFAITS

Serves 4

Prep time: 10 minutes

Cooking time: 15 minutes

Light and fruity, this parfait is certain to satisfy the vanilla lovers in your family.

2¾	cups fat-free milk
1	egg, beaten
⅓	cup sugar
3	tablespoons quick-cooking tapioca
1	fresh vanilla bean, halved lengthwise, or 1 teaspoon vanilla extract
1	pint fresh strawberries, quartered

In a medium saucepan, whisk together the milk, egg, sugar, and tapioca. If using the vanilla bean, scrape the seeds from the center directly into the saucepan. Remove from the heat and set aside for 5 minutes.

Return the pan to the stove and cook over medium heat until the pudding comes to a full boil, stirring every few minutes so the bottom doesn't burn. Remove from the heat. If using the vanilla extract, add it.

Place a piece of plastic wrap on the surface of the pudding and set side to cool for 20 minutes. Remove the plastic and stir.

Place a few strawberries on the bottom of each of 4 stem glasses. Divide half of the pudding among the glasses. Add 5 or 6 more strawberries on top of the pudding, placing the berries close to the edge of each glass. Divide the remaining pudding among the glasses and top with the remaining berries. Cover and refrigerate for 1 hour to overnight.

Per serving: 192 calories, 8 g protein, 37 g carbohydrates, 2 g total fat, 56 mg cholesterol, 1 g dietary fiber, 89 mg sodium

GRAND MARNIER–INFUSED BERRIES

Makes 10 servings (10 cups)

Prep time: 5 minutes

Cooking time: 20–30 minutes

I think fresh berries are perfect on their own, but for an extra-special treat, try this dressed-up version. If you wish, you can serve them over Orange Angel Food Cake (page 371).

2	cups sugar
1	cup Grand Marnier
1	cup dry white wine
1	cup water
	Juice of 1 orange
	Grated peel of 1 orange
8	cups mixed fresh berries (quarter strawberries if large)

In a medium saucepan, combine the sugar, Grand Marnier, wine, water, orange juice, and orange peel. Bring the mixture to a boil. Reduce the heat to medium and simmer until reduced by one-quarter. Remove from the heat and cool slightly.

Place the berries in a serving bowl. Pour in the liquid and steep for 1 hour, or until cooled. Refrigerate until ready to serve.

Per serving: 275 calories, 1 g protein, 61 g carbohydrates, 0 g total fat, 0 mg cholesterol, 4 g dietary fiber, 3 mg sodium

OATMEAL CHOCOLATE CHIP COOKIES

Makes 84

Prep time: 15 minutes

Baking time: 10–12 minutes

These chewy little cookies are packed with whole grain goodness. Using mini chocolate chips distributes the chocolate flavor throughout the cookie, so the fat content stays low.

2¼	cups rolled oats
2¼	cups whole wheat pastry flour
¾	teaspoon salt
½	teaspoon baking soda
¼	teaspoon ground cinnamon
½	cup unsalted butter, softened
1	cup packed brown sugar
½	cup maple syrup
2	eggs
1	teaspoon vanilla extract
1½	cups mini chocolate chips

Preheat the oven to 350°F. Line 2 baking sheets with parchment paper or coat with cooking spray.

In a medium bowl, combine the oats, flour, salt, baking soda, and cinnamon.

In a large bowl, beat the butter with an electric mixer on medium speed until creamy. Add the brown sugar and beat until smooth. Beat in the maple syrup. Add the eggs 1 at a time and then the vanilla, beating after each addition.

Stir the flour mixture into the butter mixture by hand until combined well. Fold in the chocolate chips.

Drop the dough by rounded teaspoons onto the prepared baking sheets about 2" apart. Bake 1 sheet at a time for 10 to 12 minutes, or until the cookies just begin to brown.

Remove the cookies from the baking sheets and cool on a wire rack.

Per cookie: 68 calories, 1 g protein, 10 g carbohydrates, 3 g total fat, 8 mg cholesterol, 1 g dietary fiber, 31 mg sodium

Oatmeal Nut Cookies: Simply substitute any variety of finely chopped nuts and 1 teaspoon grated orange peel for the chocolate chips.

CINNAMON SUGAR COOKIES

Makes 64

Prep time: 15 minutes

Baking time: 10–12 minutes

A slightly different version of this recipe appeared in my previous book, *Low-Fat Living Cookbook*. It was then, and still is, one of my family's favorite cookies. I've modified the recipe slightly, so the cookies taste even better. By using whole wheat pastry flour, you get healthy complex carbohydrates.

½	cup unsalted butter, softened
⅔	cup + 1 tablespoon sugar
½	cup brown sugar
2	eggs
¼	cup light corn syrup
1	tablespoon vanilla extract
3	cups whole wheat pastry flour or unbleached flour
1½	teaspoons baking powder
1	teaspoon + ½ teaspoon ground cinnamon
¼	teaspoon salt

Preheat the oven to 350°F. Line 2 baking sheets with parchment paper or coat with cooking spray.

In a large bowl, beat the butter with an electric mixer until creamy. Add the ⅔ cup sugar, brown sugar, eggs, corn syrup, and vanilla, beating after each addition.

In a medium bowl, stir together the flour, baking powder, 1 teaspoon cinnamon, and salt. Mix well.

Add the flour mixture to the butter mixture and mix well by hand.

In a cup, combine the remaining I tablespoon sugar and ½ teaspoon cinnamon. Mix well.

Drop the dough onto the prepared baking sheets by spoonfuls about 2" apart. Sprinkle with the cinnamon-sugar mixture.

Bake I sheet at a time for I0 to I2 minutes, or until the cookies just begin to darken. Remove from the baking sheets and cool on a wire rack.

Per cookie: 48 calories, I g protein, 8 g carbohydrates, 2 g total fat, I0 mg cholesterol, I0 g dietary fiber, 23 mg sodium

----

Smart Cooking: Whole wheat pastry flour is milled from "soft" wheat berries, which contain less gluten than the regular whole wheat flour that is made from "hard" wheat. As a result, whole wheat pastry flour is best suited for muffins, cookies, quick breads, piecrusts, and other baked goods that use baking powder or baking soda for leavening.

Although both are whole grain and loaded with essential fiber and nutrients, pastry flour is not interchangeable with regular whole wheat flour, which is best used in recipes containing yeast. Look for whole wheat pastry flour in natural food stores or in the specialty flour section of supermarkets.

LIGHT PUMPKIN CHEESECAKE

Serves I6

Prep time: 20 minutes

Baking time: I½ hours

Here's a lighter version of an autumn favorite. It makes a **great** Thanksgiving dessert.

2	ounces (about 8) gingersnap cookies or graham crackers, finely ground
2	pounds reduced-fat cream cheese, at room temperature
I½	cups sugar
2	teaspoons ground cinnamon
I	teaspoon ground ginger
½	teaspoon ground nutmeg

½	teaspoon ground allspice
¼	teaspoon ground cloves
4	eggs or I cup liquid egg substitute, at room temperature
I	15-ounce can solid-pack pumpkin
½	cup reduced-fat sour cream, at room temperature
½	cup half-and-half, at room temperature
2	teaspoons vanilla extract

Preheat the oven to 325°F.

Line the bottom of a 10" springform pan with heavy-duty foil. Assemble the pan, pulling the foil up and around the sides. With another piece of foil, wrap the outside of the pan to prevent water from leaking in.

Coat the bottom and sides of the pan with cooking spray. Sprinkle evenly with the cookie or graham cracker crumbs and set in a large roasting pan.

Bring a pot of water to a boil for a water bath.

In a medium bowl, beat the cream cheese with an electric mixer until smooth. Gradually add the sugar, cinnamon, ginger, nutmeg, allspice, and cloves. Beat on medium speed for about 3 minutes.

Add the eggs one at a time or the egg substitute, beating until just incorporated. Scrape down the sides of the bowl to make sure all the lumps of cream cheese are gone.

Stir in the pumpkin, sour cream, half-and-half, and vanilla just until incorporated. Pour the batter into the springform pan. Pour enough of the boiling water into the roasting pan to come about halfway up the sides of the springform pan. Bake for 1½ hours. Turn off the heat and leave the oven door slightly ajar for I hour longer.

Remove the pan from the water bath and cool completely on a wire rack. Remove the outer foil, cover, and refrigerate overnight before unmolding.

Per serving: 282 calories, 8 g protein, 33 g carbohydrates, I3 g total fat, 85 mg cholesterol, I g dietary fiber, 341 mg sodium

LIGHT STRAWBERRY MARBLE CHEESECAKE

Serves 16

Prep time: 25 minutes

Baking time: 2 hours

This recipe has all the rich and creamy texture of traditional cheesecake, but without all the fat.

1	3½-ounce package ladyfingers
1½	pounds fresh strawberries, washed and tops removed
2	pounds reduced-fat cream cheese, at room temperature
1½	cups sugar
1	cup reduced-fat sour cream, at room temperature
¼	cup unbleached flour
2	teaspoons vanilla extract
4	eggs or 1 cup liquid egg substitute, at room temperature

Preheat the oven to 325°F. Line the bottom of a 10" springform pan with heavy-duty foil. Assemble the pan, pulling the foil up and around the sides. With another piece of foil, wrap the outside of the pan to prevent water from leaking in.

Coat the bottom and sides of the pan with cooking spray. Arrange the ladyfingers in a single layer covering the bottom of the pan and set in a large roasting pan.

Bring a pot of water to a boil for a water bath.

Place the strawberries in a food processor or blender and puree until smooth. Using a fine strainer, strain the berries into a bowl to remove the seeds, leaving about 2½ cups of berry puree. Set aside.

In a medium bowl, beat the cream cheese with an electric mixer until smooth. Gradually add the sugar and beat on medium speed for about 3 minutes.

Reduce the speed to low and beat in the sour cream, flour, and vanilla.

Add the eggs one at a time or the egg substitute, beating until just incorporated. Scrape down the sides of the bowl to make sure all the lumps of cream cheese are gone.

Slowly pour the berry puree into the batter. Stir with a knife to create a marbleized effect.

Pour the batter into the springform pan. Pour enough of the boiling water into the roasting pan to come about halfway up the sides of the springform pan. Bake for 2 hours. Turn off the heat and leave the oven door slightly ajar for I hour longer.

Remove the pan from the water bath and cool on a wire rack. Remove the outer foil, cover, and refrigerate overnight before unmolding.

Per serving: 344 calories, II g protein, 42 g carbohydrates, 14 g total fat, 172 mg cholesterol, I g dietary fiber, 329 mg sodium

ORANGE ANGEL FOOD CAKE

Serves 10

Prep time: 30 minutes

Baking time: 45 minutes

This update on traditional angel food cake uses whole grain flour and the fresh, bright flavor of citrus. You can substitute lemon or lime for the orange, with delicious results. For a light yet elegant dessert, try serving it with Grand Marnier-Infused Berries (page 365) and a dollop of low-fat fresh or frozen vanilla yogurt.

I	cup whole wheat pastry flour or unbleached flour
½	teaspoon salt
1½	cups sugar
3	tablespoons grated orange peel
12	egg whites
I	teaspoon cream of tartar
I	teaspoon vanilla extract
4	tablespoons fresh orange juice
1¼	cups confectioners' sugar

Preheat the oven to 325°F.

In a medium bowl, combine the flour and salt. Set aside.

In a small bowl, stir together the sugar and orange peel. Set aside.

In a large bowl, beat the egg whites with an electric mixer until foamy. Add the cream of tartar, vanilla, and I tablespoon of the orange juice. Beat on high speed until soft peaks form. Gradually add the sugar mixture, beating until the peaks are stiff and glossy. Gently fold in the flour mixture.

Pour the batter into an ungreased tube pan with a removable bottom. Using a knife, cut through the batter several times to release any air bubbles.

Bake for 45 minutes, or until the top is golden brown and springy to the touch. Invert the cake onto the neck of a wine bottle and cool completely.

Run a knife along the inside edges of the pan to loosen the cake and transfer to a cake plate.

In a small bowl, combine the confectioners' sugar and the remaining 3 tablespoons orange juice. Drizzle the glaze over the top of the cake, allowing it to drip slightly down the sides.

Per serving: 234 calories, 6 g protein, 53 g carbohydrates, 0 g total fat, 0 mg cholesterol, I g dietary fiber, 183 mg sodium

MIXED BERRY PIE

Serves 9

Prep time: IO minutes

Baking time: 55–60 minutes

This dessert has such a rich and satisfying flavor that you might forget it's essentially fruit. Try serving it with low-fat frozen yogurt or ice cream.

5	cups frozen mixed berries (blueberries, raspberries, strawberries, or blackberries)
¾	cup sugar
I	teaspoon ground cinnamon
¼	cup Chambourd liqueur
6	tablespoons arrowroot or cornstarch
I	tablespoon lemon juice
I	unbaked deep-dish pie crust
I	tablespoon packed brown sugar

Line a baking sheet with foil. Place in the oven and preheat to 425°F.

In a large bowl, combine the berries, sugar, and cinnamon.

In a cup, combine the Chambourd, arrowroot or cornstarch, and lemon juice. Stir well and pour over the berries. Toss until well combined.

Spoon the berries into the pie crust and sprinkle with the brown sugar.

Bake for 15 minutes. Reduce the heat to 350°F and bake for 40 to 45 minutes, or until the filling is bubbling. Cool on a wire rack for at least 1 hour before slicing.

Per serving: 272 calories, 2 g protein, 2 g carbohydrates, 46 g total fat, 9 mg cholesterol, 3 g dietary fiber, 126 mg sodium

PEACH AND RASPBERRY PIE WITH ALMOND CRUNCH TOPPING

Serves 10

Prep time: 15 minutes

Baking time: 55–60 minutes

The fruits give this pie a perfect balance of sweet and tart. It makes a wonderful late-summer treat, when juicy peaches and fresh raspberries are readily available. Out of season, frozen fruits work just as well.

Filling

12–14	peaches, peeled and sliced into ½" wedges
1½	tablespoons lemon juice
¼	cup packed brown sugar
¼	cup sugar
3	tablespoons cornstarch or arrowroot
1½	teaspoons ground cinnamon
¼	teaspoon ground ginger
⅛	teaspoon salt
2	cups fresh raspberries (about 12 ounces)

Topping

½	cup almonds, toasted
½	cup whole wheat pastry flour or unbleached flour
3	tablespoons packed brown sugar

1	tablespoon sugar
¾	teaspoon ground cinnamon
	Pinch of salt
2	teaspoons vanilla extract
4	tablespoons unsalted butter, cut into cubes

Preheat the oven to 375°F. Lightly coat a 10″ or 11″ deep-dish pie pan with cooking spray. Line a baking sheet with foil.

To make the filling: In a large bowl, gently toss the peaches with the lemon juice.

In a small bowl, combine the brown sugar, sugar, cornstarch or arrowroot, cinnamon, ginger, and salt. Sprinkle the sugar mixture over the peaches and toss gently.

To make the topping: In a food processor, combine the almonds, flour, brown sugar, sugar, cinnamon, and salt. Mix until finely ground. Add the vanilla and butter. Pulse until the butter is cut into small crumbs.

Pour half of the peaches into the prepared pan. Add half of the raspberries. Top with the remaining peaches and then the remaining raspberries. Sprinkle with the topping and press gently.

Place the pie on the baking sheet. Bake for 55 to 60 minutes, or until the crust is lightly browned and the filling is bubbling. Cool on a wire rack before slicing.

Per serving: 227 calories, 3 g protein, 38 g carbohydrates, 8 g total fat, 12 mg cholesterol, 5 g dietary fiber, 42 mg sodium

RICOTTA CHEESECAKE CUPS

Makes 12

Prep time: 15 minutes

Baking time: 1 hour

Because you bake these cakes in single servings, they're perfect for quick and easy, high-energy snacks.

15	ounces reduced-fat ricotta cheese, softened
4	ounces Neufchatel cheese, softened
4	ounces fat-free cream cheese, softened
½	cup sugar

3	eggs
1	vanilla bean, halved lengthwise

Preheat the oven to 325°F. Line a 12-cup muffin pan with paper liners.

Fill a large pan with enough water to cover the bottom of the muffin pan but not come over the top. Place in the oven to heat.

In a large bowl, beat the ricotta with an electric mixer until creamy. Add the Neufchatel, cream cheese, sugar, and eggs. Using a sharp knife, scrape the seeds from the center of the vanilla bean directly into the bowl. After each addition, beat until smooth and creamy.

Spoon the batter into the prepared muffin pan. Place in the pan of hot water and bake for 45 minutes.

Turn off the heat and open the door slightly. Let the cheesecake cups cool for 15 minutes. Remove the pan from the water bath and cool completely on a wire rack.

Remove the cups from the pan, place on a platter, and cover lightly with plastic wrap. Refrigerate for at least 2 hours or overnight.

Per cup: 118 calories, 7 g protein, 11 g carbohydrates, 5 g total fat, 69 mg cholesterol, 0 g dietary fiber, 140 mg sodium

CHEWY PEANUT BITES

Makes 20

Prep time: 10 minutes

Baking time: 10 minutes

If you like peanuts, this just might become your new favorite snack. It's simple to make, and it contains a good amount of protein. You'll need a non-stick mini-muffin pan with 24 cups.

½	cup unsalted roasted peanuts, chopped
½	cup packed dark brown sugar
3	tablespoons whole wheat pastry flour or unbleached flour
¼	teaspoon baking powder
	Pinch of salt

I	egg
I	teaspoon vanilla extract

Preheat the oven to 350°F. Coat a mini-muffin pan with cooking spray.

In a medium bowl, combine the peanuts, sugar, flour, baking powder, and salt.

Place the egg and vanilla in a small bowl. Stir until the yolk and white are just combined. Fold the eggs into the peanut mixture until combined.

Spoon equal amounts of the batter into 20 of the muffin cups. Bake for 10 minutes, or until golden. Cool for I minute.

Using a knife, carefully lift each piece from the pan and place on a foil-lined rack to cool completely. Store in an airtight container with wax or parchment paper between layers.

Per bite: 50 calories, I g protein, 7 g carbohydrates, 2 g total fat, II mg cholesterol, 0 g dietary fiber, II mg sodium

PEANUT BUTTER BURSTS

Makes 42

Prep time: 25 minutes

Cooking time: 5–7 minutes

Packed with nutrients, these bursts make a great high-energy snack. One batch lasts for weeks when stored in a covered container in the refrigerator.

I	cup natural peanut butter
½	cup honey
½	teaspoon vanilla extract
¼	cup sunflower seeds
¼	cup pumpkin seeds or finely chopped almonds
2	cups quick-cooking oats
¼	cup chopped dates or other chopped dried fruits
¼	cup wheat germ, wheat bran, or oat bran
¼	cup warm water
4	tablespoons sesame seeds

Preheat the oven to 350°F. Line a baking sheet with parchment or wax paper.

In a large bowl, combine the peanut butter, honey, and vanilla. If necessary, heat in the microwave for 30 seconds to soften.

Place the sunflower seeds and pumpkin seeds or almonds on a baking sheet. Toast for 5 to 7 minutes, or until lightly browned.

Add the seeds; oats; dates or dried fruits; wheat germ, wheat bran, or oat bran; and water to the peanut butter mixture. Stir until blended well. The dough will be very stiff.

Roll the dough into 42 walnut-size balls. Roll each ball in the sesame seeds to coat. Place in a single layer on the prepared baking sheet and refrigerate for several hours. Store in a covered container.

Per burst: 86 calories, 3 g protein, 9 g carbohydrates, 4 g total fat, 0 mg cholesterol, I g dietary fiber, 2 mg sodium

NOTES

Chapter 1

1. CDC's 1999–2000 Health and Nutrition Examination Survey. www.cdc.gov/nchs/nhanes.htm.

2. Crister, G. *Fat Land* (Boston: Houghton Mifflin, 2003).

3. For one summary of these research findings, see: Stein, R. "Fat Cells Aren't Just Passive Blobs, Scientists Learn." *Washington Post* (Jul. 12, 2004).

4. "A Healthy Internal Clock Keeps Weight Off." Howard Hughes Medical Institute Report: *Science Daily* Apr. 24, 2005.

5. "The Metabolic Impact—Or How Your Body Works Out While You Put Your Feet Up." *Peak Performance Journal* 213(2005).

6. James, W. P., and Trayhum, P. "Thermogenesis and Obesity." *British Medical Bulletin* 37(1)(1981): 43–48; Groff, J. L., and Gropper, S. S. *Advanced Nutrition and Human Metabolism* 3rd ed. (Wadsworth Publishing, 1999).

7. See, for example: Barneys, M., et al. "Effect of Exercise and Protein Intake on Energy Expenditure." *Revista Española de Fisiologia* 4(4)(1993): 209–17.

8. Eaton, S. B., and Konner, M. "Paleolithic Nutrition: A Consideration of Its Nature and Current Implications." *New England Journal of Medicine* 312(1985): 283–89; Eaton, S. B., and Konner, M. *The Paleolithic Prescription* (New York: HarperCollins, 1988).

9. Armelagos, G. J. "Human Evolution and the Evolution of Disease." *Ethnic Disease* 1(1991): 21–25.

10. See, for example: Rossi, E. L. *The 20 Minute Break* (Palisades Gateway Publ, 1991); Smolensky, M., and Lamberg, L. *The Body Clock* (New York: Holt, 2000); Edlund, M. *The Body Clock Advantage* (Avon, MA: Adams, 2003).

11. Prochaska, J. O., Norcross, J. C., and DiClemente, C. C. *Changing for Good* (New York: William Morrow, 1994): 59 (more than 50 scientific studies cited).

12. Patterson, R. E., Haines, P. S., and Popkin, B. M. "Healthy Lifestyle Patterns of US Adults." *Preventive Medicine* 23(1994): 453–60.

13. Weaver, J. J., Morgan, B. B., Adkins-Holmes, C., and Hall, J. K. "A Review of Potential Moderating Factors in the Stress-Performance Relationship." *U.S. Naval Training Systems Center Technical Reports* 92-012(1992): 84.

14. Prochaska, Norcross, and DiClemente. *Changing for Good.*

15. Land, G. *Grow or Die: The Unifying Principle of Transformation* (New York: Wiley, 1986).

16. James, W. *Talks to Teachers* (New York: Norton, 1982 and 1950).

17. Pi-Sunyer, F. X. *Journal of the American Medical Association* Dec./Jan. 1995.

Chapter 2

1. Eaton, S. B., and Konner, M. "Paleolithic Nutrition: A Consideration of Its Nature and Current Implications." *New England Journal of Medicine* 312(1985): 283–89; Eaton, S. B., and Konner, M. *The Paleolithic Prescription* (New York: HarperCollins, 1988).

2. Eaton and Konner. *The Paleolithic Prescription*; Cordain, L., Gotshall, R. W., Eaton, S. B., and Eaton, S. B. III. "Physical Activity, Energy Expenditure and Fitness: An Evolutionary Perspective." *International Journal of Sports and Medicine* 19(1998): 328–35; Cordain, L., et al. "Plant-Animal Subsistence Ratios and Macronutrient Energy Estimations in Worldwide Hunter-Gatherer Diets." *American Journal of Clinical Nutrition* 71(2000): 682–92.

3. Colmers, W., et al. "Integration of NPY, AGRP, and Melanocortin Signals in the Hypothalamic Paraventricular Nucleus: Evidence of a Cellular Basis for the Adipostat." *Neuron* 24(1999): 155–63.

4. Hendler, S. S. *The Doctor's Vitamin and Mineral Encyclopedia* (New York: Simon & Schuster, 1990).

5. See, for example: Sapolsky, R. *Why Zebras Don't Get Ulcers* (New York: Freeman, 1998).

6. See, for example: Wurtman, J. J. *Managing Your Mind and Mood Through Food* (New York: Rawson, 1986).

7. Leibowitz, S., and Kim, T. "Impact of Galanin Antagonist on Exogenous Galanin and Natural Patterns of Fat Ingestion." *Brain Research* 599(1992): 148–52.

8. Leibowitz, S. F. Quoted in Marano, H. E. "Chemistry and Craving." *Psychology Today* (Jan./Feb. 1993): 30–36, 74.

9. Klein, S. "The War Against Obesity." *American Journal of Clinical Nutrition* 69(6)(1999): 1061–63; Moor, C. V., and Ha, E. Y. "Whey Protein Isolates." *Critical Reviews in Food Science and Nutrition* 33(6)(1993): 431–76.

10. Nash, M. "Cracking the Fat Riddle." *Newsweek* (Sept. 2, 2002): 49–55.

11. *Recent Progress in Hormonal Research* 56(2001): 359–75; *Peptides* 21(10)(Oct., 2000): 1479–85; *Nutrition Reviews* 56(9)(1998): 271–74.

12. *Diabetes Care* 22(3)(1999): 413–17.

13. *Life Sciences* 69(2001): 987–1003; *Journal of Lipid Research* 42(2001): 743–50.

14. *International Journal of Obesity and Related Metabolic Disorders* 25(1)(2001): 106–14.

15. *Journal of Neuroscience* 21(10)(2001): 3639–45; *Recent Progress in Hormonal Research* 56(2001): 359–75; *Peptides* 21(10)(Oct. 2000): 1479–85; *Nutrition Reviews* 56(9)(1998): 271–74.

16. *Nature* 385(6612)(1997): 165–68; *Pigment Cell Research* 15(1)(2002): 10–18; *Science* 278(5335)(1997): 135–38.

17. *European Journal of Pharmacology* 440(2-3)(2002): 85–98; *American Journal of Physiology* 272(Pt 1, 3)(1997): E379–384; *The Federation of American Societies for Experimental Biology (FASEB) Journal* 13(1998): 1391–96.

18. For one summary of these research findings, see: Stein, R. "Fat Cells Aren't Just Passive Blobs, Scientists Learn." *Washington Post* (Jul. 12, 2004).

19. Futagawa, N. K., et al. "Effect of Age on Body Composition and Resting Metabolism." *American Journal of Physiology* 259(1990): E233.

20. Hsieh, C., et al. "Predictors of Sex Hormone Levels Among the Elderly." *Journal of Clinical Endocrinology and Metabolism* 10(1999): 837–41.

Chapter 3

1. Zajonc, A. *Catching the Light* (New York: Bantam, 1993); see also Harvard research; *Peak Performance Journal* articles; etc.

2. Hendler, S. S. *The Oxygen Breakthrough* (New York: Pocket Books, 1989).

3. Batmanghelidj, F. *Your Body's Many Cries for Water*; nutrition and metabolism texts, etc.

4. Cailliet, R., and Gross, L. *The Rejuvenation Factor* (New York: Doubleday, 1986).

5. See, for example: Hauri, P., and Linde, S. *No More Sleepless Nights* (New York: Wiley, 1990); Darden; E. books; evolutionary biology references, etc.

6. Thayer, R. E. *Calm Energy* (New York: Oxford University Press, 2001).

7. Von Kries, R., et al. "Reduced Risk for Overweight and Obesity." *International Journal of Obesity* 24(12)(2002): 710–16.

8. Zhang, K., et al. "Sleeping Metabolic Rate in Relation to Body Mass Index and Body Composition." *International Journal of Obesity* 26(3)(2002): 376–83; Edlund, M. *The Body Clock Advantage* (Avon, MA: Adams, 2003); Mass, J. B., *Power Sleep* (New York: Villard, 1998); Jackson, F. R., et al. "Oscillating Molecules and Circadian Clock Output Mechanisms." *Molecular Psychiatry* 3(5)(1998): 381–85; Vioque, J., et al. "Time Spent Watching Television, Sleep Duration, and Obesity." *International Journal of Obesity* 24(12)(2000): 1683–88.

9. Van Cauter. In Edlund. *The Body Clock Advantage*.

10. Hendler. *The Oxygen Breakthrough*.

11. *Medicine and Science in Sports and Exercise* 17(4)(1985): 456–61.

12. Lindner, P. *Fat, Water Retention and You*. Cited in *Prevention's Lose Weight Guidebook 1992*: 16.

13. Heus, M., Heus, G., and Heus, J. *Low-Fat for Life* (Barneveld, WI: Micamar Publishing, 1994): 87.

14. Suter, P. M., Schutz, Y., and Jequier, E. "The Effect of Ethanol on Fat Storage in Healthy Subjects." *New England Journal of Medicine* 326(15)(1992): 983–87.

15. Selby, J. V., et al. *American Journal of Epidemiology* 1259(1987): 979–88; Fowman, D. T. *Annals of Clinical Laboratory Science* 18(1988): 181–89; Gerald, M. J., et al. *Diabetes* 26(1977): 780–85.

16. Morgan, E. *The Scars of Evolution* (New York: Oxford University Press, 1990).

17. Thayer. *Calm Energy.*

18. Sternberg, B. "Relapse in Weight Control: Definitions, Processes, and Prevention Strategies." In Marlatt, G. A., and Gordon, J. R., eds. *Relapse Prevention: Maintenance Strategies in the Treatment of Addictive Behaviors* (New York: Guilford Press, 1985): 521–45.

19. Linde, B., et al. *American Journal of Physiology* 256(1989): E12–E18.

20. Mirkin, G. *Getting Thin* (Boston: Little, Brown, 1983): 62–63, 84–85.

21. Studies by Callaway, W. Cited in Rodin, J. *Body Traps* (New York: Morrow, 1992): 193.

22. Harper, P. Quoted in "Burn Fat Faster." *Men's Health* (Nov. 1994): 26.

23. Schmidt, M. A. *Brain-Building Nutrition* (Berkeley, CA: Frog Books, 2001).

24. Barneys, M., et al. "Effect of Exercise and Protein Intake on Energy Expenditure." *Revista Española de Fisiologia* 4(4)(1993): 209–17.

25. Brownell, K. D., and Horgen, K. B. *Food Fight* (New York: McGraw-Hill, 2003).

26. Rechtschaffen, A. Quoted in "Overeating? Get Some Sleep." *Tufts University Diet & Nutrition Letter* 12(9)(Nov. 1994): 1–2.

Chapter 4

1. Hager, D. L. "Why Breakfast Is Important." *Weight Control Digest* 3(1)(Jan./Feb. 1993): 225–26.

2. Stamford, B. A., and Shimer, P. *Fitness without Exercise* (New York: Warner, 1990); Zak, V., Carlin, C., and Vash, P. D. *The Fat-to-Muscle Diet* (New York: Berkeley, 1988): 30; Natow, A. B., and Heslin, J. *The Fat Attack Plan* (New York: Pocket Books, 1990): 42, 165.

3. Zak, Carlin, and Vash. *Fat-to-Muscle Diet:* 30.

4. Zak, Carlin, and Vash. *Fat-to-Muscle Diet*; Stamford and Shimer. *Fitness without Exercise:* 41, 44.

5. Mark, V. H. *Reversing Memory Loss* (Boston: Houghton Mifflin, 1992): 216–17; Mark, V. H. *Brain Power* (Boston: Houghton Mifflin, 1989): 186–87; Benson, H., et al. *The Wellness Book* (New York: Birch Lane Press, 1992); Nathan, R. G., Stats, T. E., and Rosch, P. J. *The Doctors' Guide to Instant Stress Relief.* (New York: Ballantine, 1989).

6. Sedlacek, K. *The Sedlacek Technique: Finding the Calm Within You* (New York: McGraw-Hill, 1989): 14.

7. Southwestern Health Institute in Phoenix. Study cited in Powell, D. R., American Institute for Preventive Medicine, *A Year of Health Hints* (Emmaus, PA: Rodale Press, 1990): 96.

8. Wilcox, A. Study cited in "Fat Burns as Sun Rises." *Prevention* (Oct., 1986): 67.

9. Sheats, C. *Lean Bodies* (Dallas: Summit Group, 1992): 25.

10. Lamberg, L. *Bodyrhythms: Chronobiology and Peak Performance* (New York: Morrow, 1994): 42.

11. Czeisler, C. H., et al. "Bright Light Induction of Strong (Type O) Resetting of the Human Circadian Pacemaker." *Science* 244(Jun. 16, 1989): 1328–33; Czeisler, C. H., et al. "Human Sleep: Its Duration and Organization Depend on Its Circadian Phase." *Science* 210(Dec. 12, 1980); Kronauer, R., and Czeisler, C. Quoted in "Jet Lag Breakthrough." *Conde Naste's Traveler* (Sept. 1989): 35–36.

12. "Insights into the Body's Daily Clock." *Society for Neuroscience* (Nov. 3, 2004).

13. *American Journal of Epidemiology* (reported in Autumn 2003).

14. Vanderbilt University Study. Schlundt, D. G., et al. "The Role of Breakfast in the Treatment of Obesity." *American Journal of Clinical Nutrition* 55(1992): 645–51; *Obesity & Health* 6(12)(Nov./Dec. 1992): 103.

15. Hager. "Why Breakfast Is Important": 225–26.

16. Zak, Carlin, and Vash. *Fat-to-Muscle Diet:* 30.

17. Hager. "Why Breakfast Is Important": 225–26.

18. Leibowitz, S. F. Quoted in Marano, H. E. "Chemistry and Craving." *Psychology Today* (Jan./Feb. 1993): 30–36, 74.

19. Special Report. *Tufts University Diet and Nutrition Letter* 10(4)(Jun. 1992): 6.

20. Natow and Heslin. *The Fat Attack Plan:* 42; Schlundt, et al. "The Role of Breakfast in the Treatment of Obesity": 645–51.

21. Schlundt, D. G., et al. "The Role of Breakfast in the Treatment of Obesity."

22. Nester, J. E., et al. *Diabetes Care* 11(1988): 755–60.

23. *Muscle & Fitness:* Oct. 2003.

24. Lamberg. *Bodyrhythms: Chronobiology and Peak Performance:* 42; *Prevention's Weight Loss Guide 1993* (Emmaus, PA: Rodale Books, 1993): 148.

25. Jenkins, D. A., et al. *American Journal of Clinical Nutrition* 35(1982): 1339–46.

26. Stone, K. *Snack Attack* (New York: Warner, 1991): 169.

27. Callaway, W. C. *The Callaway Diet* (New York: Bantam, 1991): 192.

28. Storch, M. "Taking the Reins." *Scientific American Mind* 16(2)(May 2005): 88–89.

29. Howat, W. "Journaling to Self-Evaluation: A Tool for Adult Learners." *International Journal of Reality Therapy* 18(1999): 32¬-34.

30. "Third-Person Perspective is Helpful in Meeting Goals." Cornell University Report and comments. *Science Daily* (Apr. 14, 2005); Libby, L. K., and Eibach, R. *Journal of Personality and Social Psychology* 88(1)(2005).

31. Ibid.

Chapter 5

1. Tucker, L. A., and Friedman, G. M. "Television Viewing and Obesity in Adult Males." *American Journal of Public Health* 79(4)(1989): 516–18.

2. Gortmaker, S. L., Dietz, W. H., and Cheung, L. W. Y. "Inactivity, Diet, and the Fattening of America." *Journal of the American Dietetic Association* 90(1990): 1247–52.

3. Johnsgard, K. Quoted in *Prevention's Lose Weight Guide 1994* (Emmaus, PA: Rodale Books, 1994): 19–20.

4. Brooks, G., Fahey, T., and Baldwin, K. *Exercise Physiology: Human Bioenergetics and Its Application.* 4th ed. (New York: McGraw-Hill, 2005).

5. Ravussin, "Lean People Stand and Move More: Physiology: A Neat Way to Control Weight?" *Science* 307(2005): 530–31.

6. Levine, J. Quoted in Hellmich, N. *USA Today* Jan. 28, 2005: A1.

7. Marano, H. E. "Chemistry and Craving." *Psychology Today* (Jan./Feb. 1993): 30–36, 74.

8. Stamford, B. "Meals and the Timing of Exercise." *The Physician and Sports Medicine* 17(11)(Nov. 1989): 151.

9. Stamford B. A., and Shimer, P. *Fitness without Exercise* (New York: Warner, 1990): 44, 128; Stamford, B. "Meals and the Timing of Exercise": 151; Davis, J. M., et al. "Weight Control and Calorie Expenditure: Thermogenic Effects of Pre-Prandial and Post-Prandial Exercise." *Addictive Behavior* 14(3)(1989): 347–51; Poehlman, E. T., and Horton, E. S. "The Impact of Food Intake and Exercise on Energy Expenditure." *Nutrition Reviews* 47(5)(May 1989): 129–37.

10. Stamford and Shimer. *Fitness without Exercise:* 44.

11. Grilo, C. M., Wilfley, D. E., and Brownell, K. D. "Physical Activity and Weight Control: Why Is the Link So Strong?" *The Weight Control Digest* 2(3)(May/June 1992): 153–60; Grilo, C. M., Brownell, K. D., and Stunkard, A. J. "The Metabolic and Psychological Importance of Exercise in Weight Control." In Stunkard, A. J., and Walden, T. A., eds. *Obesity: Theory and Therapy* (New York: Raven Press, 1992); Piscatella, J. C. *Controlling Your Fat Tooth* (New York: Workman, 1991): 100–104.

12. Tremblay, A. In *International Journal of Obesity* 13(1989): 4.

13. Bailey, C. *Smart Exercise* (Boston: Houghton Mifflin, 1994): 28.

14. Grilo, Wilfley, and Brownell. "Physical Activity and Weight Control: Why Is the Link So Strong?": 53–60.

15. Pavlou, K. N., et al. "Exercise as an Adjunct to Weight Loss and Maintenance in Moderately Obese Subjects." *American Journal of Clinical Nutrition* 49(1989): 1115–23; Kayman, S., Bruvold W., and Stern J. S. "Maintenance and Relapse after Weight Loss in Women: Behavioral Aspects." *American Journal of Clinical Nutrition* 52(1990): 800–807.

16. Kayman, et al. "Maintenance and Relapse after Weight Loss in Women."

17. Walberg-Rankin, J. Quoted in *Men's Health* (Jan./Feb. 1994): 83.

18. Bartlett, S. J. "Exercise, Stress Reduction, and Overweight." *Weight Control Digest* 4(3)(May/June 1994): 353–55.

19. Moore-Ede, M. *The Twenty-Four-Hour Society* (Reading, MA: Addison-Wesley, 1993): 55–56.

20. "Just Do It, Even If It's Just a Little." *Tufts University Diet & Nutrition Letter* 11(8)(Oct. 1993): 1.

21. Moore-Ede. *The Twenty-Four-Hour Society.*

22. "Weight Loss." *Men's Health* (Mar. 2003): 44.

23. National Institutes of Health Conference on Physical Activity and Obesity, held in Dec., 1992 in Bethesda, MD. Reported in *Obesity & Health* 8(1)(Jan./Feb. 1994): 10.

24. Kirschenbaum, D. S. *The 9 Truths About Weight Loss* (New York: Henry Holt, 2000).

Chapter 6

1. See, for example: Cordain, L. *The Paleo Diet* (New York: Wiley, 2002); and Jacobs, G. D. *The Ancestral Mind* (New York: Viking, 2003).

2. *Recent Progress in Hormonal Research* 56(2001): 359–75; *Peptides* 21(10)(Oct. 2000): 1479–85; *Nutrition Reviews* 56(9)(1998): 271–74.

3. *Diabetes* 51(5)(2002): 1337–45; *Transgenic Research* 9(2)(2000): 145–54; *Endocrinology* 143(6)(2002): 1277–83, 2277–83; *Recent Progress in Hormonal Research* 56(2001): 359–75; *Peptides* 21(10)(Oct. 2000): 1479–85; *Nutrition Reviews* 56(9)(1998): 271–74; *Journal of Neuroscience* 21(10)(2001): 3639–45.

4. *European Journal of Pharmacology* 440(2-3)(2002): 85–98.

5. *Nature* 385(6612)(1997): 165–68; *Pigment Cell Research* 15(1)(2002): 10–18; *Science* 278(5335)(1997): 135–38.

6. *European Journal of Pharmacology* 440(2-3)(2002): 85–98; *American Journal of Physiology* 272(Pt 1, 3)(1997): E379–84; *FASEB Journal* 13(1998): 1391–96.

7. Holick, M. *The UV Advantage* (I Books, 2004).

8. Nash, M. "Cracking the Fat Riddle." *Newsweek* (Sept. 2, 2002): 49–55.

9. Holick, M. Interview in "Soaking Up the D's." *Nutrition Action Healthletter* 30(10)(Dec. 2003): 1–6.

10. Zajonc, A. *Catching the Light* (New York: Bantam, 1993); Harvard research, *Peak Performance Journal* articles, etc.

Chapter 7

1. Hendler, S. S. *The Oxygen Breakthrough* (New York: Pocket Books, 1989).

2. Hendler. *The Oxygen Breakthrough.*

3. Grout, P. *Jumpstart Your Metabolism* (New York: Fireside, 1998).

4. Streeter, T. In "Breathless." *Men's Health* (Apr. 2003): 82.

5. *Peak Performance Journal* 171(Oct. 2002): 1–4.

6. Daniels, L., and Worthingham, C. *Therapeutic Exercise for Body Alignment and Function* (Philadelphia: W. B. Saunders, 1977): 58.

Chapter 8

1. Boschmann, M., et al. "Water-Induced Thermogenesis." *Journal of Clinical Endocrinology and Metabolism,* 88(12): 6015–19.

2. McArdle, W. D., Katch, F. I., and Katch, V. L. *Exercise Physiology: Energy, Nutrition, and Human Performance* (Philadelphia: Lea and Febiger, 1986): 451; Hanson, P. G. *The Joy of Stress* (Kansas City: Andrews, McMeel & Parker, 1987): 27.

3. Stone, K. *Snack Attack* (New York: Warner, 1991): 145.

4. *Medicine and Science in Sports and Exercise* 17(4)(1985): 456–61.

5. European studies. Highland Springs Research, Blackford, Perthshire, Scotland.

6. Goldman, B., and Hackman, R. M. *The "E" Factor* (New York: William Morrow, 1988).

7. McArdle, Katch, and Katch. *Exercise Physiology:* 451; Swarth, J. *Stress and Nutrition* (San Diego: Health Media of America, 1986): 23; Brooks, G. A., and Fahey, T. D. *Exercise Physiology: Human Bioenergetics and Its Applications* (New York: Macmillan, 1985): 462.

8. McArdle, Katch, and Katch. *Exercise Physiology:* 451.

9. Applegate, L. *Power Foods* (Emmaus, PA: Rodale, 1991): 2.

10. Callaway, W. C. *The Callaway Diet* (New York: Bantam, 1991): 191.

11. Batmanghelidj, F. *Your Body's Many Cries for Water*; nutrition and metabolism texts, etc.

12. Heus, M., Heus, G., and Heus, J. *Low-Fat for Life* (Barneveld, WI: Micamar Publishing, 1994): 87.

13. Darden, E. *A Day-by-Day 10-Step Program* (Dallas: Taylor Publishing, 1992): 41.

14. *Journal of Clinical Endocrinology and Metabolism* 88(2004): 6015–19.

15. Darden. *Day-by-Day:* 43.

16. Blackburn, G. L. Quoted in *Prevention* (Sept. 1992): 50.

17. Miller, W. C. *The Non-Diet Diet* (Englewood, CO: Morton Publishing, 1991): 83–84.

18. Mark, V. H. *Brain Power: A Neurosurgeon's Complete Program to Maintain and Enhance Brain Fitness Throughout Your Life* (Houghton Mifflin, 1989).

19. Willett, W. *Eat, Drink, and Be Healthy* (New York: Simon & Schuster, 2001).

20. Willett. *Eat, Drink, and Be Healthy.*

21. *Peak Performance Journal* 170 (Sept. 2002): 6–7.

22. UCLA School of Medicine studies by David Heber, MD, PhD. Reported in Heber, D. *The LA Shape Diet* (Regan Books, 2003).

23. Dulloo, A. G., et al. "Efficacy of a Green Tea Extract Rich in Catechin Polyphenols and Caffeine in Increasing 24-Hour Energy Expenditure and Fat Oxidation in Humans." *American Journal of Clinical Nutrition* 70(6)(1999): 1040–45; and Dulloo, A. G., et al. "Green Tea and Thermogenesis Interactions." *American Journal of Clinical Nutrition* 24(2000): 252–58.

24. Dulloo, et al. "Efficacy of a Green Tea Extract": 1040–50.

25. Moore-Ede, M. *The Twenty-Four-Hour Society* (Reading, MA: Addison-Wesley, 1993).

26. Fordyce-Baum, M. K., et al. "Use of an Expanded-Whole-Wheat Product in the Reduction of Body Weight and Serum Lipids in Obese Females." *American Journal of Clinical Nutrition* 50(1989): 30–36; Rossner, S. D., et al. "Weight Reduction with Dietary Fibre Supplements—Results of Two Double-Blind Randomized Studies." *Acta Medica Scandinavica* 222(1988): 83–88.

27. Miller. *The Non-Diet Diet:* 75–77.

28. Selby, J. V., et al. *American Journal of Epidemiology* 125(1987): 979–88; Fowman, D. T. *Annals of Clinical Laboratory Science* 18(1988): 181–89; Gerald, M. J., et al. *Diabetes* 26(1977): 780–85; *New England Journal of Medicine* 326(1992): 983–87; *Nutrition Reviews* 50(9)(1995): 267–70; *Obesity & Health* (Nov./Dec. 1993): 107–108; *Obesity & Health* (Sept./Oct. 1993): 87–89; Laws, A., Terry, R. B., and Barrett-Connor, E. "Behavioral Covariates of Waist-to-Hip Ratio in Rancho Bernardo." *American Journal of Public Health* 80(1990): 1358–62.

29. Barneys, M., et al. "Effect of Exercise and Protein Intake on Energy Expenditure." *Revista Española de Fisiologia* 4(4)(1993): 209–17.

Chapter 9

1. *Reuters Health* (May 21, 2003).

2. Colgan, M. *Perfect Posture* (Vancouver: Apple Publishing, 2002).

3. Bhatnager, V., et al. "Posture, Postural Discomfort, and Performance."

Human Factors 27(2)(Apr. 1985): 189–99; "Remedies for a Painful Case of Terminal-itis." *US News & World Report* (Jan. 9, 1989): 60–61; Cailliet and Gross. *Rejuvenation: 52–54;* Grandjean, E. *Fitting the Task to the Man.* 4th ed. (London: Taylor and Francis, 1991): 11; Migdow, J. A., and Loehr, J. E. *Take a Deep Breath* (New York: Villard, 1986): 97; Kraus, H. *Backache, Stress and Tension* (New York: Pocket Books, 1969): 40; Imrie, D., with Dimson, C. *Good Bye to Backache* (New York: Fawcett, 1983): 128–29; Astrand, P. O., and Rodahl, K. *Textbook of Work Physiology: Physiological Bases of Exercise* (New York: McGraw-Hill, 1986): 112; Hanna, T. *The Body of Life* (New York: Knopf, 1980).

4. "Don't Be Slack About Good Posture." *University of California, Berkeley Wellness Letter* (Oct. 1986): 6.

5. Cailliet and Gross. *Rejuvenation: 56.*

6. Heller, J. and Henkin, W. A. *Bodywise* (Los Angeles: Tarcher, 1986): 92; Cailliet and Gross. *Rejuvenation: 56.*

7. Barlow, W. Quoted in *Somatics* (Spring/Summer 1987): 11.

8. Cailliet, R., and Gross, L. *The Rejuvenation Factor* (New York: Doubleday, 1986).

9. Roach, M. "Do You Fit Into Your Office?" *Hippocrates/In Health* (Jul./Aug. 1989): 44.

10. See Cailliet, R. *The Rejuvenation Strategy.* (New York: Doubleday, 1987).

11. Bhatnager, et al. "Posture, Posture Discomfort, and Performance": 189–99.

12. Riskind, J. H., and Gotay, C. C. "Physical Posture: Could It Have Regulatory or Biofeedback Effects on Motivation and Emotion?" *Motivation and Emotion* 6(3)(1982): 273–98.

13. Riskind and Gotay. "Physical Posture"; Weisfeld, G. E., and Beresford, J. M. "Erectness of Posture as an Indicator of Dominance or Success in Humans." *Motivation and Emotion* 6(2)(1982): 113–31; Wilson, E., and Schneider, C. "Static and Dynamic Feedback in the Treatment of Chronic Muscle Pain." Paper presented at the Biofeedback Society of America meeting (New Orleans, Apr. 16, 1985); Winter, A., and Winter, R. *Build Your Brain Power* (New York: St. Martin's, 1986); *The Neuropsychology of Achievement* (Sybervision Systems, Inc., Fountain Square, 6066 Civic Terrace Ave., Newark, CA 94560; 1985).

14. Imrie. *Good Bye to Backache:* 128–29.

15. Cailliet and Gross. *Rejuvenation:* 62; Hanna, T. *Somatics* (Reading, MA: Addison-Wesley, 1988); Heller, J., and Heller and Henkin. *Bodywise.*

16. Calliet, R., and Gross, L. *The Rejuvenation Factor* (Garden City, NY: Doubleday, 1987): 3–5.

17. Warfel, J. H. *The Head, Neck, and Trunk.* 4th ed. (Philadelphia: Lea & Febiger, 1973): 46.

18. Cailliet and Gross. *Rejuvenation:* 64–65.

19. Barker, S. *The Alexander Technique* (New York: Bantam, 1978): 24.

20. Cailliet and Gross. *Rejuvenation:* 127.

21. Gould, N. "Back-Pocket Sciatica." *New England Journal of Medicine* 290 (1974): 633.

22. Lettvin, M. *Maggie's Back Book* (Boston: Houghton Mifflin, 1976): 131.

Chapter 10

1. Morgan, E. *The Scars of Evolution* (New York: Oxford University Press, 1990): 80–91. Also see, for example: Hauri, P., and Linde, S. *No More Sleepless Nights* (New York: Wylie, 1990); E. books, evolutionary biology refs, etc.

2. See, for example: Cordain, L. *The Paleo Diet* (New York: Wiley, 2002); and Jacobs, G. D. *The Ancestral Mind* (New York: Viking, 2003).

3. Nybo, L., et al. *Journal of Physiology* 545(Pt. 2)(2002): 697–704.

4. A study about this was cited in a Rodale book or *Prevention* within the past two years.

Chapter 11

1. See, for example: Cordain, L. *The Paleo Diet* (New York: Wiley, 2002); and Jacobs, G. D. *The Ancestral Mind* (New York: Viking, 2003).

2. Isaacs, S. *Hormonal Power: Understanding Hormones, Weight, and Your Metabolism.* (Boulder, CO: Bull Publishing Co., 2002).

3. Isaacs, 47–48.

4. Isaacs, 52.

5. Isaacs, 60.

6. Isaacs, 79.

7. Eriksson, J., et al. "Exercise and the Metabolic Syndrome." *Diabetologia* 40(1997): 125–35.

8. *Recent Progress in Hormonal Research* 56(2001): 359–75; *Peptides* 21(10)(Oct. 2000): 1479–85; *Nutrition Reviews* 56(9)(1998): 271–74.

9. *Diabetes Care* 22(3)(1999): 413–17.

10. *Life Sciences* 69(2001): 987–1003; *Journal of Lipid Research* 42(2001): 743–50.

11. Kleiner, S. *Power Eating.* 2nd ed. (Champaign, IL: Human Kinetics, 2001).

12. *International Journal of Obesity and Related Metabolic Disorders* 25(1)(2001): 106–14.

13. For one summary of these research findings, see: Stein, R. "Fat Cells Aren't Just Passive Blobs, Scientists Learn." *Washington Post* (Jul. 12, 2004).

14. *Journal of Neuroscience* 21(10)(2001): 3639–45; *Recent Progress in Hormonal Research* 56(2001): 359–75; *Peptides* 21(10)(Oct. 2000): 1479–85; *Nutrition Reviews* 56(9)(1998): 271–74.

15. *Diabetes* 51(5)(2002): 1337–45; *Transgenic Research* 9(2)(2000): 145–54; *Endocrinology* 143(6)(2002): 2277–83; *Recent Progress in Hormonal Research* 56(2001): 359–75; *Peptides* 21(10)(Oct. 2000): 1479–85; *Nutrition Reviews* 56(9)(1998): 271–74.

16. *Nature* 385(6612)(1997): 165–68; *Pigment Cell Research* 15(1)(2002): 10–18; *Science* 278(5335)(1997): 135–38.

17. Thorpy, M., Montefiore Medical Center. "Sleep More, Weigh Less." *Men's Health* (Apr. 2003): 36.

18. *Journal of Endocrinology and Metabolism* 75(1992): 157–62.

19. *Growth Hormone and IGF Research* 8(suppl B) 1998: 127–29.

20. *Medicine and Science in Sports and Exercise* 31(12)(1999): 1748–54.

21. *Peak Performance Journal* 191(Jan. 2004): 190–92.

22. *Metabolism* 48(9)(1999): 1152–56.

23. *Journal of Clinical Endocrinology and Metabolism* 76(6)(1993): 1418–23.

24. Ladenson, P. W., et al. *Archives of Internal Medicin* 160(2000): 1573–75; Tagliaferri, M., et al. "Subclinical Hypothyroidism in Obese Patients, Relation to Resting Energy Expenditure, Body Composition, and Lipid Profile." *Obesity Research* 9(2001): 196–201

25. Hendler, S. S. *Doctor's Vitamin and Mineral Encyclopedia* (New York: Simon & Schuster, 1990).

26. Leibowitz, S., and Kim, T. "Impact of Galanin Antagonist on Exogenous Galanin and Natural patterns of Fat Ingestion." *Brain Research* 599(1992): 148–52.

27. Leibowitz, S. F. Quoted in Marano, H. E. "Chemistry and Craving." *Psychology Today* (Jan./Feb. 1993): 30–36, 74.

28. Klein, S. "The War Against Obesity." *American Journal of Clinical Nutrition* 69(6)(1999): 1061–63; Moor, C. V., and Ha, E. Y. "Whey Protein Isolates." *Critical Reviews in Food Science and Nutrition.*

29. *Journal of Nutrition* 133(2003): 243S–67S.

30. Nash, M. "Cracking the Fat Riddle." *Newsweek* (Sept. 2, 2002): 49–55.

31. Zemel, M. In *Men's Health* (Aug. 2003): 46.

32. Richard, D. "The Role of Corticotropin-Releasing Hormone in the Regulation of Energy Balance." *Current Opinion in Endocrinology and Diabetes* 199(6)(2002): 10–18.

33. Isaacs, S. *Hormonal Power*: 228

Chapter 12

1. Thayer, R. E. *Calm Energy* (New York: Oxford University Press, 2001).

2. Thayer. *Calm Energy.*

3. For introductory reading, see: Rossi, E. L. *The 20 Minute Break* (New York: TarcherPutnam, 1991); and Lamberg, L. *Bodyrhythms: Chronobiology and Peak Performance* (New York: Morrow, 1998).

4. Rossi. *The 20 Minute Break:* 35–36.

5. See, for example: Moore-Ede, M. *The Twenty-Four-Hour Society* (Reading, MA: Addison-Wesley, 1993); and Lamberg. *Bodyrhythms.*

6. Dement, W. C. Foreword to Lamberg. *Bodyrhythms:* 8.

7. See, for example: Norfolk, D., *Executive Stress* (New York: Warner, 1986); Moore-Ede. *Twenty-Four-Hour Society*; and Grandjean, E. *Fitting the Task to the Man* (New York: Taylor and Francis, 4th ed., 1988).

8. Hendler, S. S. *The Oxygen Connection* (New York: Pocket Books, 1990): 7–8.

9. See, for example: Hendler. *The Oxygen Connection*; and Fried, et al.

10. Hendler. *The Oxygen Connection:* 8, 83.

11. Cailliet, R., and Gross, L. *The Rejuvenation Strategy* (New York: Doubleday, 1987): 52.

12. Cailliet and Gross. *The Rejuvenation Strategy:* 5.

13. See, for example: Grandjean. *Fitting the Task*; and Cailliet and Gross. *The Rejuvenation Strategy.*

14. Stellman and Henifin. *Office Work:* 28. Stellman, J. M. and Henifin, M. S. *Office Work Can Be Dangerous to Your Health.* Rev. ed. (New York: Ballantine-Fawcett, 1989) or 1st ed. (New York: Pantheon, 1984).

15. See, for example: Nezer, A. M., et al. "Sense of Humor as a Moderator of the Relation Between Stressful Events and Psychological Distress: A Prospective Analysis." *Journal of Personality and Social Psychology* 54(1988): 5220–25.

16. See, for example: Kelley, R. E. *How to Be a Star at Work* (New York: Times Books, 1998); and Loehr, J. E. *Stress for Success* (New York: Times Books, 1998).

17. Hyman, J. W. *The Light Book* (Los Angeles: Tarcher, 1990); Ackerman, D. *A Natural History of the Senses* (New York: Random House, 1990).

18. Zajonc, A. *Catching the Light* (New York: Bantam, 1993); Moore-Ede. *Twenty-Four-Hour Society:* 60.

19. Sobel, D., and Ornstein, R. *Healthy Pleasures* (Reading, MA: Addison-Wesley, 1989).

20. McIntyre, I., et al. *Life Sciences* 45(1990): 327–32; *Brain/Mind Bulletin* (Jan. 1990): 7.

21. *Journal of Clinical Endocrinology and Metabolism* 88(2004): 6015–19.

22. Heus, M., Heus, G., and Heus, J. *Low-Fat for Life* (Barneveld, WI: Micamar Publishing, 1994): 87.

23. McArdle, W. D., Katch, F. I., and Katch, V. L. *Exercise Physiology: Energy, Nutrition, and Human Performance* (Philadelphia: Lea and Febiger,

1986): 451; Hanson, P. G. *The Joy of Stress* (Kansas City: Andrews, McMeel & Parker, 1987): 27.

24. Grandjean. *Fitting the Task*.

25. Janaro, R. E., et al. "A Technical Note on Increasing Productivity Through Effective Rest Break Scheduling." *Industrial Management* 30(1)(Jan./Feb. 1988): 29–33; Penc, J. "Motivational Stimulation and System of Work Improvement." *Studia-Socjologiczne* 3(102)(1986): 179–97; Foegen, J. H. "Super-Breaktime." *Supervision* 49(Oct. 1988): 9–10; Bechtold, S. E., and Sumners, D. L. "Optimal Work-Rest Scheduling with Exponential Work-Rate Decay." *Management Science* 34(Apr. 1988): 547–52; Krueger, G. P. "Human Performance in Continuous/Sustained Operations and the Demands of Extended Work/Rest Schedules: An Annotated Bibliography." *Psychological Documents* 15(2)(Dec. 1985): 27–28; Boothe, R. S. "Optimization of Rest Breaks: A Productivity Enhancement." *Dissertation Abstracts International* 45(9-A)(Mar. 1985): 2927; Gustafson, H. W. "Efficiency of Output in Self-Paced Work, Machine-Paced Work." *Human Factors* 24(4)(Aug. 1982): 395–410; Janaro, R. E., and Bechtold, S. E. "A Study of the Reduction of Fatigue Impact on Productivity Through Optimal Rest Break Scheduling." *Human Factors* 27(4)(Aug. 1985): 459–66; Okogbaa, O. G. "An Empirical Model for Mental Work Output and Fatigue." *Dissertation Abstracts International* 15(2)(Dec. 1985): 27–28; Thatcher, R. E. *Journal of Personality and Social Psychology* 52(1987): 119–25; Zarakovski, G. M., et al. "Psychophysiological Analysis of Periodic Fluctuations in the Quality of Activity Within the Work Cycle." *Human Physiology* 8(3)(May 1983): 208–20; Bechtold, S. E., et al. "Maximization of Labor Productivity through Optimal Rest-Break Schedules." *Management Science* 30(12)(Dec. 1984): 1442–48.

26. Thayer, R. E. *The Biopsychology of Mood and Arousal* (New York: Oxford University Press, 1989); Globus, G. G., et al. "Ultradian Rhythms in Human Performance." *Perceptual and Motor Skills* 33(1971): 1171–74; Kleitman, N. *Sleep and Wakefulness*. Rev. ed. (Chicago: University of Chicago Press, 1963); Kripe, D. F. "An Ultradian Rhythm Associated with Perceptual Deprivation and REM Sleep." *Psychosomatic Medicine* 34(1972): 221–34; Lavie, P., and Scherson, A. "Evidence of Ultradian Rhythmicity in 'Sleep-Ability.'" *Electroencephalography and Clinical Neurophysiology* 52(1981): 163–74; Gertz, J., and Lavie, P. "Biological Rhythms in Arousal Indicies." *Psychophysiology* 20(1983): 690–95; Orr, W., et al. "Ultradian Rhythms in Extended Performance." *Aerospace Medicine* 45(1974): 995–1000.

27. Rossi. *The 20 Minute Break*: 103.

28. Chafetz, M. *Smart for Life* (New York: Penguin, 1993).

29. Bailey, C. *Smart Exercise* (Boston: Houghton Mifflin, 1994): 28.

30. Moore-Ede. *Twenty-Four-Hour Society*: 55–56.

31. Dienstbier, R., et al. "Catecholamine Training Effects from Exercise: A Bridge to Exercise-Temperament Relationships." *Motivation and Emotion* 2(1987): 297–318.

32. Lamb, L. E. *The Weighting Game: The Truth About Weight Control* (New York: Lyle Stuart, 1988): 95–96.

33. Leveille, T. "Adipose Tissue Metabolism: Influence of Eating and Diet Composition." *Federation Proceedings* 29(1970): 1294–1301; Lukert, B. "Biology of Obesity." In Wolman, B., ed. *Psychological Aspects of Obesity: A Handbook* (New York: Van Nostrand Reinhold, 1982): 1–14; Szepsi, B. "A Model of Nutritionally Induced Overweight: Weight 'Rebound' Following Caloric Restriction." In Bray, G., ed. *Recent Advances in Obesity Research* (London: Newman, Ltd., 1978).

34. Jenkins, D. A., et al. "Nibbling Versus Gorging: Metabolic Advantages of Increased Meal Frequency." *New England Journal of Medicine* 321(4)(Oct. 5, 1989): 929–34.

35. Jones, P. J., Leitch, C. A., and Pederson, R. A. "Meal-Frequency Effects on Plasma Hormone Concentrations and Cholesterol Synthesis in Humans." *American Journal of Clinical Nutrition* 57(6)(1993): 868–74; Edelstein, S. L., et al. "Increased Meal Frequency Associated with Decreased Cholesterol Concentrations." *American Journal of Clinical Nutrition* 55(1992): 664–69.

36. Miller, W. C. *The Non-Diet Diet* (Englewood, CO: Morton Publishing, 1991): 88.

37. Leibowitz, S. F. Quoted in Marano, H. E. "Chemistry and Craving." *Psychology Today* (Jan./Feb. 1993): 30–36, 74.

38. Travell, J. G., and Simons, D. G. *Myofascial Pain and Dysfunction: The Trigger Point Manual* (Baltimore: Williams and Wilkins, Vol. I: 1983; Vol. II: 1992): 5.

39. Sola, A. E., et al. "Incidence of Hypersensitive Areas in Posterior Shoulder Muscles." *American Journal of Physical Medicine* 34(1955): 585–90.

40. Kraft, G. H., et al. "The Fibrositis Syndrome." *Archives of Physical Medicine and Rehabilitation* 49 (1968): 155–62.

41. Travell and Simons. *Myofascial Pain and Dysfunction*: 13.

42. Travell and Simons. *Myofascial Pain and Dysfunction*: 31.

43. The standard medical text in this field is *Myofascial Pain and Dysfunction: The Trigger Point Manual* by Janet G. Travell, MD, and David G. Simons, MD. These highly technical manuals, complete with several thousand scientific and medical references, are the result of decades of research by the authors, and are strongly endorsed by the author of the foreword to the first volume, René Cailliet, MD, professor and former chairman of the department of physical medicine and rehabilitation at the University of Southern California School of Medicine.

Some of the most recent studies on myofascial pain and dysfunction include: Simons, D. G. "Myofascial Pain Syndromes." *Archives of Physical Medicine and Rehabilitation* 65(9)(Sept. 1984): 561; Simons. D. G. "Myofascial Pain Syndromes: Where Are We? Where Are We Going?" *Archives of Physical Medicine and Rehabilitation* 69(3 Pt. 1)(Mar. 1988): 207–12; Simons, D. G. "Familial Fibromyalgia and/or Myofascial Pain Syndrome?" *Archives of Physical Medicine and Rehabilitation* 71(3)(Mar. 1990): 258–59; Simons, D. G. "Trigger Point Origin of Musculoskeletal Chest Pain." *Southern Medical Journal* 83(2)(Feb. 1990): 262–63; Smythe, H. "Referred Pain and Tender Points." *American Journal of Medicine* 81(3A)(Sept. 29, 1986): 7–14; Fisher, A. A. "Documentation of Myofascial Trigger Points." *Archives of Physical Medicine and Rehabilitation* 69(4)(Apr. 1988): 286–91; Mennell, J. "Myofascial Trigger Points as a Cause of Headaches." *Journal of Manipulative and Physiological Therapeutics* 11(2)(Apr. 1989): 63–64; Friction, J. R. "Myofascial Pain Syndrome." *Neurological Clinics* 7(2)(May 1989): 413–27; Campbell, S. M. "Regional Myofascial Pain Syndromes." *Rheumatic Diseases Clinics of North America* 15(10)(Feb. 1989): 31–44.

44. Referred to as *ischemic compression* in Travell and Simons. *Myofascial Pain and Dysfunction*: 87.

45. Travell and Simons. *Myofascial Pain and Dysfunction*: 18.

Chapter 13

1. Williams, R. Quoted in "Natural Weight Control." *Prevention* (Jul. 1994): 134.

2. *Obesity Research* 1(3)(1993): 206–22.

3. Berg, F. S. "Risks Focus on Visceral Obesity, May Be Stress Linked." *Obesity & Health* 7(5)(Sep./Oct. 1993): 87–89.

4. Rebuffe-Scrive, M. Quoted in *Prevention* (Jul. 1994): 136.

5. *International Journal of Obesity* 17(1993): 597–604.

6. Berg. "Risks Focus on Visceral Obesity": 87–89.

7. See for example: Hendler. *The Oxygen Breakthrough*; Nathan, Staats, and Rosch. *The Doctors' Guide to Instant Stress Relief*; and Fried, R. *The Breath Connection* (New York: Plenum, 1991).

8. Ghinassi, F. "Coping With Stress and Eating." *The Weight Control Digest* 4(2)(Mar./Apr. 1994): 335–38.

9. Rookus, M. A., et al. "Changes in Body Mass Index in Young Adults in Relation to Number of Life Events Experienced." *International Journal of Obesity* 12(1988): 29–39.

10. Sternberg, B. "Relapse in Weight Control: Definitions, Processes, and Prevention Strategies." In Marlatt, G. A., and Gordon, J. R., eds. *Relapse Prevention: Maintenance Strategies in the Treatment of Addictive Behaviors* (New York: Guilford Press, 1985): 521–45.

11. Linde, B., et al. *American Journal of Physiology* 256(1989): E12–E18.

12. Elias, M. "Hostility, Anxiety May Hold Key to Heart Attack." *USA Today* (Apr. 15, 1994).

13. Stoney, C. American Psychosomatic Society Meeting. Quoted in Elias, M. "Hostility, Anxiety."

14. Nathan, R. G., Staats, T. E., and Rosch, P. J. *The Doctors' Guide to Instant Stress Relief* (New York: Ballantine, 1989): xxiii and 4.

15. Bartlett, S. J. "Exercise, Stress Reduction and Overweight." *Weight Control Digest* 4(3)(May/June 1994): 353–55.

16. Daniel, M. "Opiate Receptor Blockade by Naltrexone and Mood State After Physical Activity." *British Journal of Sports Medicine* 26(1992): 111; Raglin, J. "Exercise and Mental Health." *Sports Medicine* 9(1990): 323.

17. King, A. C., Taylor, C. B., Haskell, W. L. "Effects of Differing Intensities and Formats of 12 Months of Exercise Training on Psychological Outcomes in Older Adults." *Health Psychology* 12(1993): 292–300.

18. Dienstbier, R. "Arousal and Physiological Toughness: Implications for Mental and Physical Health." *Psychological Bulletin* 96(10)(1989): 84–100; "The Toughness Response." *Advances* 7(1)(1990): 6–7.

19. Thayer, R. E. *Calm Energy* (New York: Oxford University Press, 2001). Based on extensive research and more than 100 scientific studies.

20. Seligman, M. E. P. *What You Can Change and What You Can't* (New York: Ballantine, 1995); Amen, D. *Change Your Brain, Change Your Life* (New York: Three Rivers Press, 1999).

21. Ljungdahl, L. "Laugh If This Is a Joke." *New England Journal of Medicine* 261(1989): 558; Dillon, K. M., et al. "Positive Emotional States and Enhancement of the Immune System." *International Journal of Psychiatry in Medicine* 15(1)(1985–1986): 13–18; Eckman, P., et al. "Autonomic Nervous System Activity Distinguishes Among Emotions." *Science* 221(1983): 1208–10; Berk, A. L. S., et al. *Clinical Research* 36(1988): 121 and 435A; Berk, A. L. S., et al. *FASEB Journal* 2(1988): A1570.

22. Grilo, C. M., and Schiffman, S. "Longitudinal Investigation of the Abstinence Violation Effect in Binge Eaters." *Journal of Consulting and Clinical Psychology* 62(1994): 611–19. Grilo, C. M., Wilfley, D. E., Jones, A., et al. "The Social Self, Body Dissatisfaction, and Binge Eating in Obese Females." *Obesity Research* 2(1994): 24–27.

23. Lefcourt, H. M., and Martin, R. A. *Humor and Life Stress* (New York: Springer-Verlag, 1986); Nezu, A. M., et al. "Sense of Humor as a Moderator of the Relation Between Stressful Events and Psychological Distress: A Prospective Analysis." *Journal of Personality and Social Psychology* 54(1988): 520–25.

24. Williams, R., and Williams, V. *Anger Kills* (New York: Times Books, 1993); Eliot, R. S. *From Stress to Strength* (New York: Bantam, 1994); Eliot,

R. S., and Breo, D. *Is It Worth Dying For?* (New York: Bantam, 1989); Tavris, C. *Anger: The Misunderstood Emotion* (New York: Simon and Schuster, 1982).

25. Watsom, M., Greer, S., Rowden, L., Gorman, C., et al. *Psychological Medicine* 21(1991): 51–57; Seligman, M. E. P. *Learned Optimism* (New York: Knopf, 1991): 167–78.

26. Eliot, R. S. *From Stress to Strength* (New York: Bantam, 1994).

27. Lazarus, R. S. *American Psychologist*, 30(1975): 553–61; DeLongis, A., et al. "Relationship of Daily Hassles, Uplifts, and Major Life Events to Health Status." *Health Psychology* 1(1982): 119–36; Kanner, A. D., et al. "Comparison of Two Modes of Stress Measurement: Daily Hassles and Uplifts Versus Major Life Events." *Journal of Behavioral Medicine* 4(1981): 1–39.

28. Zillman, D. "Mental Control of Angry Aggression." In Wegner, D., and Pennebaker, J. S., eds. *Handbook for Mental Control* (New York: Prentice Hall, 1993).

29. Hendler, S. S. *The Oxygen Breakthrough* (New York: Simon and Schuster, 1989).

30. "Breathing Linked to Personality." *Psychology Today* (Jul. 1983): 109; Teich, M., and Dodeles, G. "Mind Control: How to Get It, How to Use It, How to Keep It." *Omni* (Oct. 1987): 53–60.

31. Ekman, P., Levenson, R. W., and Friesen, W. V. "Autonomic Nervous System Activity Distinguishes Among Emotions." *Science* (Sep. 16, 1983): 1208–10; Greden, J., et al. *Archives of General Psychiatry* 43(1987): 269–74; Teich and Dodeles, "Mind Control"; Zajonc, R. B. "Emotion and Facial Efference: A Theory Reclaimed." *Science* 228 (4695) (Apr. 5, 1985): 15–21.

32. Riskind, J. H., and Gotay, C. C. "Physical Posture: Could It Have Regulatory or Biofeedback Effects on Motivation and Emotion?" *Motivation and Emotion* 6(3)(1982): 273–98.

33. See, for example: Nadler, G., and Hibino, S. *Breakthrough Thinking* (Rocklin, CA: Prima Publishing, 1990); and Nadler, G., and Hibino, S., with Farrell, J. *Creative Solution Finding* (Rocklin, CA: Prima Publishing, 1995).

34. Winter, A., and Winter, R. *Build Your Brain Power* (New York: St. Martin's, 1986): 70.

35. Kannel, W. B. Quoted in Maleskey, G. "What It Means When You're Short of Breath." *Prevention* (Dec. 1985): 75.

36. Nathan, Staats, and Rosch. *The Doctors' Guide to Instant Stress Relief*: 50.

37. Funk, E. "Avoiding Altitude Sickness." *Summit County Journal* (Breckenridge, CO: Jan. 12, 1978): 7.

38. Hendler. *The Oxygen Breakthrough*.

39. Nathan, Staats, and Rosch. *The Doctors' Guide to Instant Stress Relief*: 56–58.

40. Ghinassi. "Coping with Stress and Eating": 335–38.

41. Kubey, R., and Csikszentmihalyi, M. *Television and the Quality of Life: How Viewing Shapes Everyday Experience* (Hillsdale, NJ: Erlbaum, 1990); Kubey, R., and Csikszentmihalyi, M. "Watching TV Makes People Feel Worse, 13-Year Study Finds." *New Brunswick, NJ Morning Call* (May 1, 1990): A-3.

42. "Television Trance Slows Metabolism." *Environmental Nutrition* 15(6)(Jun. 1992): 1; Report to the Society of Behavioral Medicine by Robert C. Klesges, PhD, Memphis State University.

43. Foreyt, J. Quoted in "Natural Weight Loss." *Prevention* (Jan. 1994): 117.

44. King, G. A., Polivy, J., and Herman, P. C. "Cognitive Aspects of Dietary Restraint: Effects on Person Memory." *International Journal of Eating Disorders* 10(3)(May 1991): 313–21.

Chapter 14

1. Rossi, L. *The 20 Minute Break* (Los Angeles: Tarcher, 1992).

2. Moore-Ede, M. *The Twenty-Four-Hour Society* (Reading, MA: Addison-Wesley, 1993); Wyman, J. W. *The Light Book* (Los Angeles: Tarcher, 1990).

3. Miller, E. E. *Software for the Mind* (Berkeley: Celestial Arts, 1988); Sheikh, A. A., ed. *Imagery: Current Theory, Research, and Application* (New York: Wiley Interscience, 1984); Marks, D. F., ed. *Theories of Image Formation* (New York: Brandon House, 1986); Suinn, R. M. *Seven Steps to Peak Performance* (Lewiston, NY: Hans Huber Publishers, 1986).

4. Kaplan, R. "The Role of Nature in the Context of the Workplace." *Landscape and Urban Planning* 26(1993): 193–201; *Mental Medicine Update* 2(2)(Fall, 1993).

5. Mackoff, B. *The Art of Self-Renewal* (Los Angeles: Tarcher, 1992).

6. Imber-Black, E., and Roberts, J. *Rituals for Our Time* (New York: HarperCollins, 1992); O'Neil, J. R. *The Paradox of Success* (New York: Tarcher/Putnam, 1993).

7. deBono, E. *Serious Creativity* (New York: HarperCollins, 1993).

8. Ziv, A., and Gadish, O. "Humor and Marital Satisfaction." *Journal of Social Psychology* 129(1990): 759–68.

9. Wurtman, J. J. *Managing Your Mind and Mood Through Food* (New York: HarperCollins, 1987); Chafetz, M. *Smart for Life* (New York: Penguin, 1993); Lamberg, L. *Bodyrhythms: Chronobiology and Peak Performance* (New York: Morrow, 1994).

10. Nagler, W. *The Dirty Half Dozen* (New York: Warner, 1991): 47–48.

11. Liebman, B. "The Last Supper?" *Nutrition Action Health Letter* 21(4)(May, 1994): 6–7; American Heart Association's 20th Science Forum. January 17–20, 1993. Report in *Environmental Nutrition* 16(3) (Mar. 1993): 1.

12. Kenney, J. Quoted in "Natural Weight Control." *Prevention* (Jul. 1994): 133.

13. "Better to Eat Ze Main Meal Earlier?" *Tufts University Diet & Nutrition Letter* 11(4)(Jun. 1993): 1.

14. University of Minnesota study. Proceedings of the Tenth International Congress on Nutrition.

15. Lipetz, P. *The Good Calorie Diet*. (New York: HarperCollins, 1994): 66. Wolever, T. M. S., et al. *American Journal of Clinical Nutrition* 48(1988): 1041–47.

16. Clouatre, D. *The Complete Guide to Anti-Fat Nutrients* (San Francisco: Pax Publishing, 1993): 106.

17. Smith, A. F. Cited in DeAngelis, T. "On a Diet? Don't Trust Your Memory." *Psychology Today* (Oct. 1989): 12.

18. Brownell, K. D. *The LEARN Program for Weight Control* (Dallas: The Learn Education Center, 1991): 15.

19. Streit, K. J., et al. "Food Records: A Predictor and Modifier of Weight Change in a Long-Term Weight Loss Program." *Journal of the American Dietetic Association* 91(1991): 213–16.

20. Wurtman. *Managing Your Mind and Mood Through Food*; Chafetz, M. *Smart for Life* (New York: Penguin, 1993); Lamberg. *Bodyrhythms*.

21. Wolfe, J. *What to Do When He Has a Headache* (New York: Warner, 1992).

22. *British Journal of Nutrition* 91(2004): 991–95.

23. Lejuene, M. P., et al. "Effect of Capsicum on Substrate Oxidation and Weight Maintenance in Human Subjects." *British Journal of Nutrition* 90(3)(2003): 651–59.

24. Simonson, M. Quoted in *Prevention's 1992 Weight Loss Guide* (Emmaus, PA: Rodale Books, 1992): 133.

25. *Tufts University Diet and Nutrition Letter* 9(4)(Jun. 1991): 1–2.

26. Ferber, C., and Cabanac, M. "Influence of Noise on Gustatory Affective Ratings and Preference for Sweet or Salt." *Appetite* 8(1987): 229–35; McCarron, A., and Tierney, K. J. "The Effect of Auditory Stimulation on the Consumption of Soft Drinks." *Appetite* 13(1989): 155–59; Roballey, T. C., et al. "The Effect of Music on Eating Behavior." *Bulletin of the Psychonomic Society* 23(1985): 221–22.

27. Brandon, J. E. *Health Values* (May/June 1987); "What Is a Slender Eating Style?" *Obesity & Health* 3(2)(Feb. 1989): 4.

28. *Prevention's 1992 Weight Loss Guide* (Emmaus, PA: Rodale Books, 1992): 133.

29. Spiegel, T. A., Wadden, T. A., and Foster, G. D. "Objective Measurement of Eating Rate During Behavioral Treatment of Obesity." *Behavior Therapy* 22(1991): 61–67.

30. Rolls, B. J., Fedoroff, I. C., Guthrie, J. F., and Laster, L. J. "Foods with Different Satiating Effects in Humans." *Appetite* 15(1990): 115–20.

31. Davis, J. M., et al. "Weight Control and Calorie Expenditure: Thermogenic Effects of Pre-Prandial and Post-Prandial Exercise." *Addictive Behaviors* 14(1989): 347–51; Gleeson, M. "Effects of Physical Exercise on Metabolic Rate and Dietary-Induced Thermogenesis." *British Journal of Nutrition* 47(1982); Bielinski, et al. "Energy Metabolism during the Postexercise Recovery in Man." *American Journal of Clinical Nutrition* 42(1985); Darden. *A Day-by-Day 10-Step Program* (Dallas: Taylor Publishing, 1992): 75; Clouatre. *The Complete Guide to Anti-Fat Nutrients:* 107.

32. Stamford, B. Quoted in "Natural Weight Control." *Prevention* (Apr. 1993): 67.

33. Davis, et al. "Weight Control": 347–51.

34. Roffers, M. "Nutrition Myths." *Medical Self-Care* (Mar./Apr. 1986): 52.

35. Stamford, B. "What Time Should You Exercise?" *The Physician and Sportsmedicine* 14(8)(Aug. 1986): 162.

36. Stamford. "Meals and the Timing of Exercise"; Roffers. "Nutrition Myths."

37. Duncan, J., Cooper Institute for Aerobics Research in Dallas. Study cited in *Prevention* July 1994; Blair, S. N., Kohl, H. W., and Gordon, N. F. "Physical Activity and Health: A Lifestyle Approach." *Medicine, Exercise, Nutrition, and Health* 1(1)(1992): 54–57; Blair, S. N., Kohl, H. W., and Barlow, C. E. "Physical Activity, Physical Fitness, and All-Cause Mortality in Women: Do Women Need to Be Active?" *Journal of the American College of Nutrition* 12(4)(1993): 368–71; Pate, R. R., et al. "Physical Activity and Public Health." *Journal of the American Medical Association* 273(5)(1995): 402–407.

38. "Natural Weight Control." *Prevention* (Apr. 1993): 67.

39. *European Journal of Applied Physiology* 86(2002): 411–17.

40. *Prevention's Weight Loss Guide 1993* (Emmaus, PA: Rodale Books, 1993): 166.

41. Hauri, P., and Linde, S. *No More Sleepless Nights* (New York: Wylie, 1992).

42. Hagerman, F. C. Quoted in "Natural Weight Loss." *Prevention* (Mar. 1994): 70.

Chapter 15

1. Von Kries, R., et al. "Reduced Risk for Overweight and Obesity." *International Journal of Obesity* 24(12)(2002): 710–16.

2. Zhang, K., et al. "Sleeping Metabolic Rate in Relation to Body Mass Index and Body Composition." *International Journal of Obesity* 26(3)(2002): 376–83; Edlund, M. *The Body Clock Advantage* (Avon, MA: Adams, 2003);

Mass, J. B., *Power Sleep* (New York: Villard, 1998); Jackson, F. R., et al. "Oscillating Molecules and Circadian Clock Output Mechanisms." *Molecular Psychiatry* 3(5)(1998): 381–85; Vioque, J., et al. "Time Spent Watching Television, Sleep Duration, and Obesity." *International journal of Obesity* 24(12)(2000): 1683–88.

3. Van Cauter, E. In Edlund, M. *The Body Clock Advantage.*

4. Department of Nutrition and Dietetics at King's College, University of London. Study cited in Bricklin, M. "Train Your Body to Trim Your Tummy." *Prevention* (May 1994): 51.

5. National Sleep Foundation poll, 2002.

6. University of Chicago research cited in Weintraub, A. "I Can't Sleep." *Business Week* (Jan. 26, 2004).

7. Barnard, N. *Food for Life* (New York: Harmony Books, 1993): 114.

8. "Overeating? Get Some Sleep." *Tufts University Diet & Nutrition Letter* 12(9)(Nov. 1994): 1–2.

9. Rechtschaffen, A. Quoted in "Overeating? Get Some Sleep."

10. "Why You Need Your Zs." *Men's Fitness* (Sept. 2003): 53.

11. "Sleep Loss Boosts Appetite, Weight Gain." University of Chicago Medical Center. *Annals of Internal Medicine* Dec. 7, 2004.

12. Sleep 27(2004): 661–66.

13. *Archives of Internal Medicine* 165(2005): 25–30; paper presented at North American Association for the Study of Obesity, Nov. 2004.

14. "Overeating? Get Some Sleep." *Tufts University Diet & Nutrition Letter.*

15. *USA Today* (Feb. 9, 2004): 1D.

16. Darden, E. *A Day-by-Day 10-Step Program* (Dallas: Taylor Publishing, 1992): 77.

17. To learn more about deep, healthy sleep, see:

• *Easing Into Sleep,* an audiocassette program by Dr. Emmett E. Miller (Source, P.O. Box W, Stanford, CA 94309; 415-328-7171). Features two excellent listening options: "Put the Day to Rest" and "Escape from Insomnia."

• *No More Sleepless Nights* by Peter Hauri, PhD, and Shirley Linde, PhD (New York: Wiley, 1990). An informative book by the director of the Mayo Clinic Insomnia Program and codirector of the Sleep Disorders Center at the Mayo Clinic.

• For medical information on sleep treatments and the addresses and telephone numbers of accredited sleep disorders centers, contact: American Sleep Disorders Association, 604 2nd Street SW, Rochester, MN 55902. Telephone: 507-287-6006.

18. Shapiro, C. M., et al. "Fitness Facilitates Sleep." *European Journal of Applied Physiology* 53(1984): 1–4; Baekland, F., Downstate Medical Center, NY, 1966 study; and Shapiro, C., and Zloty, R. B., University of Manitoba

studies; both reported in Mirkin, G., *Dr. Gabe Mirkin's Fitness Clinic* (Chicago: Contemporary Books, 1986).

19. Sewitch, D. "Slow Wave Sleep Deficiency Insomnia: A Problem in Thermo-Down Regulation at Sleep Onset." *Psychophysiology* 24(1987): 200–15; Perl, J. *Sleep Right in Five Nights* (New York: Morrow, 1993): 232–33.

20. *Sleep* 22(1999): 891–98.

21. Hauri and Linde. *No More Sleepless Nights* (New York: Wiley, 1990): 130–31.

22. Horne, J. A., et al. *Sleep* 10(1987): 383–92; Willensky, D. "Hints for Sound Sleep." *American Health* (May 1992): 50.

23. Perl, J. *Sleep Right in Five Nights* (Reading, MA: Addison-Wesley, 1993): 213.

24. Darden. *Day-by-Day*: 81–82.

25. *Nature* 401(1999): 36–37.

26. Karklin, A., Driver, H. S., and Buffenstein, R. "Restricted Energy Intake Affects Nocturnal Body Temperature and Sleep Patterns." *American Journal of Clinical Nutrition* 59(1994): 346–49.

27. Edelberg, D. *The Healing Power of Vitamins, Minerals, and Herbs* (Readers Digest, 1999).

28. Mohr, C. *Men's Health* (Mar. 2004): 107.

29. *Journal of Nutrition* 133(2003): 2525–65; 2495–2515; 2455–85; 2575–2605; 2685–2705.

30. Lamberg, L. "The Boy Who Ate His Bed . . . And Other Mysteries of Sleep." *American Health* (Nov. 1990): 56.

31. Perl. *Sleep Right in Five Nights*: 205.

32. Broughton, R. "Performance and Evoked Potential Measures of Various States of Daytime Sleepiness." *Sleep* 5(Suppl. 2)(1982); Dotto, L. *Asleep in the Fast Lane* (Toronto: Stoddart Pub., 1990): 138; Hauri, P. "Behavioral Treatment of Insomnia." *Medical Times* 107(6)(1986); Regestein, Q. R. "Practical Ways to Manage Insomnia." *Medical Times* 107(6)(1986): 19–23.

33. Hauri. "Behavioral Treatment of Insomnia": 36–47; Regestein. "Practical Ways to Manage Insomnia": 19–23.

34. Perl. *Sleep Right in Five Nights*: 195, 209.

Chapter 16

1. "Go Hard." Study reported in *Men's Health* (Aug. 2003): 118.

Chapter 17

1. Kirschenbaum, D. S. *The 9 Truths About Weight Loss* (New York: Henry Holt, 2000).

2. Bailey, C. *Fit or Fat* (Boston: Houghton Mifflin, 1976).

3. Stamford, B. A., and Shimer, P. *Fitness without Exercise* (New York: Warner, 1991): 71.

4. Evans, W. Quoted in "Bodybuilding for the Ninetics." *Nutrition Action Health Letter* (June 1992): 1–7.

5. *European Journal of Applied Physiology* 86(2002): 411–17.

6. *Medicine and Science in Sports and Exercise* 34(2002): 1793–1800.

7. Wilmore, J. In "Ask the Expert." *The Weight Control Digest* 1(5)(Jul./Aug.1991); Westcott, W. L. "Exercise Sessions Can Make the Difference in Weight Loss." *Perspective* 13(1987): 42–44; Westcott, W. *Strength Fitness* (Dubuque, IA: Wm C. Brown Co., 3rd edition, 1991): 3, 74–75; Westcott, W. L. "Strength Training: How Much Is Enough?" *IDEA Today* (Feb. 1991): 33–35; Westcott, W. L. "The Magic of 'Fast Fitness': They Enjoy It More and Do It Less." *Perspective: The Journal of Professional Directors of YMCAs* (January 1992):14–16; Wilmore, J. H. "Alterations to Strength, Body Composition and Anthropometric Measurements Consequent to 10-Week Weight Training Program." *Medicine and Science in Sports and Exercise* 6(1974): 133–38; Westcott, W. L., Toomey, K., and Doherty, A. "Strength Training, Body Composition, and Spot Reducing." (1992).

8. Evans, W. Cited in "Fat to Firm at 40-Plus." *Prevention* (Aug. 1994): 59–63, 136.

9. Evans. Quoted in "Bodybuilding for the Nineties": 5.

10. Fiatarone, A., et. al. "High-Intensity Strength Training in Nonagenarians: Effect on Skeletal Muscle." *Journal of the American Medical Association* 263(1990): 3029–34; see also: Evans and Rosenberg. *Biomarkers.*

11. Westcott. "Exercise Sessions"; Westcott. *Strength Fitness.*

12. Westcott. "Strength Training: How Much Is Enough?": 33–35; Westcott. "The Magic of 'Fast Fitness'."

13. Lamb, L. E. *Weighting Game: The Truth About Weight Control* (New York: Lyle Stuart, 1988): 147–48.

14. Drinkwater, B. Quoted in Hogan, C. "Strength." *American Health* (Nov. 1988): 55–59.

15. Boyden, T. W., et al. "Resistance Exercise Training Is Associated with Decreases in Serum Low-Density Lipoprotein Cholesterol Levels in Premenopausal Women." *Archives of Internal Medicine* 153(1)(Jan. 11, 1993): 97–100.

16. *European Journal of Applied Physiology* 86(2002): 411–17.

17. *Medicine and Science in Sports and Exercise:* June 2002; *Food and Fitness Advisor.* (Cornell Medical School) (Sept. 2002): 2.

18. *Archives of Internal Medicine* 164(2003): 31–39.

19. Rothenberg, B., and Rothenberg, O. *Touch Training for Strength* (Champaign, IL: Human Kinetics, 1995).

Chapter 18

1. Cailliet, R. *Understand Your Backache* (Philadelphia: F. A. Davis, 1984): 118–21; Mensendieck, E. M. *Look Better, Feel Better* (New York: Harper and Row, 1954): 48.

2. Loehr, J. *Stress for Success* (New York: Crown Business, 2000).

3. Katzmarzyk, P., et al. *Journal of Medicine and Science in Sports and Exercise* (May 2002).

4. Katch, F. I., et al. "Effects of Sit Up Exercise Training on Adipose Tissue Cell Size and Activity." *Research Quarterly for Exercise and Sport* 55(1984): 242–47; Clark, N. "Sit-Ups Don't Melt Ab Flab." *Runner's World* (Mar. 1985): 32.

5. Sharkey, B. J. *Physiology of Exercise* (Champaign, IL: Human Kinetics, 1984): 336; Cailliet. *Understand Your Backache:* 122–24; and Cailliet, R., and Gross, L. *The Rejuvenation Strategy* (Garden City, NY: Doubleday, 1987).

6. Westcott, W. L. Quoted in *Shrink Your Stomach in Nothing Flat* (Emmaus, PA: Rodale Press, 1994): 15.

7. Darden, E. *Living Longer Stronger* (New York: Perigee/Putnam, 1995): 54.

8. *Journal of Strength and Conditioning Research* 15(4): 480–85.

9. Daniels, L., and Worthingham, C. *Therapeutic Exercise for Body Alignment and Function* (Philadelphia: W.B. Saunders, 1977): 77; Yessis, M. "Kinesiology." *Muscle & Fitness* (Feb. 1985): 18–19, 142.

10. Lamb, L. E. *The Weighting Game: The Truth About Weight Control* (New York: Lyle Stuart, 1988): 201.

11. "What's the Best Ab Exercise Ever?" *Men's Health* (Nov. 2003): 126.

12. Lagerwerff, E. B., and Perlroth, K. A. *Mensendieck Your Posture and Your Pains* (New York: Anchor/Doubleday, 1973): 148–50; Yessis, M. "Back in Shape." *Sports Fitness* (Jun. 1986): 46, 76; Yessis, M. "The Midsection: Your Essential Link." *Sports Fitness* (Apr. 1985): 91–93; Daniels and Worthingham. *Therapeutic Exercise:* 59.

13. Cailliet. *Understand Your Backache:* 116.

Chapter 19

1. Evans, W., and Rosenberg, I. H. *Biomarkers: The 10 Determinants of Aging You Can Control.* (New York: Simon & Schuster, 1991): 119.

2. Fiatarone, M. Quoted in *Prevention* (Feb. 1992): 55.

3. *Medicine and Science in Sports and Exercise* 33(2001): 196–200.

Chapter 20

1. Cailliet, R. *Understand Your Backache* (Philadelphia: F. A. Davis, 1984); Cailliet, R. *The Rejuvenation Strategy* (New York: Doubleday, 1987); White, A. A. III. *Your Aching Back* (New York: Bantam, 1984); Imrie, D., and

Barbuto, L. *The Back Power Program* (New York: Wiley, 1990); Swezey, R. L., and Swezey, A. M. *Good News for Bad Backs* (New York: Knightsbridge, 1990).

Chapter 21

1. Studies by Callaway, W. Cited in Rodin, J. *Body Traps* (New York: Morrow, 1992): 193.

2. Harper, P. Quoted in "Burn Fat Faster." *Men's Health* (Nov. 1994): 26.

3. *International Journal of Obesity* 28(2004): 653–60.

4. *International Journal of Obesity* 58(7) (2004): 1071–77.

5. Moore-Ede, M. *The Twenty-Four-Hour Society* (Reading, MA: Addison-Wesley, 1993): 55–56; Blair, S. N. *Living with Exercise* (Dallas: American Health Publishing, 1991); Stamford, B., and Porter, S. *Fitness without Exercise* (New York: Warner, 1991).

6. Lamb, L. E. *The Weighting Game: The Truth About Weight Control* (New York: Lyle Stuart, 1988): 56.

7. Lamb. *The Weighting Game:* 95–96.

8. Leibowitz, S. F. Quoted in Marano, H. E. "Chemistry and Craving." *Psychology Today* (Jan./Feb. 1993): 30–36, 74.

9. Jenkins, D. A., et al. "Nibbling versus Gorging: Metabolic Advantages of Increased Meal Frequency." *New England Journal of Medicine* 321(14)(1989): 929–34.

10. Leveille, T. "Adipose Tissue Metabolism: Influence of Eating and Diet Composition." *Federation Proceedings* 29(1970): 1294–1301; Lukert, B. "Biology of Obesity." In Wolman, B., ed. *Psychological Aspects of Obesity: A Handbook* (New York: Van Nostrand Reinhold, 1982): 1–14; Szepsi, B. "A Model of Nutritionally Induced Overweight: Weight 'Rebound' Following Caloric Restriction." In Bray, G., ed. *Recent Advances in Obesity Research* (London: Newman, Ltd., 1978).

11. Mirkin, G. *Getting Thin* (Boston: Little Brown, 1983): 62.

12. Jenkins, et al. "Nibbling Versus Gorging": 929–34.

13. Jones, P. J., Leitch, C. A., and Pederson, R. A. "Meal-Frequency Effects on Plasma Hormone Concentrations and Cholesterol Synthesis in Humans." *American Journal of Clinical Nutrition* 57(6)(1993): 868–74; Edelstein, S. L., et al. "Increased Meal Frequency Associated with Decreased Cholesterol Concentrations." *American Journal of Clinical Nutrition* 55(1992): 664–69.

14. Lamb. *The Weighting Game.* "There are millions of people in the United States who are suffering from *undernutrition*—a simple lack of calories because they have been on unwise diets . . . ," says Dr. Lamb, cardiologist and medical consultant to the President's Council on Physical Fitness. "As metabolism slows, there is less demand for oxygen. . . . fatigue is the single most commonly experienced symptom by individuals on a diet overly restricted in calories."

15. Rossi, E. L., with Nimmons, D. *The 20 Minute Break* (Los Angeles: Tarcher, 1991): 122–23.

16. Chafetz, M. *Smart for Life* (New York: Penguin, 1993).

17. Norfolk, D. *Executive Stress* (New York: Warner, 1986).

18. Grandjean, E. *Fitting the Task to the Man* (London: Taylor and Francis, 1988).

19. Podell, R. N. *The G-Index Diet* (New York: Warner, 1993): 262.

20. *Obesity & Health* 3(2)(Feb. 1989): 4; Brandon, J. E. *Health Values* (May/June 1987).

21. Blackburn, G. Cited in *Environmental Nutrition* 16(2)(Feb. 1993): 1.

22. Ornish, D. *Eat More, Weigh Less* (New York: HarperCollins, 1993): 43.

23. McDougall, J. A. *The McDougall Program for Maximum Weight Loss* (New York: Dutton, 1994): 73.

24. Hallfrisch, J. "Metabolic Effects of Dietary Fructose." *FASEB Journal* 4(1990): 2652; Roongpisuthpong, C. *Diabetes Research and Clinical Practice* 14(1991): 123.

25. McDougall. *The McDougall Program for Maximum Weight Loss*: 64.

Chapter 22

1. Barneys, M., et al. "Effect of Exercise and Protein Intake on Energy Expenditure." *Revista Española de Fisiologia* 4(4)(1993): 209–17.

2. Gibala, M. J. "Dietary Protein, Amino Acid Supplements, and Recovery from Exercise." *Sports Science Exchange* 87(15)(4)(2002).

3. Levenhagen, D. L., et al. "Post-Exercise Nutrient Intake Timing in Humans Is Critical to Recovery of Leg Glucose and Protein Homeostasis. *American Journal of Physiology, Endocrinology and Metabolism* 280(2001): E982–E993.

4. *Peak Performance Journal* 191(Jan. 2004): 190-192.

5. Kleiner, S. *Power Eating.* 2nd ed. (Champaign, IL: Human Kinetics, 2001); *Journal of the American College of Nutrition* 21(1)(2001): 55–61; *International Journal of Obesity and Related Metabolic Disorders* 23(3)(1999): 287–92; *European Journal of Clinical Nutrition* 53(6)(1999): 495–502; *European Journal of Clinical Nutrition* 52(7)(1998): 482–88.

6. "More Protein Boosts Fat Loss, Preserves Muscle." *Muscle Media* (Sept. 2002): 141.

7. Wurtman, J. J. *Managing Your Mind and Mood Through Food* (New York: Rawson, 1988).

8. *Growth Hormone and IGF Research* 8(suppl B) 1998: 127–29.

9. *Medicine and Science in Sports and Exercise* 31(12)(1999): 1748–54.

10. *American Journal of Clinical Nutrition* 62(1)(1995): 93–103.

11. *Medicine and Science in Sports and Exercise* 19(Supplement 5)(1987): S1578–S166; *American Journal of Clinical Nutrition* 62(1)(1995): 93–103.

12. Ratto, T. "The New Science of Weight Control." *Medical Self-Care* (Mar./Apr. 1987): 29.

13. Manson, J. E. et al. "Body Weight and Longevity." *Journal of the American Medical Association* 257(3)(Jan. 1987): 353–58.

14. Kleiner. *Power Eating*

15. *Journal of Nutrition* 133(2003): 243S–267S.

16. Zemel, M. In *Men's Health* (Aug. 2003): 46.

17. *Men's Health* (Aug. 2003): 126.

18. Willett, W. *Eat, Drink, and Be Healthy* (New York: Simon & Schuster, 2001): 105.

19. American Dietetic Association News Release, May 24, 2004.

20. Cordain, L. *The Paleo Diet* (New York: Wiley, 2002); Pratt, S. *SuperFoods Rx* (New York: William Morrow, 2004).

21. *American Journal of Clinical Nutrition* 70(suppl)(1999): 451S–458S; *Nutrition Reviews* 59(2)(2001): 52–55.

22. *Peak Performance Journal* 191(Jan. 2004): 190–92.

Chapter 23

1. Barnard. *Food for Life*: 96; Rodin, J. "Comparative Effects of Fructose, Aspartame, Glucose, and Water Preloads on Calorie and Macronutrient Intake." *American Journal of Clinical Nutrition* 51(1990): 428–35.

2. *Nutrition Reviews* 62 (2004): 1–17.

3. World Health Organization Expert Committee on Cardiovascular Disease. *Prevention of Coronary Heart Disease*. WHO Technical Report Series, No. 678 (Geneva, 1982): 12.

4. Story, J. *Federation Proceedings* 41(Sept. 1982): 2797.

5. Elias, A., et al. *General Pharmacology* 15(6)(1984): 535; Offenbacher, E., et al. *Diabetes* 29 (11)(Nov. 1980): 919.

6. Draser, B., and Irving, D. *British Journal of Cancer* 27(1973): 167–72; Hems, G. *British Journal of Cancer* 37(1978): 974–82; Hems, G., and Stuart, A. *British Journal of Cancer* (3)(1975): 118–23.

7. Shell, E. R. "It's Not the Carbs, Stupid." *Newsweek* (Aug. 5, 2002): 41.

8. Shell. "It's Not the Carbs, Stupid."

9. *American Journal of Clinical Nutrition* 76(2002): 721–29.

10. Miller, W. C. *The Non-Diet Diet* (Englewood, CO: Taylor Publishing, 1993): 75–77.

11. Aronne, L. Quoted in O'Neill. *The New York Times* (Feb. 8, 1995): C6.

12. Fordyce-Baum, M. K., et al. "Use of an Expanded-Whole-Wheat Product in the Reduction of Body Weight and Serum Lipids in Obese Females." *American Journal of Clinical Nutrition* 50(1989): 30–36; Rossner, S. D., et al. "Weight Reduction with Dietary Fibre Supplements—Results of Two Double-Blind Randomized Studies." *Acta Medica Scandinavica* 222(1988): 83–88.

13. Kenney, J. Quoted in "Natural Weight Loss." *Prevention* (Sept. 1992): 52; Blundell, J., Burley, V. J., Cotton, J. R., et al. "Dietary Fat and the Control of Energy Intake: Evaluating the Effects of Fat on Meal Size and Post Meal Satiety." *American Journal of Clinical Nutrition* 57(suppl)(1993): 772S–78S.

14. Anderson, J. W. "Medical Benefits of High-Fiber Intakes." *The Fiber Factor* (Quaker Oats Co., Chicago, IL, Aug. 1983); Anderson, J. W. *Plant Fiber in Foods* (Lexington, KY: CF Diabetes Research Foundation, Inc., 1986); Kinosian, B. P., and Eisenberg, J. M. "Cutting into Cholesterol." *Journal of the American Medicine Association* 259(15)(Apr. 15, 1988); Kirby, "Oat Bran."

15. Weininger, J., and Briggs, G. M. "Nutrition and Diabetes." *Nutrition Update* (New York: John Wiley and Sons, 1985): 59–60.

16. Connor S. L., and Connor, W. E. *The New American Diet* (New York: Simon and Schuster, 1986): 38; Alabaster, O. *The Power of Prevention* (New York: Fireside, 1985): 127.

17. Anderson. *Plant Fiber.*

18. Henry, C. J. K., and Emergy, B. "Effect of Spiced Food on Metabolic Rate." *Human Nutrition: Clinical Nutrition* 40C(1986): 165–68.

19. *Men's Health* (Aug. 2003): 126.

20. Schiffman, S. "The Use of Flavor to Enhance the Efficacy of Reducing Diets." *Hospital Practice* 21(7)(1986): 44H–44R; Quebec studies cited in Bricklin, M., ed. *Prevention's Lose Weight Guidebook* (Emmaus, PA: Rodale Press, 1992): 64; Henry and Emergy. "Effect of Spiced Food on Metabolic Rate": 165–68.

21. Willett, W. *Eat, Drink, and Be Healthy* (Simon & Schuster, 2002): 94.

22. *Food and Fitness Advisor* (Cornell Medical School) (Feb. 2003): 8.

23. Willett, W. *Eat, Drink, and Be Healthy* (New York: Simon & Schuster, 2001): 94.

24. Barnard, N. *Food for Life* (New York: Harmony, 1994); Cordain, L. *The Paleo Diet* (New York: Wiley, 2002): 85.

25. See, for example: Heber, D. *What Color Is Your Diet?* (New York: Regan Books, 2002); and Joseph, J. A. *The Color Code* (New York: Hyperion, 2003).

26. *American Journal of Preventive Medicine* 20(2)(2001): 1124–29; *Nutrition in Clinical Care I* (1998): 6–12.

27. Pratt, S., and Matthew, K. *SuperFoods Rx* (New York: William Morrow, 2004): 140.

Chapter 24

1. Stark, R. E. T. Quoted in "Good, Better, Best Weight Loss Ideas from the American Society for Bariatric Physicians." *Prevention* (Jan. 1988): 35–41; 115–24.

2. For one summary of these research findings, see: Stein, R. "Fat Cells Aren't Just Passive Blobs, Scientists Learn." *Washington Post* (Jul. 12, 2004).

3. Willett, W. *Eat, Drink, and Be Healthy* (Simon & Schuster, 2002): 57.

4. Miller, W. C. *The Non-Diet Diet* (Englewood, CO: Taylor Publishing, 1993): 77.

5. Drewnowski, A. *Environmental Nutrition* 16(10)(Oct. 1993): 6; Oscai, L.B. et al. "Effects of Dietary Sugar and of Dietary Fat on Food Intake and Body Fat Content in Rats." *Growth* 5(1987): 64–73; Oscai, L. B., and Miller, W. C. "Dietary-Induced Severe Obesity: Exercise Implications." *Medicine and Science in Sports and Exercise* 18(1)(1985): 6–9; Oscai, L. B., et al. "Effect of Dietary Fat on Food Intake, Growth, and Body Composition in Rats." *Growth* 48(1984): 415–24.

6. Bouchard, C. "The Response to Long-Term Overfeeding in Identical Twins." *New England Journal of Medicine* 322(1990): 1477–82.

7. Wurtman, J. J. *Managing Your Mind and Mood Through Food* (New York: HarperCollins, 1987).

8. Barnard, N. *Food for Life* (New York: Harmony Books, 1993): 129.

9. Wurtman, J. Quoted in "Peak Performance Brain Food." *Omni Longevity* 2 (6)(Apr. 1988): 67.

10. *Metabolism* 47(1998): 106–12.

11. *Men's Health Muscle* (Spring 2004): 79.

12. *International Journal of Obesity Research* 21(1997): 637–43; *Journal of Nutrition* 120(1990): 544–52; *American Journal of Clinical Nutrition* 69(1999): 890–97; *American Journal of Clinical Nutrition* 70(1999): 817–25.

13. See, for example: *British Journal of Nutrition* 83(2000): S59–S66; *Annual Review of Nutrition* 19(1999): 63–90; *American Journal of Clinical Nutrition* 70(1999): 566–71; *Biochimie* 79(1998): 95–99; *Journal of Biological Chemistry* 275(2000): 30749–30752; *Journal of Nutrition* 128(1998): 923–26.

14. *International Journal of Obesity* 26(2002): 814–21.

15. *American Journal of Clinical Nutrition* 75(2002): 213–20.

16. Ullis, K. *The Hormone Revolution Weight Loss Plan* (Avery Press, 2003).

17. *American Journal of Clinical Nutrition* 66(5)(1997): 1264–76.

18. Ornish, D. *Dr. Dean Ornish's Program for Reversing Heart Disease* (New York: Random House, 1990): 25.

19. Kendall, A., Levitsky, D. A., Strupp, B. J., and Lissner, L. "Weight Loss on a Low-Fat Diet." *American Journal of Clinical Nutrition* 53(1991): 1124–29.

20. Levitsky, D. Quoted in "Low-Fat Diets Really Work, Without Reducing Food Intake, Cornell Study Finds." *Cornell University News Service* (Apr. 29, 1991).

21. "Are You Eating Right? What 68 Nutrition Experts *Really* Think About Diet and Health." *Consumer Reports* (Oct. 1992): 644–53; Hallfrisch, J., et al. "Modification of the United States' Diet to Effect Changes in Blood Lipids and Lipoprotein Distribution." *Atherosclerosis* 57(2-3)(Nov. 1985): 179–88;

Connor, S. L., and Connor, W. E. *The New American Diet* (New York: Simon and Schuster, 1986); Alabaster, O. *The Power of Prevention* (New York: Fireside, 1985): 87–88, 107.

22. Ornish, D. *Eat More, Weigh Less* (New York: HarperCollins, 1993): 20.

23. Astrup, A., and Raben, A., Bricklin, M *European Journal of Clinical Nutrition* 32(1992): 611–20; Ekwyn, D. H., et al. *American Journal of Clinical Nutrition* 46(1979): 1597–1611.

24. Blundell, J. E., and Bruley, V. J. In *Progress in Obesity Research*. Oomura, Y., et al., eds. (London: John Libbey, 1990): 453–57.

25. Rolls, B. J., Fedoroff, I. C., Guthrie, J. F., and Laster, L. J. "Foods with Different Satiating Effects in Humans." *Appetite* 15(1990): 115–20.

Chapter 25

1. Mirkin, G. *Getting Thin* (Boston: Little, Brown, 1983): 62–65, 195; Darden. E. *A Day-by-Day 10-Step Program* (Dallas: Taylor Publishing, 1992): 26.

2. Schiffman, S. "The Use of Flavor to Enhance the Efficacy of Reducing Diets." *Hospital Practice* 21(7)(1986): 44H–44R.

3. Schiffman, S. "The Use of Flavor to Enhance the Efficacy of Reducing Diets": 44H–44R; Quebec studies cited in Bricklin, M., ed. *Prevention's Lose Weight Guidebook* (Emmaus, PA: Rodale Press, 1992): 64.

Chapter 26

1. Williams, R. *Biochemical Individuality* (New York: Keats, 1984).

2. Thayer, R. E. *Calm Energy* (New York: Oxford University Press, 2001).

Chapter 27

1. Howat, W. "Journaling to Self-Evaluation: A Tool for Adult Learners." *International Journal of Reality Therapy* 18(1999): 32–34.

2. Restak. *Mozart's Brain and the Fighter Pilot* (New York: Harmony Books, 2001).

3. Polivy, J., and Herman, C. P. *International Journal of Eating Disorders* 26(1999): 434–37.

4. *Peak Performance Journal* 195 (Apr. 2004): 2.

5. Howatt, W. A., "Journaling to Self-Evaluation: A Tool for Adult Learners": 32–34.

6. Deci, E. *Intrinsic Motivation and Self-Determination in Human Behavior* (Kluwer Academic Publishers, 1985).

Chapter 28

1. See, for example: Seligman, M. E. P. *What You Can Change and What You Can't* (New York: Ballantine Books, 1995).

2. Claxton, G. *Wise Up: The Challenge of Lifelong Learning* (New York: Bloomsbury, 1999).

3. Gershon, M. D. *The Second Brain* (New York: HarperCollins, 1999).

4. Gershon. *The Second Brain*; Blakeslee, S. "Complex and Hidden Brain in Gut Makes Stomachaches and Butterflies." *New York Times* (Jan. 23, 1996).

5. See, for example: Armour, J., and Ardell, J., eds. *Neurocardiology* (New York: Oxford University Press, 1994); Childre, D., and Martin, H. *The HeartMath Solution* (New York: HarperCollins, 1999); Institute of HeartMath; 800-450-9111; www.heartmath.org.

6. See, for example: Childre, D., and Cryer, B. *From Chaos to Coherence* (Boston: Butterworth Heinemann, 1999); Armour, J. A. "Anatomy and Function of the Intrathoracic Neurons Regulating the Heart." In Zucker, I. H., and Gilmore, J. P., eds. *Reflex Control of the Circulation* (Boca Raton, FL: CRC Press, 1991); Cantin, M., and Genest, J. "The Heart as an Endocrine Gland." *Clinical and Investigative Medicine* 9(4)(1986): 319–27.

7. See, for example: Childre and Cryer. *From Chaos to Coherence*.

8. See, for example: Pribram, K. H., and Rozman, D. "Early Childhood Development and Learning: What New Research About the Brain and Heart Tell Us." White House Conference on Human Development and Learning, San Francisco, 1997; Pribram, K. H., ed. *Brain and Values* (Mahwah, NJ: Lawrence Earlbaum, 1998).

9. Armour, J. "Neurocardiology: Anatomy and Functional Principles." In McCraty, R., Rozman, D., and Childre, D. *HeartMath: A New Biobehavioral Intervention for Increasing Coherence in the Human System* (Amsterdam: Harwood Academic Publishers, 1999).

10. See, for example: Langhorst, P., Schultz, G., and Lambertz, M. "Oscillating Neuronal Network of the 'Common Brain System.'" In Miyakawa, K., et al. *Mechanisms of Blood Pressure Waves* (Tokyo: Japan Scientific Societies Press, 1984): 257–75.

11. Telegdy, G. "The Action of ANP, BNP, and Related Peptides on Motivated Behavior." *Reviews in the Neurosciences* 5(4)(1994): 309–15; see also: Pert, C. A. *The Molecules of Emotion* (New York: Scribner, 1997).

12. See, for example: Epictetus. *The Art of Living* (HarperSanFrancisco, 1995); and Aurelius, M. *Meditations* (New York: Knopf, 1992).

13. See, for example: Song, L., Schwartz, G., and Russek, L. "Heart-Focused Attention and Heart-Brain Synchronization: Energetic and Physiological Mechanisms." *Alternative Therapies in Health and Medicine* 4(5)(1998): 44–62.

14. McCraty, R., Atkinson, M., and Tiller, W. A. "New Electrophysiological Correlates Associated with Intentional Heart Focus." *Subtle Energies* 4(3)(1995): 251–68; see also: Lynch, J. J. *The Language of the Heart* (New York: Basic Books, 1985).

15. For an overview, see: Damasio, A. R. *Descartes' Error: Emotion, Reason, and the Human Brain* (New York: Grosset/Putnam, 1995); and Damasio, A. R. *The Feeling of What Happens* (New York: Harcourt Brace, 1999).

INDEX

Underscored references indicate boxed text. **Boldface** references indicate illustrations.

A

Abdominal fat
  muscle toning and, 99, 168
  protein and, 213
  stress and, 99, 105, 123–24
  suggestions for, 99
Abdominal muscles
  crunches and, 178
  guidelines for toning, 179–80
  as health indicator, 177
  toning exercises
    abdominal vacuum, 180
    elbow-to-knee curl-up, 182
    exhalation towel roll-up, 181–82
    lean-back tone-up, 178
    reverse trunk rotation, 183–84
    for transpyramidalis, 181
    for transverse abdominis, 180–81
    twisting exhalation roll-up, 183
Activity. *See* Physical Activity
Adenosine triphosphate (ATP)
  biological role of, 5–6
  breathing and, 71, 110
Adiponectin, 28, 100–101
Adrenal gland, 105
Adrenaline. *See* Epinephrine
Aerobic exercise
  high-intensity intervals, 161–62
  stairs for, 162
  using
    elliptical trainers, 163
    stairclimbers, 163
    stationary cycles, 163
    treadmills, 163
Aging
  muscle toning and, 166–68
  posture and, 88

Agouti
  appetite and, 28, 101
  fat storage and, 69
  Vitamin D and, 69
Alcohol intake
  excessive, as "off" switch,
    35–36
  fat gain and, 83
Aldosterone, dehydration and, 35
Alertness
  posture and, 88
  protein and, 213
  taking breaks for, 109
Almonds, benefits of, 217
Alpha-linolenic acid, 234
Amino acids, essential
  beans and, 218
  in diet, 211–12
Ancestral forebears
  activity patterns of, 9–10
  gender and body fat, 29–30
  lifestyle of, 8–10, 8–10
  metabolic physiology of, 7–8,
    19
  overeating and, 240
  sunlight and, 67
  temperature adjustments of,
    94
  trimness of, 8–9
  winter fat storage and, 67
Anger
  cancer and, 128
  fat metabolism and, 124
Antioxidants, in
  berries, 227
  colored vegetables, 230
  spinach, 231

Appetite
  blood sugar and, 203
  stimulation
    agouti and, 28, 101
    cortisol and, 105
    ghrelin and, 101
    sweeteners, 82–83
  suppression
    melanocortin and, 101
    water intake and, 80
  very low fat diets and, 237
Apples, before meals, 220
Arm toning exercises
  arm curl, 192–93
  biceps curls, 172
  lateral raises, 171, 174
  one-arm extension, 175
  upper arm extension, 193
ATP
  biological role of, 5–6
  breathing and, 71, 110
Atrial peptide, 265
Attention shifting, for stress, 134
Avocados, 236, 238

B
Back strength stretches
  back arch, 196
  pelvic tilt, 197
  seated lower-back stretch, 197
  single knee-to-chest lift, 196
  torso rotation, 195
Balance and flexibility
  importance of, 194
  stretches for
    back strength, 195–97
    neck flexibility, 195
Basal metabolic rate, 36–37
Beans, 218, 227
Beds, choosing, 155–56
Berries, as carb power food, 227
Beverages, energy-boosting, 82–83
Bloating, stress and, 105
Blood fats. See Triglyceride levels

Blood sugar
  alcohol and, 35–36
  appetite and, 203
  carbohydrates and, 21
  evening arguments and, 141
  fiber and, 224
  glycemic load and, 224–26
  large meals and, 202–3
  oats and, 230
  snacks and, 116
  very low fat diets and, 237
Blueberries, 227
Body heating, passive, 155
Body, listening to, 262–65
Brain
  in the gut, 263–64
  in head, 262–63
  in the heart, 264–65
Breakfast
  benefits of, 48, 50–52
  exercising before, 46
  food ideas for, 49, 51, 52
  hormonal balance and, 98–99
  protein for, 98–99
  shakes, 49
  skipping, as "off" switch, 34, 48
Breaks
  cues you need a break, 108–9
  meal and snack times as, 208
  techniques for
    essential breaks, 114–18
    strategic pause, 110–14
  ultradian rhythms and, 107–8
  in the workplace, 205
Breathing
  for healthier blood, 133
  as "on" switch, 71–74
  oxygen and, 71–72, 110
  posture and, 86
  PowerLung device, 74
  shallow, as "off" switch, 35
  as step in
    instant calming, 129
    strategic pause, 110–11

for stress relief, <u>124</u>, 131–32
techniques for
    deep breathing, 10–11, 132, <u>133</u>
    rib elasticity, 73–74
Broccoli, as carb power food, 227
Burgers, tips for, 239

C

Caffeine
    avoiding before bedtime, 156
    excessive, as "off" switch, 35
    fat burning and, 80–81
Calcitrol, 27, 69, 104–5
Calcium
    calcitrol and, 27, 69, 104–5
    fat burning and, 104–5
    Vitamin D and, 69
Calm energy, as "on" switch, 106–21
Calories count, 240–42
Cancer
    breast, carbohydrates and, 221
    tomatoes and, 231
Canola oil, <u>236</u>
Cantaloupe, as carb power food, 227
Capsicum, for weight loss, <u>145</u>
Carbohydrates. *See also* Sugar
    biological role of, 220–21
    complex
        benefits of, 222–23
        as energy source, 219–20
        fiber and, <u>224–25</u>
        protein and, 213
        weight loss and, 223
    glycemic load
        foods chart, <u>228–29</u>
        as nutritional tool, 224–26
    low, dehydration and, <u>77</u>
    power foods, 227, 230–31
    simple, effects of, <u>83</u>, 219–21
    starchy, early in day, 99
    types of, 219–20
Cardiovascular exercise. *See* Aerobic
    exercise
Catecholamines, 140–41

CCK
    foods that maximize, 104
    hunger and, 26, 104
    slow eating and, 144
Cells, fat
    expansion of, 4
    hormones and, 100–101
    insulin levels and, 21–22,
        202–3
    large meals and, 202
    overeating and, 241–42
Chairs, ergonomics of, 91–92
Change, personal
    as choice, 18
    commitment and, <u>73</u>
    developing skills for, <u>15</u>
Cheese, low-fat, for protein, 217
Chicken, 216, 236
Children
    evening unwinding and, 140
    as natural break takers, 109
Chocolate, bedtime and, 156
Cholecystokinin (CCK)
    foods that maximize, 104
    hunger and, 26, 104
    slow eating and, 144
Cholesterol
    bad dietary fats and, 233
    foods for
        garlic and onions, 227
        nuts, 217
    simple carbohydrates and, 221
    small frequent meals and, 204
Chromium, sucrose and, 221
Chronobiology, 107
Coenzyme Q_{10}, spinach and, 231
Coffee
    avoiding before bedtime, 156
    metabolism and, 80–81
Cool downs, after toning, 189
Cortisol
    abdominal fat and, <u>99</u>, 105, 123
    appetite and, 105
    sleep deficiency and, 102

Cortisol *(cont.)*
    small frequent meals and, 204
    stress and, 23–24, 36, 108, 123
Cottage cheese, 157, 217
Cravings, food. *See also* Appetite
    fruit to quash, <u>220</u>
    galanin and, 104
    goal-setting for, 260
    sugars and, <u>222</u>
    water intake and, 80
Crunches, 178
Cycles, stationary, for workouts,
    163

D

Daily energy wave, tracking, 251
Dairy
    choosing low-fat, 239
    fat loss and, 104–5
    as protein source, 216–17
    for sleep, 157
Dehydration
    fat deposits and, 78
    low-carb diets and, <u>77</u>
    as "off" switch, 35
    physiological effects of, 76–77
Desserts
    delaying, after diner, 146–47
    suggestions for, 147, 239
Diabetes
    fiber and, <u>224</u>
    simple carbohydrates and, 221
Diets
    failure of, 3
    restrictive, 16
    slow-wave sleep and, 156
    typical vs. Meta-Stat, **12**
Direct Pressure Therapy (DPT), 121
Disaccharides, 220
Dopamine, 24, 25
DPT, 121
Dynamic resistance (DR), 171–72
Dynamic visualized tension (DVT),
    171–76, 178

E

Eating. *See also* Meals
    frequently, 100–101, 201–2
    overeating, as "off" switch, 37
    for soul nourishment, 208
Eating plan, MSOn
    components of
        calories count, 240–42
        good fats, 232–39
        mealtime principles, 201–10
        proper protein, 211–18
        right carbohydrates, 219–31
    guidelines for, 206, 208
    health benefits of, 201–5
    menu suggestions, 208–10
    mix of nutrients for, 205
    recipes (*See the recipe index*)
    success map for, 250
Edamame, for protein, 217
EFAs, 234–36
Eggs, organic or free-range
    for omega-3 fatty acids, 236
    as protein source, 216
Emotions
    negative, as "off" switch, 36
    posture and, 88
    power of, 265
Energy
    breathing and, 110
    calm, in the mornings, 42–43, <u>44–45</u>
    complex carbohydrates and,
        219–20
    eyes and, 112
    fluid intake for, 80, <u>82–83</u>
    inspiration and, 117–18
    snacks for, <u>207</u>
    starter program for, 253
    sunlight for, 67–68
    wave, daily, 251
Enteric nervous system, 263–64
Enzymes, fat-burning, 61, 115
Epinephrine
    abdominal fat and, 123
    stress and, 23–24, 108, 123

Essential fatty acids (EFAs)
    biological role of, 234
    foods that contain, 235–36
    forms of, 234–35
Estrogen, metabolism and, 29–30
Evening
    dining suggestions for, 142–47, <u>146</u>
    light and, <u>138</u>, 140
    overeating during, <u>144</u>
    postmeal exercise, 147–49
    predinner snacks, 140–42, <u>141</u>
    routine, optimal, 142–49
    staying active, 140
    unwinding, 139–40
    as vulnerable time, 136–37
    workplace transition to, 137–38
Evolution. *See* Ancestral forebears
Exercise. *See also* Physical activity
    coolness during, <u>95</u>
    goal-setting for, 259–60
    guilt-based, 16
    intense
        as "off" switch, 34–35
        tension and, 126
    leptin levels and, 101
    nutrition after
        for HGH production, 103
        protein benefits, 103, <u>212</u>
    for stress reduction, 125–26
Exercises. *See* Muscle toning; Stretches
Expression, stress and, 129–30
Eyes
    focus shifts, for energy, 112
    "lightening" to reduce stress, 129–30
    as light harvesters, 113
Eyestrain, reducing, 112

F
Families, activity levels of, 63
Fat, body
    abdominal (*See* Abdominal fat)
    burning (*See also* Metabolism)
        dairy foods for, 104–5
        exercise after eating for, 148

fluid intake and, 113–14
green tea and, 81, 83
hormones, 20–30
muscles toning and, 165–66
cells
    expansion of, 4
    insulin levels and, 21–22
    large meals and, 202
    overeating and, 241–42
gain, due to stress, 24
insulin levels and, 21–22
large meals and, 202
loss (*See* Weight loss)
Fat, dietary
    bad fats
        combined with sugar, 233
        consequences of, 233–34
        as "off" switch, 37
    calculating target intake, 238
    good fats
        essential fatty acids, 234–36
        monounsaturated oils, <u>236</u>
        optimal daily intake, 236–39
    popular beliefs about, 232
    strategies for trimming, 238–39
    types of, 232–33
    very low, in diet, 237
Fatigue
    bad dietary fats and, 234
    fluid intake and, 80
    simple carbohydrates and, 223
Fatty acids. *See* Essential fatty acids;
        Free fatty acids
Fiber
    complex carbohydrates and, 223,
        <u>224–25</u>
    foods high in
        beans, 218
        fruit, <u>220</u>
    optimal daily intake,
        <u>224–25</u>
    types of, <u>225</u>
Fish, 215–16
Fish oil, for fat burning, 100

Flexibility, stretches for
  back strength, 195–97
  neck flexibility, 195
Fluid intake. *See also* Water intake
  benefits of, 75–76, 114
  beverages
    for energy, 82–83
    green tea, 81, 83
    list of energy-boosting, 82–83
    protein shakes, 49, 83–84
    sodas, 222
  body fat and, 78–79, 113–14
  cravings and, 79–80
  for energy, 80
  low carbohydrates and, 77
  as "on" switch, 75–84
  soups for, 84
  as step in strategic pause, 113–14
  weight loss and, 78–79
Food labels, sugars and, 221
Foods
  alternatives to high-fat, 238–39
  carb power foods, 227, 230–31
  colored, health benefits of, 231
  fat-free, 241
  flavorful, thermic effect of, 242
  glycemic load of, 228–29
  for HGH production, 103
  high in protein, 25
  high in tryptophan, 25
  protein-rich, 145, 215–18
  spicy, 145, 226
  stress and choice of, 124
  vegetables, cruciferous, 30
Free fatty acids
  caffeine and, 81
  fluid intake and, 78
  muscle toning and, 115–16
  physical activity and, 61
Free-running, on weekends, 157
French fries, 239
French people, heart disease and,
  143
Fructose, cravings and, 222

Fruit
  colored, health benefits of, 231
  dried, 206–7
  for fiber, 220
  glycemic load of, 228
  whole, fresh, 208, 220
Fruit juice, 208
Fullness at meals. *See* Satiety

G
Galanin
  biological role of, 25–26, 104
  foods that increase, 104
Garlic, as carb power food, 227
Genetics. *See* Ancestral forebears
Genome, human, 7, 19
Ghrelin
  appetite and, 101
  meal skipping and, 28, 100–101
  sleep and, 153
Glucagon
  insulin and, 22–23
  metabolic role of, 22
  protein and, 83, 213
Glycemic index, 225, 226
Glycemic load
  foods chart, 228–29
  as nutritional tool, 224–26
Glycogen, body fat and, 21–22
Goals
  characteristics of good
    believable, 256
    challenging, 256
    emphasize development,
      256–57
    measurable, 256
    positive, 255–56
  creating your own, 261
  formula for achieving, 255–58
  importance of, 254–55
  measurement of, 258
  mechanisms for achieving, 258
  momentum and, 258–59
  obstacles to, 257

sample goals, 259–61
success map for, 249
Goitrogens, 104
Grains, whole
    as carb power food, 227, 230
    for omega-3 fatty acids, 236
Gum chewing, 62
Gut instincts, 263–64

H
Habits, changing, 17–18
Head
    brain, 262–63
    centering exercise for, 89–90
    forward position of, 87
    head nod exercise, 89, 111
    posture and, 111
Heart brain, 264–65
Heart disease
    bad dietary fats and, 233
    foods to prevent
        nuts, 217
        tomatoes, 231
    simple carbohydrates and, 221
Hepatic gluconeogenesis, 24
HGH
    body fat storage and, 29
    protein and, 213
    role of, 101–2
    stimulating production of, 29,
        102–3
High fructose corn syrup, 222
Hormones, *See also specific kinds*
    abdominal fat and, 99
    balancing, for optimal health,
        97–105
    biological role of, 20–21
    heart brain and, 264–65
    as master regulators, 19–30
    sleep and, 153
Hormone-sensitive lipase (HSL), 23
Human Growth Hormone (HGH)
    body fat storage and, 29
    protein and, 213

    role of, 101–2
    stimulating production of, 29,
        102–3
Humor. *See* Laughter and humor
Hunger. *See also* Appetite
    CCK and, 26
    distinguishing from thirst, 79–80
    ghrelin and, 28, 100–101
    posture and, 85
Hydration. *See* Fluid intake
Hypoglycemic reactions, 22

I
ICS, 129–31
Inactivity
    as energy drain, 111–12
    longevity and, 63
    as "off" switch, 34
    weight and, 55–56
Inspiration, for energy, 117–18
Instant calming sequence (ICS),
    129–31
Instincts, power of, 262–65
Insulin
    abdominal fat and, 99
    artificial sweeteners and, 206
    biological role of, 21
    dietary tips for stabilizing, 98–100
    fat cells and, 22, 202–3
    foods affecting
        alcohol, 35–36
        carbohydrates, 21–22, 223
        dietary fats, 234
        oats, 230
        sports drinks, 100
        sugary, fatty foods, 233
    hypoglycemic reactions, 22
    lipoprotein lipase and, 22
    meal size and frequency, 202–4
    overeating and, 241–42
    sleep and, 152
    stress and, 36
Intelligence, distributed, 263, 265
Intestinal brain, 263–64

K

Kashi, 230
Ketosis, 223

L

Laughter and humor
  in evening routine, 140
  ideas for maximizing, 128
  metabolism and, 112–13
  physical benefits of, 113, 127
  for stress reduction, 127–28
Legs
  hyperextension of, 93
  toning exercises
    hip raise, 186
    modified knee bend, 184–85
    seated leg extension, 185
    standing calf raise, 187
    standing leg raise, 185–86
Leptin
  advice for optimizing, 100–101
  exercise and, 101
  light and, 68–69, 101
  metabolic role of, 27
  sleep and, 153
Light
  bright
    for evening vigor, 138
    as "on" switch, 67–70
    as step in strategic pause, 113
    upon waking, 47
  dim, as "off" switch, 35
  hormones and, 68–69
  sunlight
    for energy and fat loss,
      67–68
    healthy exposure to, 69–70
    leptin and, 101
    upon waking, 47–48
    Vitamin D and, 69
Linolenic acid, 234
Lipoprotein lipase (LPL)
  insulin levels and, 22
  physical activity and, 60–61
  stress and, 36
  sugary, fatty foods and, 233
Lower-body toning
  abdominal exercises
    abdominal vacuum, 180
    elbow-to-knee curl-up, 182–83
    exhalation Towel roll-up, 181–82
    lean-back tone-ups, 178
    reverse trunk rotation, 183–84
    transpyramid toner, 181
    TVA ab tightener, 180–81
    twisting exhalation roll-up, 183
  guidelines for, 178–80
  leg exercises
    hip raise, 186
    modified knee bend, 176, 184–85
    seated leg extension, 185
    standing calf raise, 187
    standing side leg raise, 185–86
    step-ahead, 176
    toe raise, 175
Lycopene, 231
Lysine, 218

M

Meals
  caloric size of, 206
  eat-and-move technique, 59
  eating slowly, 144, 146, 242
  in the evening
    delaying dessert, 146–47
    eating early, 142–43
    rethinking, 143–44
  followed by activity, 203
  large, fat gain and, 202–3
  satiety, 213, 242
  skipping, as "off" switch, 36–37
  small and frequent
    cognitive function and, 205
    guidelines for, 206, 208
    health benefits of, 201–5
    hormonal response to, 101
  time of, weight loss and, 143
  tips for satisfying, 146

Melanocortin, 69, 101
Melatonin, sleep and, 26–27
Memory, vital, <u>205</u>
Metabolism
  affected by
    breathing, 71–74
    caffeine, 81
    fluid intake, 75–84
    green tea, 81, 83
    light, 67–70
    meal frequency, 100–101, 201–2
    muscle tone, 164–66
    posture, 85–93
    protein, 212
    spicy foods, <u>145</u>, <u>226</u>
    TV watching, 55–56
    water intake, 76
  ATP and, 5–6
  mitochondria and, 4–5
  physiology of, 5–6
  typical diet vs. Meta-Stat, **12**
Meta-Stat approach
  as lifestyle rhythm, 245, 248
  sample starter programs, 252–53
  success map
    chart, <u>246–47</u>
    guide to using, 249–52
    as personal tool, 248–49
  switches (*see* Switches)
  timing of, 12–15
  vs. guilt-driven approaches, 16–17
MetLife height/weight tables, 214
Milk, warm, for sleep, 157
Mindset, cultivating, 53–54
Mitochondria
  breathing and, 72
  omega-3 fatty acids and, 235
  role of, in metabolism, 4–5
Monosaccharides, 220, 237
Mood, serotonin and, 25
Mornings
  keys to
    bright light, 46–48, <u>47</u>
    calm energy, 42–43

    cultivate mindset, 53–54
    a good breakfast, 48–52, <u>49</u>, <u>51</u>
    muscle toning, 43–46
    self-regulation, 53
  one-touch relaxation for, <u>44–45</u>
  as "on" switch, 41–54
  starting wrong, as "off" switch, 34
Movement. *See* Physical activity
Muscles, *See also specific muscles*
  loss of, and body fat, 167–68
  trigger points and, 118–21
Muscle tone
  assessing, <u>167</u>
  as factor in metabolism, 6
Muscle toning
  aging and, 166–68
  in daily life, 170–71, <u>184</u>
  in essential breaks, 115–16
  exercises for
    abdominals, <u>178</u>, <u>180</u>, 180–84
    arms, 190–93
    legs, 184–87
    shoulders, <u>165</u>, 190–92
  goal-setting for, 260
  HGH production and, 29, 103
  within an hour of waking, 43–46
  importance of, 164–66
  keys to success, 168–69
  metabolism and, 6
  the MSOn workout, 164–97
  pace of, <u>169</u>
  peak focus for, <u>170</u>
  as postmeal exercise, 149
  resting metabolic rate and, 166
  for stress reduction, 115–16
Music, at meals, <u>146</u>, 208

N

Nature, as energizer, 138
Neck flexibility stretch, 195
Neurotransmitters. *See* Dopamine; Norepinephrine

Nissan Thermos Insulated Water Bottle, <u>79</u>

Norepinephrine
  biological role of, 24
  chocolate and, 156
  green tea and, 83
  tyrosine and, 25
Nutrition. *See* Eating plan, MSOn
Nuts
  for omega-3 fatty acids, 236
  for protein, 217–18

O

Oats
  for breakfast, 230
  as carb power food, 227, 230
  instant oatmeal, 230
Oils, vegetable
  olive, for metabolism, <u>236</u>
  omega-3 fatty acids and, 235
  on salad, 238–39
Olive oil, <u>236</u>
Omega-3 fatty acids
  biological role of, 234–35
  eggs, organic, 216
  foods that contain, 235–36
  salmon and fatty fish, 215, 235
  spinach, 231
  in vegetable oils, 235
Omega-6 fatty acids, 234–35
Onions, as carb power food, 227
Oranges, as carb power food, 230
Organic foods
  chicken, 216
  eggs, 216
Overeating
  as "off" switch, 37
  risks of, 240–42
Overweight
  bad dietary fats and, 233
  breakfast and, 48
  as epidemic, 17–18
  TV watching and, 55–56

P

Pasta
  refined, weight gain and, 223
  whole grain, 230
Pause, strategic, for renewal, 110–14
Peppers, hot, for weight loss, <u>145</u>
Physical activity. *See also* Exercise; Muscle toning
  action ideas, 65–66, <u>162</u>
  after meals, <u>59</u>
  benefits of, 57
  body fat storage and, 60–61
  before breakfast, 46
  in the evenings, 37
  fat burning and, 61, 115
  as human nature, 56–57
  ideas for, 63–66
  intense
    as "off" switch, 34–35
    tension and, 126
  longevity and, 63
  in the morning, 43–46
  as "on" switch, 55–66
  as part of daily regime, 58–60
  postmeal, benefits of, 148–49
  psychological benefits of, 62–63
  for sleep quality, 154–55
  starter program for, 253
  in strategic pause, 111–12
  timing of, and metabolism, 13–15, **14**
  weight loss and, 61–62
Pleasure, for renewal, 150
Polysaccharides, 220, 237
Portion control
  for meals and snacks, 206
  nuts and, 217
Posture
  aging and, 88
  breathing and, 86
  chair sitting and, 91–92
  emotions and, 88
  head position and, <u>89</u>, 89–90, <u>111</u>
  health problems and, 86–87

in instant calming sequence, 130
as learned form, 87
mental alertness and, 88
as "on" switch, 85–93
poor, as "off" switch, 35
slumped
   breathing and, 111
   commonality of, 86–87
   as "off" switch, 36
   at work, <u>139</u>
in strategic pause, 111
stress and, 130
techniques for, 10–11, 88–93, <u>139</u>
tension and, 93
PowerLung, 74
Prolactin, sleep and, 26–27
Protein
   after workouts, <u>212</u>
   amino acids and, 211–12
   benefits of, 212–13
   best food choices for, 215–18
   breakfast shakes, <u>49</u>
   for dinner, 145
   hunger and, 26
   insufficient, as "off" switch, 37
   insulin levels and, 98–99
   in the MSON eating plan, 211–18
   optimal daily intake, 214–15
   oxygen and, 83
   shakes, <u>49</u>, 83–84
   tyrosine and, 25
Pumpkin, as carb power food, 230
Pushups, for muscle toning, 44–46

R
Reading position, 92
Recipes. *See* the recipe index
Recordkeeping, for weight control, <u>144</u>
Referred pain, 118
Relaxation, one-touch, <u>44–45</u>
Republic of Tea teas, <u>82</u>
Resistance training. *See* Muscle toning
Rest. *See* Sleep

Resting metabolic rate
   muscle loss and, 167
   muscle toning and, 166
Rice, white, weight gain and, 223

S
Salads, tips for, 238–39
Salmon, wild
   for omega-3 fatty acids, 235
   as protein source, 215
Sandwiches, healthy, 239
Satiety
   complex carbohydrates and, 223
   eating slowly and, 242
   meal composition and, 213
   sugars and, <u>222</u>
Seafood, 215–16
Seasonings, spicy, <u>145</u>, <u>226</u>
Seeds, pumpkin or sunflower, 236
Selenium
   multivitamins for, 103
   oats as source of, 230
   T3 synthesis and, 23
Self-regulation, 53
Serotonin
   artificial sweeteners and, 206
   biological role of, 25
   high-glycemic carbohydrates and, 25
   sleep and, 157
   stress and, 24
   tryptophan and, 25
   turkey and, 157
Sex hormones
   improving balance of, 30
   metabolic role of, 29–30
Sex, nutrition and, 145
Shakes, protein, <u>49</u>, 83–84
Shoulders, toning exercise for, <u>165</u>
Sitting properly, advice for, 91–92
Skillpower vs. willpower, <u>15</u>
Sleep
   bedtime nutrition and, 156–57
   cool temperature and, 96, 156
   HGH production during, 29, 102

Sleep *(cont.)*
hormones and, 153
impact of, on health, 152
lack of, as "off" switch, 38
metabolism and, 151–52
as "on" switch, 151–58
postmeal exercise and, 149
preparing for, 154
strategies for improving, 154–58
on weekends, 157–58
weight control and, 152–53
Smiling, stress and, 130
Snacks
caloric size of, 206
energy-boosting, 207
fatty, 104
fruits as, 220
for increased metabolism, 116
pre-bedtime suggestions for, 157
stashing healthy choices, 206
by time of day
afternoon, 116–17, 205
evening, 99
midmorning, 204
predinner, 140–42, 141
Soda, 222
Soup
caloric intake and, 141, 146, 238
hunger satisfaction and, 84, 146
spicy, for weight loss, 145
Soy foods, 217, 230
Spicy seasonings, 145, 226
Spinach, as carb power food, 231
Sports drinks, 100
Stairclimber, for workouts, 163
Starvation response, 36
Strength training. *See* Muscle toning
Stress
abdominal fat and, 99, 105, 123–24
bloating and, 105
control, as "on" switch, 122–35
cortisol and, 36, 105
food habits and, 124
goal-setting for, 261

hormonal response to, 23–24
lipoprotein lipase and, 36
posture and, 130
starvation response to, 36
techniques for handling
30-second neutralizers, 131–35
breathing, 124, 129, 131–32
detachment, 126–27
humor, 127–28
instant calming sequence, 129–31
mind-escape word, 132–34
muscle toning, 115–16
physical activity, 125–26
positive self-talk, 135
quick tips, 135
shifting attention, 134
social support, 134–35
stress log, 126
turn TV off, 134
testosterone loss due to, 30
uncontrolled, as "off' switch, 36
Stretches for balance and flexibility,
194–97
Success map
chart, 246–47
guide to using, 249–52
as personal tool, 248–49
Sucrose, chromium and, 221
Sugar
appetite and, 82–83
combined with bad fats, 233
consumption, in the U.S., 22, 221
cravings and, 222
food labels and, 221
metabolism and, 82–83
as "off" switch, 37
satiety signals and, 222
types, blood sugar and, 221
Sunlight. *See* Light
Superobesity, TV watching and, 56
Sweeteners
appetite and, 82–83, 206
artificial, 83, 206
natural, 82–83

Switches
  "off" switches overview, 34–38
  "on" switches
    activity momentum, 55–66
    breathing for oxygen,
      71–74
    cool temperature, 94–96
    evening routines, 136–50
    fluid intake, 75–84
    hormone balance, 97–105
    light, 67–70
    morning routines, 41–54
    overview of, 32–33
    posture, 85–93
    quality rest, 151–58
    staying calm, 106–21
    stopping stress, 122–35
  success map for, 249–50
  for thermogenesis, 7

T

T3
  biological role of, 23
  foods that inhibit, 104
  as master of metabolism, 103
  selenium and, 103
Teas
  green, 81, 83
  list of energy-boosting, 82–83
Tempeh, for protein, 217
Temperature
  cool
    as "on" switch, 7, 94–96
    seeking, 95
    while exercising, 95
  too warm
    metabolic slowing and, 94
    as "off" switch, 36
Tension
  chronic, 36, 118–21
  defined, 106
  impaired alertness and, 109
  influence on posture, 93
  taking regular breaks, 107–9

  techniques for
    essential breaks, 114–18
    one-touch relaxation, 44–45
    the strategic pause, 110–14
    tension scan, 107
    trigger points, 118–21, 120
  ultradian rhythms and, 107–8
Testosterone
  metabolic role of, 29–30
  switches to increase, 30
Thermogenesis
  composition of meals and, 204
  flavorful food and, 242
  green tea and, 83
  metabolic role of, 6
  omega-3 fatty acids and, 235
  protein and, 212
Thirst, 79–80. *See also* Dehydration
Thyroid gland
  hormones, 23, 103–4
  metabolic role of, 23, 103
Tofu, for protein, 217
Tomatoes, as carb power food,
  231
Trainers, elliptical, for workouts,
  163
Trans fatty acids, 233
Treadmill, for workouts, 163
Trigger points
  causes of, 119
  direct pressure therapy for, 121
  how to find, 120
  referred pain and, 118
Triglyceride levels
  fruit sugar and, 208
  good dietary fats and, 234
  physical activity and, 61
  simple carbohydrates and, 221
Triiodothyronine (T3)
  biological role of, 23
  foods that inhibit, 104
  as master of metabolism, 103
  selenium and, 103
Tryptophan, 25

Turkey
  for omega-3 fatty acids, 236
  as protein source, 216
  for sleep, 157
TV watching
  metabolism in girls and, 134
  obesity and, 55–56
  stress and, 134
Tyrosine, 25

U

Ultradian rhythms, 107–8
Upper body toning
  additional weight for, 190
  eccentric motion, 190
  exercises
    arm curl, 192–93
    chest and shoulder raise, 191
    chest cross, 173, 192
    modified pushups, 174, 190–91
    rope pull, 173
    upper arm extension, 193
  guidelines for, 188–89

V

Vegetables
  colored, health benefits of, 231
  cruciferous, fat burning and, 30
  optimal daily intake of, 231
Visualizations for
  mind-escape word cue, 133
  stress, 135
  workplace transition, 137–38
Vitamin D
  body fat and, 69–70
  dairy products for, 70

W

Walking
  heterolateral pattern of, 93
  postmeal, benefits of, 148–49
  posture techniques for, 92–93
Warm ups, before toning, 188
Water intake. *See also* Fluid intake
  appetite and, 80

benefits of, 75–76, 79, 114
body fat and, 113–14
for energy, 80
ice water
  calories and, 78
  keeping on hand, 79
  metabolism and, 75, 114
in strategic pause, 113–14
weight loss and, 78–79
Water retention. *See* Bloating
Weekends, sleep habits on, 157–58
Weight, ideal, 214–15
Weight loss. *See also* Metabolism
  fluid intake and, 78–79
  new science of, 3–18
  recordkeeping and, 144
  spicy food for, 145, 226
  starter program for, 252–53
Willpower vs. skillpower, 15
Women
  body fat and, 29
  muscle toning and, 168
Word, as mind-escape, 132–34
Workout, MSOn
  components of
    aerobic activity, 161–63
    daily muscle tone-ups, 164–74
    strength training, 180–93
    stretches, 194–97
  overview of, 160
  recap of, 250
  success map for, 250
Workplace
  breaks, performance and, 205
  tips for loosening up, 139
  transitioning from, 137–38

Y

Yogurt
  sleep and, 157
  for weight loss, 216–17

Z

Zinc, testosterone and, 30

RECIPE INDEX

A

Almonds
  Almond Crunch Topping, 373–74
  Vanilla Almond Protein Shake, 49
Apples
  Beet and Apple Salad with Cheese and
    Walnuts, 287
  Bran Muffins with Apples and Pecans,
    282–83
Apricots
  Pistachio-Crusted Chicken with Goat
    Cheese and Apricot-Sherry
    Sauce, 328–29
Asian-style recipes
  Asian Cashew Shrimp with Brown
    Rice, 337–38
  Asian Jicama Slaw, 295
  Chicken and Vegetable Fried Rice,
    355–56
  Curried Yellow Pea and Sweet Potato
    Soup, 318–19
  Indonesian Coconut-Crusted Chicken
    Tenders, 327
  Peanut Dipping Sauce, 328
  Peanut Soba Noodles, 356–57
  Shrimp and Vegetable Fried Rice, 356
  Tofu Egg Drop Soup with Vegetables,
    323–24
Avocados
  choosing ripe, 277
  Quick and Easy Homemade
    Guacamole, 277

B

Bacon, turkey
  Cannellini Bean and Bacon Soup,
    307–8
Barley
  Creamy Chicken and Barley Soup,
    314–15
Basil
  Cream of Roasted Tomato-Basil Soup,
    319–20
Beans
  black
    Basic Black Beans, 353–54

    Black Bean Soup with Lime, 304–5
    Spicy Black Beans, 354
  lentils
    Duck and Lentil Stew, 316–17
    Mediterranean Lentil Salad, 298–99
    Roasted Chicken Breasts with
      Lentil Ragout, 330–31
    Tuscan Lentil Soup, 308–9
  mixed
    Southwestern Three-Bean Salad, 301–2
  substituting canned for dried, 306
  white (Cannellini, navy or great
    Northern)
    Broccoli and White Bean Puree, 354
    Broccoli Rabe and White Bean
      Soup, 305–6
    Cannellini Bean and Bacon Soup,
      307–8
    Farfalle with Sausage and White
      Beans, 334–35
    Seafood and White Bean Chili,
      309–10
    Tuscan White Bean Spread, 275
    White Beans and Tomatoes, 350–51
Beets
  Beet and Apple Salad with Cheese and
    Walnuts, 287
Berries
  blueberries
    Blueberry Creamsicle Protein
      Shake, 49
    Blueberry Walnut Biscotti, 361–62
  mixed
    Grand Marnier-Infused Berries, 365
    Mixed Berry Pie, 372–73
  raspberries
    Chocolate-Raspberry Tapioca
      Parfaits, 363
    Peach and Raspberry Pie with
      Almond Crunch Topping, 373–74
  strawberries
    Light Strawberry Marble
      Cheesecake, 370–71
    Strawberry Sunrise Protein Shake, 49
    Strawberry-Vanilla Tapioca
      Parfaits, 364

Biscotti
  Blueberry Walnut Biscotti, 361–62
Black beans. *See* Beans
Blueberries. *See* Berries
Bran, wheat
  Bran Muffins with Apples and Pecans,
    282–83
Bread crumbs, cooking tip, 359
Breads. *See also* Pretzels
  Bran Muffins with Apples and Pecans,
    282–83
  High-Pro Energy Bread, 279–80
  Multigrain Cloverleaf Rolls, 280–81
  sweet
    Old Fashioned Gingerbread
      Muffins, 284
    Pumpkin Cranberry Loaf, 281–82
Breakfast protein shakes, 49
Broccoli
  Broccoli and Italian Sausage Frittata,
    335–36
  Broccoli and White Bean Puree, 354
  Chicken and Broccoli with Tortellini,
    326–27
Broccoli rabe
  Broccoli Rabe and White Bean Soup,
    305–6

C

Cakes. *See also* Cheesecakes
  Orange Angel Food Cake, 371–72
Calamari
  Marinated Seafood Salad, 296–97
  tentacles, about, 297
Cannellini beans. *See* Beans
Caribbean-style recipes
  Caribbean Grilled Turkey Breast, 333
  Caribbean Jerk Chicken Pita Wraps, 325
Cashews
  Asian Cashew Shrimp with Brown
    Rice, 337–38
Casseroles
  Roasted Root Vegetable Casserole, 358
Cheese
  cheddar
    Cheddar-Filled Multigrain Soft
      Pretzels, 286
  cream cheese
    Light Pumpkin Cheesecake, 368–69

Light Strawberry Marble
    Cheesecake, 370–71
  goat
    Beet and Apple Salad with Cheese
      and Walnuts, 287
    Pistachio-Crusted Chicken with
      Goat Cheese and Apricot-Sherry
      Sauce, 328–29
  mozzarella
    Green Bean, Tomato, and Fresh Moz-
      zarella Salad with Pasta, 290–91
  ricotta
    Ricotta Cheesecake Cups, 374–75
Cheesecakes
  Light Pumpkin Cheesecake, 368–69
  Light Strawberry Marble Cheesecake,
    370–71
  Ricotta Cheesecake Cups, 374–75
Chicken
  entrées
    Caribbean Jerk Chicken Pita
      Wraps, 325
    Chicken and Broccoli with
      Tortellini, 326–27
    Indonesian Coconut-Crusted
      Chicken Tenders, 327
    Pistachio-Crusted Chicken with
      Goat Cheese and Apricot-Sherry
      Sauce, 328–29
    Roasted Chicken Breasts with
      Lentil Ragout, 330–31
    Sautéed Chicken Breasts with
      Porcini Mushrooms, 331–32
  salads
    Chopped Chicken Salad, 288
    Roasted Chicken Salad with Mango
      and Pistachios, 299–300
  sauce for
    Wild Mushroom Ragu, 276
  sausage
    Broccoli and Italian Sausage
      Frittata, 335–36
    Farfalle with Sausage and White
      Beans, 334–35
  sides
    Chicken and Vegetable Fried Rice,
      355–56
  soups
    Chicken Chipotle Chili, 313–14

Creamy Chicken and Barley Soup, 314–15

Grandma's Chicken Noodle Soup, 317–18

Chickpeas
Roasted Garlic Hummus, 271
Thick and Zesty Gazpacho, 322–23

Chili
Chicken Chipotle Chili, 313–14
Seafood and White Bean Chili, 309–10

Chocolate
Chocolate-Raspberry Tapioca Parfaits, 363
dark vs. light, cooking tip, 363
Oatmeal Chocolate Chip Cookies, 366–67

Chowders
Butternut Squash and Crab Chowder, 310–11
Seafood Chowder, 312–13

Clams
Seafood and White Bean Chili, 309–10
Seafood Chowder, 312–13

Cookies
Blueberry Walnut Biscotti, 361–62
Cinnamon Sugar Cookies, 367–68
Oatmeal Chocolate Chip Cookies, 366–67
Oatmeal Nut Cookies, 367

Corn
Fresh Corn Salsa, 278

Coulis, about, 343

Crab
Butternut Squash and Crab Chowder, 310–11
Marinated Seafood Salad, 296–97

Cranberries
Pumpkin Cranberry Loaf, 281–82

Cucumbers
hothouse, about, 273
Tzatzkiki spread, 273

Curries
Curried Yellow Pea and Sweet Potato Soup, 318–19

D
Dips. See also Spreads
Fresh Corn Salsa, 278
Peanut Dipping Sauce, 328

Quick and Easy Homemade Guacamole, 277
Tuscan White Bean Spread, 275

Duck
Duck and Lentil Stew, 316–17

E
Eggplant
Roasted Eggplant Spread, 270

Eggs
Broccoli and Italian Sausage Frittata, 335–36
Tofu Egg Drop Soup with Vegetables, 323–24

F
Fish
halibut
Halibut on a Bed of Spinach with White Beans and Tomatoes, 350–51
salmon
Fresh Salmon Cakes, 343–44
Roasted Salmon in Parchment with Lemon and Dill, 341
Smoked Salmon-Wrapped Scallops with Blood Orange-Saffron Coulis, 342–43
sauces for
Sweet Mustard-Lime Sauce, 345–46
Wild Mushroom Ragu, 276
swordfish
Marinated Swordfish with Lemon Risotto and Garlic Green Beans, 348–49
tuna
Fresh Tuna Cakes with Sweet Mustard-Lime Sauce, 344–45
Mediterranean Tuna Steaks with Orzo, 346–47
white fish, any
Seafood and White Bean Chili, 309–10
Sole in Sherry Butter Sauce, 351–52

Flour
whole wheat, (See Breads)
whole wheat pastry, about, 368

Frittatas
Broccoli and Italian Sausage Frittata, 335–36

Fruit, See specific kinds

G

Garbanzo beans. *See* Chickpeas
Ginger
  grating, equipment for, 338
  Old Fashioned Gingerbread Muffins,
    284
Goat cheese
  Beet and Apple Salad with Cheese and
    Walnuts, 287
  Pistachio-Crusted Chicken with Goat
    Cheese and Apricot-Sherry
    Sauce, 328–29
Grains, whole. *See* Barley; Breads
Greek-style recipes
  Greek Chopped Salad, 289
  Tzatzkiki spread, 273
Green beans
  Garlic Green Beans, 349
  Green Bean, Tomato, and Fresh
    Mozzarella Salad with Pasta,
    290–91
  Marinated Swordfish with Lemon
    Risotto and Garlic Green Beans,
    348–49

H

Halibut
  Halibut on a Bed of Spinach with White
    Beans and Tomatoes, 350–51
Herbs
  Sachet d'epices, making, 331

I

Icing
  Cinnamon Icing, 362
Italian-style recipes
  entrées
    Broccoli and Italian Sausage
      Frittata, 335–36
  salads
    Italian Chopped Salad, 291
    Italian Country Rice Salad, 292–93
    Italian Insalata Mista, 293–94
  soups
    Italian Tomato-Bread Soup, 320–21
    Tuscan Lentil Soup, 308–9
  spreads
    Sicilian Caponata, 274–75
    Tuscan White Bean Spread, 275

J

Jicama
  about, 295
  Asian Jicama Slaw, 295
  Jicama Slaw, 294–95

K

Kitchen equipment
  kitchen shears, 329
  microplanes, 338

L

Lentils. *See* Beans

M

Mango
  Roasted Chicken Salad with Mango
    and Pistachios, 299–300
Meatballs, vegetarian, 272
Mediterranean-style recipes
  Mediterranean Lentil Salad, 298–99
  Mediterranean Tuna Steaks with
    Orzo, 346–47
  Roasted Eggplant Spread, 270
Menu suggestions, daily, 208–10
Mexican-style recipes
  Black Bean Soup with Lime, 304–5
  Chicken Chipotle Chili, 313–14
  Fresh Corn Salsa, 278
  Jicama Slaw, 294–95
  Seafood and White Bean Chili,
    309–10
  Southwestern Three-Bean Salad, 301–2
Microplanes, for grating, 338
Middle Eastern-style recipes
  Roasted Garlic Hummus, 271
Mozzarella cheese
  Green Bean, Tomato, and Fresh Moz-
    zarella Salad with Pasta, 290–91
Muffins
  Bran Muffins with Apples and Pecans,
    282–83
  Old Fashioned Gingerbread Muffins,
    284
Mushrooms
  Creamy Chicken and Barley Soup,
    314–15
  Sautéed Chicken Breasts with Porcini
    Mushrooms, 331–32
  Wild Mushroom Ragu, 276

Mustard
  Pan-Seared Jumbo Prawns in Dijon
    Mustard Sauce, 340
  Sweet Mustard-Lime Sauce, 345–46

N

Nuts
  cashews
    Asian Cashew Shrimp with Brown
      Rice, 337–38
  peanuts
    Peanut Dipping Sauce, 328
    Peanut Soba Noodles, 356–57
  pecans
    Bran Muffins with Apples and
      Pecans, 282–83
    Peaches Praline Protein Shake, 49
  pistachios
    Pistachio-Crusted Chicken with
      Goat Cheese and Apricot-Sherry
      Sauce, 328–29
    Roasted Chicken Salad with Mango
      and Pistachios, 299–300
  walnuts
    Beet and Apple Salad with Cheese
      and Walnuts, 287

O

Oats
  Oatmeal Chocolate Chip Cookies,
    366–67
  Oatmeal Nut Cookies, 367
Olives
  Kalamata Olive Spread, 269
Oranges
  blood, about, 343
  Orange Angel Food Cake, 371–72
  Smashed Orange-Ginger Sweet
    Potatoes, 359
  Smoked Salmon-Wrapped Scallops
    with Blood Orange-Saffron
    Coulis, 342–43

P

Parfaits
  Chocolate-Raspberry Tapioca Parfaits,
    363
  Strawberry-Vanilla Tapioca Parfaits,
    364

Parmesan rinds, in soup, 306
Pasta
  entrées
    Chicken and Broccoli with
      Tortellini, 326–27
    Farfalle with Sausage and White
      Beans, 334–35
    Mediterranean Tuna Steaks with
      Orzo, 346–47
    Seared Scallops with Lemon and
      Capers, 338–39
  salads
    Green Bean, Tomato, and Fresh
      Mozzarella Salad with Pasta,
      290–91
    Shrimp and Pasta Salad with Snow
      Peas, 300–301
  sauce for
    Wild Mushroom Ragu, 276
  side dishes
    Peanut Soba Noodles, 356–57
  soups
    Grandma's Chicken Noodle Soup,
      317–18
Pastry flour, whole wheat, about,
  368
Peaches
  Peach and Raspberry Pie with
    Almond Crunch Topping,
    373–74
  Peaches Praline Protein Shake, 49
Peanuts
  Chewy Peanut Bites, 375–76
  Peanut Butter Bursts, 376–77
  Peanut Dipping Sauce, 328
  Peanut Soba Noodles, 356–57
Pears
  Wild Rice and Sweet Potato Salad
    with Pear Vinaigrette, 302–3
Pecans
  Bran Muffins with Apples and Pecans,
    282–83
  Peaches Praline Protein Shake, 49
Peppers, red
  Roasted Red Pepper Coulis, 360
Pies
  Mixed Berry Pie, 372–73
  Peach and Raspberry Pie with Almond
    Crunch Topping, 373–74

Pistachios
  Pistachio-Crusted Chicken with Goat
    Cheese and Apricot-Sherry
    Sauce, 328–29
  Roasted Chicken Salad with Mango
    and Pistachios, 299–300
Poultry. *See* Chicken; Turkey
Pretzels
  Cheddar-Filled Multigrain Soft
    Pretzels, 286
  Multigrain Soft Pretzels, 285–86
Pumpkin
  Light Pumpkin Cheesecake, 368–69
  Pumpkin Cranberry Loaf, 281–82

R

Rapini. *See* Broccoli rabe
Raspberries. *See* Berries
Relishes
  Sicilian Caponata, 274–75
Rice
  brown, how to cook, 356
  in entrées
    Asian Cashew Shrimp with Brown
      Rice, 337–38
    Marinated Swordfish with Lemon
      Risotto and Garlic Green Beans,
      348–49
  salads
    Italian Country Rice Salad, 292–93
    Wild Rice and Sweet Potato Salad
      with Pear Vinaigrette, 302–3
  side dishes
    Chicken and Vegetable Fried Rice,
      355–56
    Lemon Risotto, 348
    Shrimp and Vegetable Fried Rice, 356
Ricotta cheese
  Ricotta Cheesecake Cups, 374–75
Risotto
  Lemon Risotto, 348
Rolls
  Multigrain Cloverleaf Rolls, 280–81

S

Sachet d'epices, making, 331
Salads
  Asian Jicama Slaw, 295
  Beet and Apple Salad with Cheese and
    Walnuts, 287

Chopped Chicken Salad, 288
Greek Chopped Salad, 289
Green Bean, Tomato, and Fresh
    Mozzarella Salad with Pasta,
    290–91
Italian Country Rice Salad, 292–93
Jicama Slaw, 294–95
Marinated Seafood Salad, 296–97
Mediterranean Lentil Salad, 298–99
Roasted Chicken Salad with Mango
    and Pistachios, 299–300
Shrimp and Pasta Salad with Snow
    Peas, 300–301, 300–301
Southwestern Three-Bean Salad,
    301–2
Wild Rice and Sweet Potato Salad
    with Pear Vinaigrette, 302–3
Salmon
  Fresh Salmon Cakes, 343–44
  Roasted Salmon in Parchment with
    Lemon and Dill, 341
  Smoked Salmon-Wrapped Scallops
    with Blood Orange-Saffron
    Coulis, 342–43
Salsas
  Fresh Corn Salsa, 278
Sandwiches. *See* Wraps
Sauces
  Peanut Dipping Sauce, 328
  Roasted Red Pepper Coulis, 360
  Sicilian Caponata, 274–75
  Sweet Mustard-Lime Sauce,
    345–46
  Wild Mushroom Ragu, 276
Sausage, chicken or turkey
  Broccoli and Italian Sausage Frittata,
    335–36
  Farfalle with Sausage and White
    Beans, 334–35
Scallops
  Marinated Seafood Salad, 296–97
  Seafood and White Bean Chili,
    309–10
  Seafood Chowder, 312–13
  Seared Scallops with Lemon and
    Capers, 338–39
  Smoked Salmon-Wrapped Scallops
    with Blood Orange-Saffron
    Coulis, 342–43

Seafood. *See also* Fish
Asian Cashew Shrimp with Brown
Rice, 337–38
Marinated Seafood Salad, 296–97
Pan-Seared Jumbo Prawns in Dijon
Mustard Sauce, 340
Seafood and White Bean Chili,
309–10
Seafood Chowder, 312–13
Seared Scallops with Lemon and
Capers, 338–39
Smoked Salmon-Wrapped Scallops
with Blood Orange-Saffron
Coulis, 342–43
Seasonings
Sachet d'epices, making, 331
Sesame seed paste. *See* Tahini
Shakes, protein
Blueberry Creamsicle, 49
Peaches Praline, 49
Strawberry Sunrise, 49
Vanilla Almond, 49
Shears, kitchen, about, 329
Sherry
Pistachio-Crusted Chicken with Goat
Cheese and Apricot-Sherry
Sauce, 328–29
Sole in Sherry Butter Sauce, 351–52
Shrimp
chilis and chowders
Seafood and White Bean Chili,
309–10
Seafood Chowder, 312–13
entrées
Asian Cashew Shrimp with Brown
Rice, 337–38
Pan-Seared Jumbo Prawns in Dijon
Mustard Sauce, 340
salads
Marinated Seafood Salad, 296–97
side dishes
Shrimp and Vegetable Fried Rice,
356
Side dishes
Basic Black Beans, 353–54
Broccoli and White Bean Puree, 354
Chicken and Vegetable Fried Rice,
355–56
Garlic Green Beans, 349

Mediterranean Lentil Salad, 298
Peanut Soba Noodles, 356–57
Roasted Root Vegetable Casserole,
358
Smashed Orange-Ginger Sweet
Potatoes, 359
Spinach and Garlic Sauté, 350–51
White Beans and Tomatoes, 350–51
Slaws
Asian Jicama Slaw, 295
Jicama Slaw, 294–95
Snacks. *See also* Spreads
Chewy Peanut Bites, 375–76
Peanut Butter Bursts, 376–77
Savory Spinach Balls, 272
Snow peas
Shrimp and Pasta Salad with Snow
Peas, 300–301
Soba noodles, about, 357
Sole
Sole in Sherry Butter Sauce, 351–52
Soups. *See also* Stews
Black Bean Soup with Lime, 304–5
Broccoli Rabe and White Bean Soup,
305–6
Butternut Squash and Crab Chowder,
310–11
Cannellini Bean and Bacon Soup,
307–8
Chicken Chipotle Chili, 313–14
Cream of Roasted Tomato-Basil Soup,
319–20
Creamy Chicken and Barley Soup,
314–15
Curried Yellow Pea and Sweet Potato
Soup, 318–19
Grandma's Chicken Noodle Soup,
317–18
Italian Tomato-Bread Soup, 320–21
Seafood and White Bean Chili,
309–10
Seafood Chowder, 312–13
Thick and Zesty Gazpacho, 322–23
Tofu Egg Drop Soup with Vegetables,
323–24
Tuscan Lentil Soup, 308–9
Soy protein powder, for shakes, 49
Spanish-style recipes
Thick and Zesty Gazpacho, 322–23

Spinach
    Halibut on a Bed of Spinach with
        White Beans and Tomatoes,
        350–51
    Savory Spinach Balls, 272
    Spinach and Garlic Sauté, 350–51
Split peas, yellow
    Curried Yellow Pea and Sweet Potato
        Soup, 318–19
Spreads. *See also* Dips
    Kalamata Olive Spread, 269
    Roasted Eggplant Spread, 270
    Roasted Garlic Hummus, 271
    Sicilian Caponata, 274–75
    Tuscan White Bean Spread, 275
    Tzatzkiki spread, 273
    Wild Mushroom Ragu, 276
Squash
    Butternut Squash and Crab Chowder,
        310–11
Squid. *See* Calamari
Stews
    Duck and Lentil Stew, 316–17
Strawberries. *See* Berries
Sweet potatoes
    Curried Yellow Pea and Sweet Potato
        Soup, 318–19
    Smashed Orange-Ginger Sweet
        Potatoes, 359
    Wild Rice and Sweet Potato Salad
        with Pear Vinaigrette, 302–3
Swordfish
    Marinated Swordfish with Lemon
        Risotto and Garlic Green Beans,
        348–49

T
Tahini
    Roasted Garlic Hummus, 271
Tapioca
    Chocolate-Raspberry Tapioca Parfaits,
        363
    Strawberry-Vanilla Tapioca Parfaits,
        364
Terra Stix, about, 288
Tofu
    Tofu Egg Drop Soup with Vegetables,
        323–24

Tomatoes
    in salads
        Fresh Corn Salsa, 278
        Green Bean, Tomato, and Fresh
            Mozzarella Salad with Pasta,
            290–91
    soups
        Cream of Roasted Tomato-Basil
            Soup, 319–20
        Italian Tomato-Bread Soup, 320–21
        Thick and Zesty Gazpacho, 322–23
Toppings
    Almond Crunch Topping, 373–74
    Grand Marnier-Infused Berries, 365
Tuna
    Fresh Tuna Cakes with Sweet
        Mustard-Lime Sauce, 344–45
    Mediterranean Tuna Steaks with
        Orzo, 346–47
Turkey
    bacon
        Cannellini Bean and Bacon Soup,
            307–8
        Caribbean Grilled Turkey Breast, 333
    sausage
        Broccoli and Italian Sausage
            Frittata, 335–36
        Farfalle with Sausage and White
            Beans, 334–35

V
Vegetables, *See also specific vegetables*
    Roasted Root Vegetable Casserole,
        358
Vegetarian meatballs, 272

W
Walnuts
    Beet and Apple Salad with Cheese and
        Walnuts, 287
Wraps
    Caribbean Jerk Chicken Pita Wraps,
        325

Y
Yams. *See* Sweet potatoes
Yogurt
    Tzatzkiki spread, 273